IN THE SHADE
OF AN ACACIA TREE

MEMOIRS OF A HEALTH OFFICER
IN AFRICA: 1945–1959

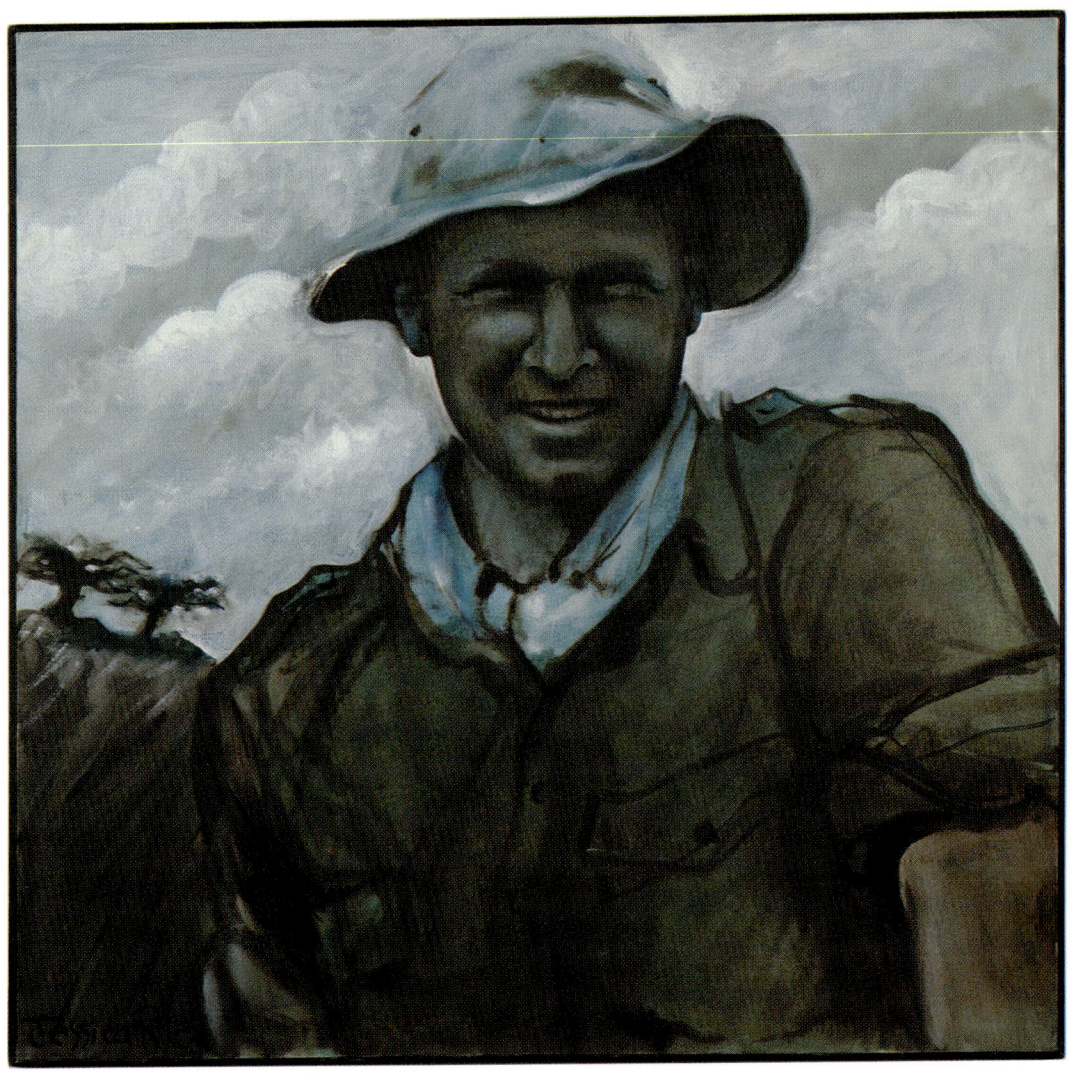

Oil painting of Frank Lambrecht by his daughter, Jessica Rice. Used with her permission.

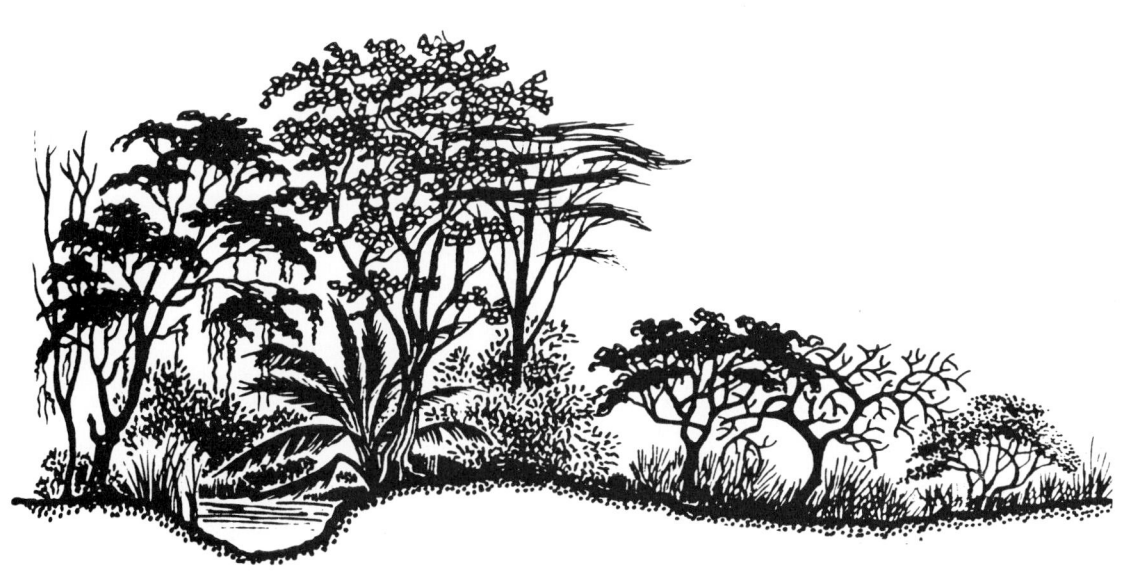

In The Shade of an Acacia Tree:

Memoirs of a Health Officer in Africa, 1945–1959

FRANK L. LAMBRECHT

American Philosophical Society
Independence Square   Philadelphia
1991

Memoirs of the
AMERICAN PHILOSOPHICAL SOCIETY
*Held at Philadelphia
For Promoting Useful Knowledge
Volume 194*

Copyright © 1991 by the American Philosophical Society

*Library of Congress Catalog Card Number 90–56110
International Standard Book Number 0–87169–194–9
US ISSN 0065–9738*

Dedicated to those who share the memories: Dora, Winifred, Jessica and Richard; and to those I may never meet again: Mutima and many others who served me well.

IN THE SHADE OF AN ACACIA TREE

Foreword—Ward H. Goodenough	xi
* Preface	xiii

Part I: In the Shadow of the Rain Forest — 1

* Introduction	3
* The Journey	12
* The Land of the Two Rivers	26
* "See You at Pawa"	46
* Much about Soap and Termites	64
* The Hippocratic Oath	70
* Basiani and Beyond	83
* Of Hunting	89
* The Bachelors of the Nepoko	103
* First Letters Home	112
* Family Reunion	129
* Settling Down	134
* Missionaries, Religious and Others	145
* The Mountains of the Moon	150
* Pulling Up Stakes	161

Part II: The Winds of the Savanna — 169

* Home on the Lake	171
* A Touch of Malaria	189
* "A Thousand Hills and Seven Volcanoes"	198
* Camp on the Malagarasi	208
* Old Shinyanga	222

Part III: Return to the Forest — 229

* Return to Africa	231
* Seven Years in the Land of Seven Volcanoes	245
* Camp on the Epulu River	261
* Years of Adventure	268
* Irangi	277
* More about Irangi	286
* Royal Hunting Party	305

Part IV: In the Shade of an Acacia Tree   317

* Where the Antelopes Roam   319
* Those Mutara Days   338
* Notes on an Overland Journey, Dar-es-Salaam to Lake Kivu   358
* Camp at Lake Tshohoha   366
* "The Lords of the Jungle"   373
* The Last Camp   378
* The Last Safari   392
* Farewell to Africa   407

Epilogue   411

Index   416

Illustrations

Frontispiece: Oil painting of Frank Lambrecht by his daughter, Jessica Rice. Used with her permission.

Part I

1. (Ma)Budu woman pounding manioc.
2. (Ma)Budu woman and baby showing elongated cranium.
3. Mangbetu woman's hairdo in the shape of a basket.
4. Mangbetu women wearing the traditional "negbe."
5. Hair dressing (Ma)Budu style.
6. (Ma)Budu Chief Kotinai in full dress.
7. (Ma)Budu Chief Karume, surrounded by his wives.
8. Capita Basiani and his youngest wife.
9. (Ma)Budu Chief Ndabani in traditional outfit.
10. Makakaru—famous Pawa termite exterminator with two termite queens.
11. and 12. Budu orchestra in full swing.
13. The author and Mutima ready for the hunt.
14. The author meeting a friend in a bush camp.
15. Dora with Winnie and Jessie.
16. Tipoy (carrier chair) safari in the bush.
17. A Mangbetu chief traditionally outfitted.
18. Budu army.
19. Assault on a termite mound.
20. Mangbetu Chief Ebandrumbi.
21. Brick-making works at Pawa, 1945.
22. Leper camp at Pawa, 1946.
23. Mrs. Lambrecht and Mrs. Cordier with gorilla. Used with permission of The National Geographic Society

Part II

1. Rudahigwa II, King of Ruanda, with Jessie and Winnie.
2. Main center of I. R. S. A. C.
3. Dr. Ignace Vincke showing the technique of malaria research.
4. The author explaining his correlation maps.
5. Jessie at the memorial for C. F. M. Swynnerton.
6. Memorial for C. H. N. Jackson.
7. and 8. The snake that almost got away.

9. The author's first buffalo hunt.
10. Bark canoe on the Malagarasi River.

Part III

1. Marcel Chardome at Utu with a young gorilla.
2. Swinging bridge spanning the Luo River near Irangi.
3. Dora and Richard on the rope bridge.
4. Our self-made ferry.
5. The platform in the Irangi forest.
6. One of the mosquito workers sorting live mosquitos.
7. Tsetse search along the Oso River.
8. The witch doctor of Oso village.
9. Oso village.
10. Princess Liliane and King Leopold in Utu.
11. Princess Liliane, King Leopold and the vanden Berghes.
12. King Leopold at I. R. S. A. C.
13. Gorillas fleeing capture.
14. *Glossina vanhoofi* resting on a tree trunk.
15. Richard at Lwiro inspecting vegetables.
16. Bolobo village.

Part IV

1. Mutara villagers wait for blood samples to be taken.
2. Camp Biharagu at Lake Tshohoha.
3. Ferry across the Nyawarongo River.
4. Our faithful Land-Rover.
5. A group of Maasai people.
6. Jessie in serious conversation with one of the Maasai.
7. Sketch of some Maasai by Jessica Rice. Used with her permission.

Sketches by Jessica Rice. Used with her permission.

1. General view of the Congo Red Cross Hospital at Pawa.
2. Window and kerosene lamp in author's home in Pawa.
3. Typical road in Kibali, Ituri.
4. Cotton shed built by COTONEPO.

Four maps of the Belgian Congo.

FOREWORD

By Ward H. Goodenough

In this autobiographical account of the years he studied the behavior and ecology of tsetse flies in what were then the Belgian colonies of Congo and Ruanda-Urundi, Frank Lambrecht documents colonial life and the conditions under which the research in which he played a major pioneering role was conducted.

His years in Africa began immediately after World War II and ended shortly before the Belgian colonies there became the politically independent countries of Zaire, Rwanda, and Burundi. Lambrecht draws heavily on the diaries he kept and letters he wrote. There is an immediacy and freshness to his account, revealing things as he saw them, understood them, and felt about them at the time. He shows in many ways what life in a variety of different settings was like for Belgian colonials during that time, including the never ending difficulties with housing and transportation. He does not question the social arrangements between Europeans and Africans, but describes events and relationships in a manner that accepts them for what they were, without apology. The result is a faithful picture from the colonial perspective, valuable as such.

His first posting was to a very isolated area in the eastern Congo's tropical forest. We get glimpses of the boredom, the progressive reclusiveness of some, the need to establish relationships with local people that would be emotionally rewarding but at the same time respect the constraints of the colonial social code. The highhanded behavior of some contrasts with the considerate behavior of others. There was no hesitation to invade privacy with police power in order to find people suffering from leprosy. There were the visiting high brass in the colonial administration who wanted to have their pictures taken with lepers to show how brave they were in the performance of duty. Of interest, too, is the great contrast of life in the isolated outposts with life in the towns, especially the highland towns, where resident colonials sought to replicate as closely as possible the amenities of home. Lambrecht comments on how cut off he was from Africans when he was resident in the towns by comparison with the much freer interactions with them he had enjoyed at the isolated posts.

Noteworthy is Lambrecht's observation that people who, like himself, found the experience of life in the more isolated areas to be rich and meaningful, could not communicate about it with people who had never experienced it. Townspeople in the colonies and the people at home in Belgium who had never experienced that kind of life tended to show only perfunctory interest in hearing about it and could not comprehend what little they heard. All they really wanted was to have their stereotypes confirmed so as to be free to concentrate on what was most immediate in their own lives where they were. Thus we get another glimpse of how it is that dependent peoples are almost invariably at the mercy of policy decisions regarding their welfare by people who are uncomprehending of and indifferent to hearing about the realities of their situation.

Lambrecht's diaries deal at length with the gross logistics of his research on tsetse flies. The facilities were often inadequate and make-shift. What comes through is the enormously important role of locally trained Africans in the gathering of the field data, especially the data that had to be collected systematically on a daily basis. The success of Lambrecht's work owed much to his including in it on a long term basis the Africans who shared with him an understanding of its importance and an interest in its being done well.

Historians of science need to have pictures of the conditions under which great pioneering researches are done. In this regard, Lambrecht's chronicle is a welcome contribution.

PREFACE

Historic accounts are to be read keeping in mind the spirit of the times in which they took place.

The colonial period was the logical result of western expansionism in the wake of merchant fleets that circled the globe in search of goods and markets at established trading posts and protected harbors in their zones of operation. While in the sixteenth century North American expansion evolved into the permanent occupation by an independent government, the colonial territories in Africa remained attached to their mother country's ruling power. Exceptions were South Africa and the short-lived Ian Smith's Rhodesia.

Colonial Africa thrived for a short while and helped carve today's African independent countries out of ill-defined empires and warring tribes.

The colonial governments in British Africa included many career officials who had served previously in India or other parts of the British Empire. The territories of Uganda and Kenya saw the immigration, early in the century, of "trekkers" from South Africa who came with the intention of permanently settling in areas suitable for agricultural development. The French had a long colonial tradition and seemed bent on making their African territories part of "La Metropole." Also with a long colonial tradition, the Portuguese territories were governed as part of the motherland. For the Belgians it was an unprecedented experience to inherit a colonial possession eighty times the size of the mother country through the act of a single signature. It was a challenge that was met with courage and determination.

With today's attitudes, it may be difficult to comprehend the aspiration and passion of those Europeans who opted to serve in the African colonies, not to rule but to teach; not to exploit but to explore; not for gain but for glory; not to oppress but for opportunity.

Before them lay a land immense, diverse, challenging and flying the national flag. In the 30's and 40's the tropics still portrayed some of the most mysterious regions of the earth, not yet available to the "ordinary" mortal. Many went with no definite career in mind. While a contract read "health officer" or "administrative agent," the former could find himself in charge of a territory the size of a province while the administrator might very well be running a regional vaccination campaign. Titles were a cover-up for what Churchill once defined as "blood, sweat and tears." But they loved it. It was a dream come true.

We went, most of us, "to try it out"; many made it a career. We loved the country and, at times, hated it. We liked the natives without motivation for close friendship. We counted the months separating us from our next home leave but even more eagerly the weeks until we were due back.

When the national flag came down for the last time we knew we had lost a world. We knew that whatever the virtues of "independence," the land would never be the same. Not for us.

* * *

During the war years, while working towards my degree in tropical medicine, I became an assistant in the laboratory of protozoology under Professor Louis vanden Berghe, at the Institute of Tropical Medicine in Antwerp. When at the end of the war I was offered a position as Health Officer in Africa the debate between Dora and me was only a formality, still it made us believe that we had discussed this important turn in our life in a reasonable fashion. To escape the memories of five years of war and moral imprisonment tipped the balance if it ever needed tipping. I left for the Congo in August of 1945 at the age of thirty.

At first we lived in the tropical rain forest. Still full of the marvels of the colorful microorganisms I had studied not so long ago, I didn't loose a single opportunity to make bloodsmears of monkeys and other animals. Many hours I sat among the giant trees waiting for monkeys to swing by. I sent monkey bloodsmears and pieces of their liver to Professor Rodhain, director of the Tropical Institute. I collected ticks and other insects, and mailed boxes of materials to my old entomology professor.

One day I caught two large tsetse flies. Back came the exciting news that they belonged to the species *Glossina tabaniformis*, a new record for that part of Africa. My first scientific discovery!

Was this the start of my commitment to tsetse research? I distinctly remember how in the fourth grade we used a textbook on hygiene showing in the section on tropical ailments a picture of a tsetse fly. That picture left a lasting impression in me, but was temporarily pushed into the background to make room for things more important at that age, such as the next soccer match.

It was the forest and the large bands of red-tail monkeys (*Cercopithecus ascanius*) that tickled the strands of my scientific interest. If they carried malarial parasites could I find the site of development outside the blood stream cycle (exo-erythrocytic cycle)? Something to take back home! At that time I was still thinking of a one-term (e.g. three years) career, not realizing that I had already been "hooked."

Near the end of my three-years' term with the Congo Red Cross, and wondering whether I should accept the offer for another term with them, I received a proposal from Dr. vanden Berghe to join him in his newly founded I.R.S.A.C. Institute ("Institut pour la Recherche Scientifique en Afrique Centrale"). I accepted eagerly.

As fate would have it, my first research project was on malaria under the supervision of Dr. I. Vincke famous for his discovery of *Plasmodium berghei*. Two years later Mr. Paul Harroy, Vice-Governor of the Congo and Governor of Ruanda-Urundi, in consultation with Dr. vanden Berghe, appointed me to carry out a medical survey in Mosso Valley, Urundi. This large region of fertile land was only sparsely populated, the people decimated by diseases, in particular by malaria and sleeping sickness. It would be an ideal area for the relocation of the overpopulated highlands—people and livestock—if the valley could be made salubrious.

The mentioning of sleeping sickness brought forth the image of my fourth grade textbook. Suddenly my vision became clear, my path well defined, I threw myself heart and soul into glossina-trypanosome research and made it the highlight of my tropical career.

It was during my work in the Mosso that I learned my trade as "glossinologist." [I never lost my fascination for the wriggling mosquito larvae, however, and malaria and other mosquito-borne parasitic diseases became part of my Mosso survey.] *Glossina morsitans*, a typical tsetse of the woodland savannas, was the local tsetse fly species. I was soon to recognize its characteristic buzzing sound, its darting movements, and its painful sting. Zaghi, a Baluba from the Katanga Province, was my trusted assistant. Together with the fly-scout teams, we endured many tsetse bites.

I loved our self-made camp in the pleasant Brachystegia-Isoberlina woodland on the banks of the mysterious Malagarasi River: the lovely coolness of the early mornings as I strolled with the flyboy team to check the tsetse traps; the excitement when we found wriggling trypanosomes in the salivary glands of dissected tsetses or in the blood of experimental guinea pigs or in an occasional antelope shot for meat. When we found a large tsetse, *Glossina brevipalpis,* until then unknown in these regions, it looked as if each day promised new thrills and discoveries.

The information gathered during the Mosso survey (1951–53), was included in the Ten-Year Plan of the Ruanda-Urundi Territories. The Mosso resettlement itself, however, was postponed when other urgent projects took priority and I was called to carry out similar medical surveys in Mutara, Ruanda (1954–56) and Bugesera, Urundi (1957–59).

* * *

As the years rolled by, I became increasingly aware of Africa's magnificent and unique but delicately balanced ecology and that, through my tsetse flies work—aimed ultimately at their elimination—I was part of the forces out to destroy it.

* * *

We returned to Africa many more times. Each time I relived the elation I experienced during my first days in the Congo: of belonging and being part of the tropical environment, of smelling the rain forest, of feeling the soft winds of the savanna, of walking among the steaming huts of an African village, of thrilling at the sight of a herd of elephants, and of resting in the shade of an acacia tree.

The memories linger on. . . .

Part I

In the Shadow of the Rain Forest

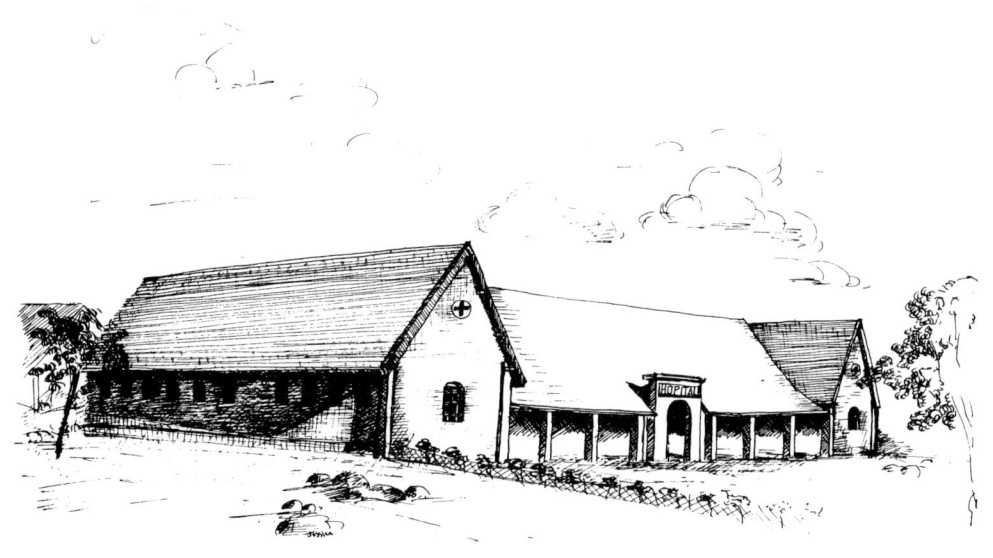

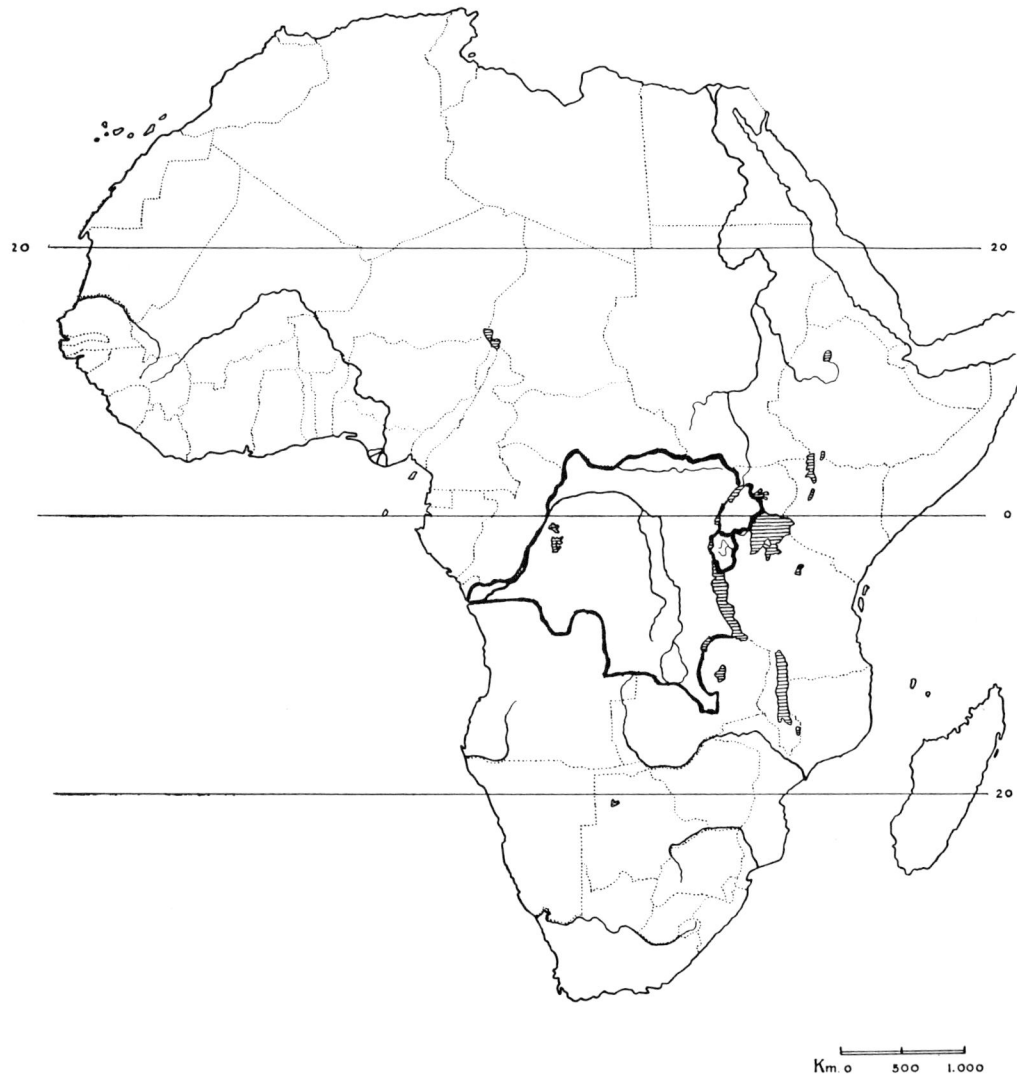

The Belgian Congo

Introduction

As I write these hesitant lines, I have in front of me two small, solid, curved ivory tusks, highly worn on the outside curves. They used to belong to a *Hylochoerus minertzhageni iturinesis*, the giant forest hog, the first big animal I hunted in the Ituri forest of Central Africa, forty-five years ago.

Recollections of this and later events are fading and may be lost altogether if not put on paper before old age erases them forever. Why bother at all? Ever since as a boy of eleven I accompanied my father, first engineer of the tankship *Ampetco*, on a voyage to New York and back to Antwerp, I have felt the urge to leave a record of my adventures which at that time—1926—seemed extraordinary.

I was born in Barry Island, South Wales, in 1915 in the house of Frank Bryan a minister who was to be my godfather. My mother and my two teen-age sisters had moved to Barry when my father, serving in an allied submarine supplyship, was stationed at Barry Dock at the start of World War I. Here the family remained until my father was released from war duty in 1921.

If I can believe my memory, my first recollection of any kind is a vague vision of the pebble beach shore and the bare, wind-swept stark boulders that bordered a low, flat plateau. My first sense of insecurity occurred when I became trapped inside the metal enclosure used to protect young trees. Somehow I had managed to squeeze myself between the bars but was unable to reverse the process. To the cries of my two sisters, two policemen came to the rescue and got me out.

Two years after the end of the war my father was retransferred to Antwerp, his ship's base port. Antwerp would become my adopted hometown for many years to come. I was now six years old, time to start grammar school. However, my spatter of Flemish mixed with 50 percent or so of English was deemed unacceptable to start grammar school. It was suggested that I "do" kindergarten, which would prepare me to enter grammar school the coming fall. As I was an extremely shy boy, my first contact with an "alien" environment was particularly alarming. I profoundly disliked to be among strange faces, to be spoken to by unknown people whose words sounded different from the ones

I knew. My strong averseness started with the sight of the massive yellow entrance door of the school, a threshold beyond which, I felt, lay hidden pitfalls which I would have to face alone. So strong was this sense of fear that even today I can set my mind to recall the impression of fright at the sight of the school's entrance. Often, as I reached the door, my panic became so great that I had to turn back for home or, more often, to lose myself among the crowd of the marketplace in the big square opposite the school. It would not be long before I was spotted by one of my sisters sent out to check after I had been reported missing a first time by the principal. After an unequal struggle I was led back through the hateful door. Once inside, my fear dissipated, but I always felt detached from the other children, almost like a stranger, as indeed I was during those first months. I remember the sandbox in which we were allowed to play occasionally and the row of purple violets which I thought glorious. I shall never forget the smell of the pea-and-onion soup, which seemed to be considered a primary source of energy for growing boys and girls, and the musty smell of the wooden square blocks we were given to play with. I recall how the other children laughed at me because I could not pronounce the letter "r" as they did. In spite of this handicap, or perhaps because of it, I was chosen to play the solo part of a singing sailor in a mock rocking boat during a presentation of the local PTA group. My first performance was deemed so hilarious that I was chosen for another solo presentation, that of a blacksmith. And as the curtain rose, there I stood in a leather apron in front of a real anvil and hammer. My loud hammering brought enthusiastic applause from the audience, but was really an effort on my part to mask my stumbling lyrics.

Whatever else they did to me, the six months at the kindergarten qualified me for grammar school. I was enrolled the following September, on my way to a proper education.

I did not learn to know my father well—most of the time he was at sea. When he returned from his long voyages, he felt like a kind of overseer checking to find if I had behaved well during his absence. He was not very communicative, and I was a very shy boy. The only time we were together for any length of time was during the one-month's journey to New York and back in the good ship *Ampetco*, where as first engineer, my father, somehow, had managed to get me mustered on board as cabin boy. Two years later my mother died, still very young, and I went to live with my newly married sister. This, more than ever, severed the paternal bond. When, on different occasions, I went to visit my father when his ship had docked, we had nothing to say to each other. I would sit on his bunk, and he would try not to seem busy although I felt he was when, during the short time in port, he was responsible, besides his other duties, for coaling or oiling and for any repairs that had to be made while the ship was in port. A few days later his ship would sail and I would forget that I had a father.

He lost three ships. One sank in the Mediterranean where he swam for six hours before he was picked up. Once his ship was torpedoed during World War I and he was rescued by a destroyer. And during one of his first trips as an apprentice-fisherman the small trawler went down in a severe storm, but the entire crew was rescued by a coast patrol boat. My father never mentioned that day when he saved the ship and many of the crew, no doubt. I got the story from my mother when I was still very young. A fire had broken out in the stokehole fed by a leaking oil valve. Everyone had fled when the flames spread to most of the engine room. The only way to stop the inferno that threatened to engulf the whole ship was to close the valve. Feeling responsible for that part of the ship, my father volunteered to do so. He ordered one of his men to keep him covered with water from the fire hose while he went naked into the inferno where he managed to stop the leak. This limited the blaze to a small area and it was put out with hand extinguishers.

It is somewhat embarrassing to boast about my father's proficiencies. Recognition often comes after death, unfortunately. While at sea he, as first engineer, had no watches to do and as long as everything ran smoothly, had plenty of leisure time. So he took up oil painting. Precise and patient, and with a wonderful sense of color-mixing, he became a master in copying classical works of the Flemish and Dutch schools from museum postcards. One appreciates that with the restricted view of the world through a porthole, his choice of subjects seemed well founded. His reproductions came extremely close to the originals except for size and freshness of paint. He must have made several dozen such paintings. Where are they now? Given away to friends, shipmates and harbor captains. Very few ended up in our own family. My younger sister salvaged a huge 5 by 8 foot beautiful reproduction of the "Reading of the Forbidden Bible" (Spanish Inquisition); I have a delightful, mellow interior of a sheep stable.

When I was still very young, my father at one time decided to stay at home to start a mechanics shop that soon became known for its precision work. I remember visiting the shop after school and playing in an old automobile, shifting gears and pulling the handbrake, both of which were operated by outside levers. But when an important deal with an Antwerp drydock company fell through, my father seized the opportunity to return to sea, to the great grief of my mother, no doubt.

My father was a marvelous mechanic. He loved to work with copper. One of his masterpieces was a small chess table made from solid brass, the checkerboard composed of precisely inlaid squares of yellow and red copper. He had an inventive mind and once put together for a distant relative, a manufacturer of gingerbread cookies, a complicated piece of machinery that automatically packed and wrapped the finished product. This was in 1926! Had he gone on in this line, he would have become a wealthy man. But he loved the sea!

My father had taught himself to play the banjo and the mandolin. I recall how, during rare family gatherings, he skillfully handled the popular arias of that time. I was amazed and slightly embarrassed because I knew my father only as an austere disciplinarian. The lively tunes he played somehow did not fit my mind's image of him.

As far as I can go back into the family tree on my father's side, all my male ancestors were fishermen operating from the North Sea coast near Ostend. My grandfather was still at sea when he was sixty, but a fall into the fishhold broke his hip and left him with a bad limp. Unfit for further sailing, he started a grocery store in one of Ostend's main streets. Even till this day I can remember the shop's homey smell of gunny sacks and roasted coffee and of the various cheeses displayed in big chunks on the marble counter.

Due to circumstance, I did not go to say goodbye to my father retired and living in the country when, at the age of thirty, I left for Africa on my first three years' tour. We parted as we had lived, genetically linked, subconsciously loving, socially unattached. He died one year later at the age of seventy-one. We remained strangers till the end in spite of the exchange of his and my last letter in which we desperately searched to express our mutual affection.

My mother died at the age of forty-eight, in great pain after a long illness. I was thirteen. Vivid in my mind was her very dark complexion: dark eyes and black hair, common to a large section of the Antwerp population—due, it was said, to a genetic leftover from the long Spanish occupation in the past of this part of the Flemish lowlands. She had a gentle but rather sad face. Hers was not a happy life—as I much later realized—with my father away most of the time—especially when my younger sister married at the age of twenty-four, my older sister having left home several years earlier. During the years that followed, my father sailed with a Far-East company on voyages that lasted up to six months. When his ship *Indier* put in, it was only for a week at the most. How dreadfully long the days and nights must have seemed to my mother living with a 12-year-old boy in a two-story house with only the ground floor and two bedrooms on the top floor fully furnished, with all the other rooms empty and devoid of active family life. What a miserable existence it must have seemed to her, waiting most of the year for a husband increasingly estranged from a depleted family, my mother hoping, in vain, for a more meaningful life, my father committed to the sea.

At times we lived in great poverty when the arrival of father's paycheck was delayed—for reasons I never found out—and the payments for gas and coal bills took priority, with daily meals reduced to the strict necessity for survival. These were the times when empty bottles were collected, newspapers and magazines were bundled and old clothes gathered for sale to the junkman. After these periods of great frugality, times of abundance would follow. One of the first things my mother would do was to take me to the pastry shop and let me eat any kind in any amount of sweets I fancied. My favorites were chocolate eclairs. But in the face of all this abundance my appetite, to my great regret, failed and I usually managed to eat no more than three.

On my mother's side I can only remember my grandfather, a tall, erect man with a bushy moustache. He, too, had a limp. His was the result of an accident during the building of a railroad where he was supervisor of a work team. Grandmother had died young and I never met her. Grandfather lived all by himself, passing his time with cut-out carpentry of small shelves, birdcages and similar trivia. But when he started making low footstools from heavy oak, his popularity with the family soared to new heights. Soon his handiwork was to be found in every household of his nearby or remote family. We had three of the beautiful stools. I had my favorite on which I used to sit during winter evenings in front of the coal stove, eating cocoa powder mixed with sugar and reading the adventures of Nick Carter or Buffalo Bill while the water kettle on top of the range sang its dreamy song. All three stools are gone, dispersed during multiple moves and changes in the family. I am sure they are in use somewhere because they are indestructible.

When I was ten, a change in my environment occurred which may have sharpened my love for exploration and for the natural sciences. We moved from a strictly city apartment ambiance to the more open suburban area at the southern outskirts of Antwerp. The move was almost ritual: never since I can remember did my parents, and I later in life, remain longer than three years in the same place. As if guided by migratory instinct, we kept to our three-year cycle whether through fate or by desire.

Our new place was only a short walk from the open spaces of the fortification complex, built in the nineteenth century, that surrounded Antwerp on all land-sides, the river Scheldt making up the rest of the defense system. The fortified city was considered impregnable until modern warfare made a mockery of its elaborate defense system. At the time my friends and I roamed the area, a start had been made towards the removal of the now obsolete, large number of fortifications and underground structures covered by hundred-foot-high mounds, surrounded by hundred-foot-wide moats. Not a few drownings occurred in these waterways during the summer months! The half-demolished ramparts and underground casemates were, of course, a marvelous playground for ten-year-olds. We had our own hidden passages that led to underground chambers where we held "secret meetings" by the light of a candle. These and other activities were not without danger and I shudder at the remembrance of some of our exploits. Dared by my friends, I once crossed on top of a two-brick-wide ledge of a very high wall, part of a kind of hangar, over a length of about fifty feet with a sheer drop on either side of perhaps thirty feet. What made the feat particularly perilous was the slanted mat of slippery dry grass that covered the top of the ledge. The worst part came at the far end of the wall when I had to turn around and face a return journey that seemed twice as long and ten times more dangerous. During the demolition of the mounds a stage was reached where half of some had been removed leaving half high domes, from the top of which we leaped to see who dared to jump the farthest. In my own group of friends we only deplored one broken arm. By miracle, no one broke a neck. In the dark gray, sandy soil deep inside the mounds we found hundreds of shark's teeth—the mounds had been built from sediment dredged from the river Scheldt.

We formed the inevitable soccer team, in which I played goalkeeper. My taste in sports later included tennis and field hockey. When I was ten, my father gave me a small bicycle which he had custom-made, perhaps the first children's bike in the country. And although my indoor family life was minimal, my numerous outdoor activities made it seem unimportant, and I can say that I lived a happy boyhood.

After Mother died, I went to live with my married sister. This changed my life in many ways. First, the days of uncertainties were over, the loneliness of an empty house replaced by a cozy household. Bottle-collection became a thing of the past; food was always plentiful. Above all, it changed completely the future conduct of my life. Destined by family tradition to become a sailor, and without even considering another career, I started inquiring about enrollment at the Naval Academy, hoping to sail one day with the schoolship *Comte Smet de Nayer*. For reasons of his own, but probably considering his own broken family life, my father opposed my choice of going to sea, saying that if I persisted he would see to it that I got the worst ship so that I would be disgusted from the start. His opposition did not affect me greatly. I considered it a mere hurdle to my aspirations, believing that his disapproval was only a token restraint of the same kind, and with the same effect as when *his* father had objected to *his* going to sea. What affected me much more were the dialogs with my brother-in-law, a chemical engineer, who cunningly introduced me to the fascination of chemistry. I have always admired the sciences greatly, enhanced by the reading of books by Jules Verne. It did not take too long for me to consider being a chemist as an attractive alternative to life at sea. And so, for the first time in my family tradition, the call of the sea was forsaken for the appeal of the chemist's crucible.

From then onwards, so it seems, events followed like a chain reaction. I got my degree in chemistry. I was drafted in the Belgian Army (infantry). A knee injury, caused earlier while playing hockey, brought me into the military hospital where my knowledge in chemistry got me a temporary job in the diagnostic laboratory. There I met a chemist who, later during the German occupation, managed to get me appointed to one of the laboratories of the Institute for Tropical Medicine, thereby reducing the probabilities for me to be "recruited" to work in factories in Germany. This brings me to the war years. But before that, another important event took place. I married Dora Mangin, a lovely girl, who for long had shared a close friendship with me and my best friend.

When, on 10 May 1940, Hitler invaded the lowlands, our first daughter was four months old. Obeying the government order that all men up to the age of 35 had to retreat to France, I had to leave Dora and the baby. After many hazards I arrived eventually in Bordeaux. Here, deciding that I could go no farther south before the German Army did, I went to the harbor looking for a ship to cross the channel. As I arrived at the docks, I saw a ship leave that would be the last, I was told, since all shipping from Bordeaux had been ordered to be stopped. At that moment, an air-raid alarm sounded. The dock area was forceably evacuated and I resumed my journey south.

Meanwhile, Dora, the baby and Dora's parents had also decided to leave Antwerp, hoping that the Germans would be stopped and turned around somewhere in France. Dodging bombardments and suffering long traffic jams of military convoys mixed with west European evacuees, indiscriminate targets for airplane strafing and dive-bombing, they arrived in southern France at the time when General Petain signed France's surrender.

The way Dora's family and, later, my sister's family and I found each other during those confusing times was rather clever. Before leaving, Dora and I had agreed to mail letters to the address of a restaurant in France where we had dined a year before, asking the owner to forward them to the other's address. He did, bless his soul. The result was that we found each other in southern France near the end of May. By then, all of France and western Europe was under German occupation and eventual routes of escape were blocked. There seemed nothing else to do but to return to Antwerp.

Four long, anxious years followed with dashed hopes as the Allies lost ground on all fronts until the turn came in October 1942 when, our ears glued to the clandestine radio, the familiar voice pronounced those unforgettable words: "This is the BBC morning news, Bruce Selfridge reading it: the Eighth Army has broken through at El Alamein. Rommel is in full retreat."

And while the one thousand bomber squadrons roared overhead to demolish the Rhineland's heavy industries and weapons factories, I sat down to study for my diploma in tropical medicine.

The Journey

Towards the end of March 1945, the inhabitants of Antwerp cautiously accepted the idea that for them the war was over. On 4 September 1944, Montgomery's Second Army had swept across northern Belgium and, after a battle that lasted only a few days, had liberated the great port of Antwerp. The sudden rush of the British 11th Armored Division and the gallant efforts of the Belgian underground army had taken the Germans by surprise and thwarted their plan to destroy the harbor installations. Antwerp's hugh 1,000-acre harbor area, warehouses, cranes, bridges, four miles of wharves and quays, locks and drydocks, rolling stock and, unbelievably, even the electrically controlled sluice gates had been seized intact. Henceforth, Antwerp became a major Allied supply line that fed the Allied Armies in their liberation of the rest of western Europe and total victory, still nine months away. As such, it also became, together with London, a prime target for the brutal German V-bombings. The first V-2 rocket bomb hit Antwerp on the morning of Friday, October 13. A second came down in the afternoon—followed the next day by several V-1's, the flying bombs. Antwerp was back in the war. And so it went until, on 27 March 1945, the last V-bomb came down in the Antwerp area, ending the eight-month-long bombardment.

About that time I was summoned by Professor Rodhain, then director of the Institute of Tropical Medicine. I had been working at the Institute for the last three years as a part-time volunteer and had taken courses in tropical diseases, concluding successfully with a "Diploma of Tropical Medicine and Hygiene" (D.T.M. & H.) I had speculated that the umbrella would help keep me out of the scrutiny of the German occupation authorities' in search for technicians sent to work in Germany. With my British birth certificate I was, furthermore, in a somewhat precarious position should I ever be arrested or questioned. I had taken the precaution of hiding my British passport—I was too proud to burn it—wrapped in oil-cloth inside a tin can in a hole in the backyard.

"I have an interesting job opportunity for you," said Professor Rodhain, never wasting time, "the Congo Red Cross is in immediate need of a health officer in its Pawa Medical Center. I have talked to Dr. Gillet and he wants you to see him in his Brussels office; here is the address."

I was dumbfounded, completely bewildered—speechless for a while. Professor Rodhain, dean of the very select world of tropical diseases experts, was proposing *me* for a position in Africa, the ink on my diploma barely dry?

"But," I blurted out, "I had no intention of going to Africa."

He looked at me through the thick glasses of his pince-nez with an icy stare that would have frozen the bacteria in the peri dishes lining his worktable, his white goatee quivering impatiently.

"Then why the devil did you enroll and get a degree?" he wanted to know, his voice sharp as a well-honed microtome knife.

"I was interested in the subject," was all I could say, thunderstruck.

Three days later I was in the Congo Red Cross headquarters in Brussels, discussing and getting briefed in what the job would embrace; wages, family allowances, pension, living conditions, medical certificates, and so on. They would send me the final contract to be signed. I would have to wait for transport, still scarce at the moment because the war in the Far East was still being fought. Neither was it possible to foresee when my wife and two children would be able to join me.

My wife and I talked it over. I had always dreamed of going to the tropics, a young boy's dream probably shared at that time by other boys of my generation, and later enhanced when I started reading books such as Muspratt's *My South Sea Island*. My previous attempt at "escaping civilization" by going to sea having floundered through my choice of becoming a chemist instead, this new opportunity seemed like another offer by fate that could not be ignored.

I went to see Professor Rodhain.

"I accept the Red Cross job," I mumbled humbly.

"Of course," he said, "the only way to go. Good luck, you will enjoy the experience."

I did.

As soon as I had signed my contract, I became busy selecting my outfit. This is the stage of evolution in the life of a new colonial officer during which he is especially vulnerable to the ploys of "Colonial Outfitters & Merchandise." Spotted from the moment he opens the door, the "green" colonial is confronted by the head sales clerk, who "from personal experience" (Bas-Congo, you know) or that of one of his uncles (just back from his second tour) or his nephew (now with OTRACO), recites a long list of bare essentials if one wishes to survive the next three years.

"Absolutely essential, sir," said the man with a slight limp ("a charging rhino," he volunteered—I learned later that charging rhinos seldom leave people with just a limp), pointing to an odd, long and narrow trunk.

"What for," I wanted to know. He hesitated.

"It is called *malle-épée*. It has the exact length of a regulation army sabre. But, of course, it can be used for packing any other long object, such as a gun," he added satisfactorily, having found a solution to my terse question.

Sensing my dislike for the *malle-épée*, he pointed to another odd-shaped trunk.

"*Malle-bain*," he announced, "absolutely vital in the tropics. When you take off the lid, it becomes a comfortable bathtub so terribly appreciated after a long march out in the bush. When not in use as such, it provides plenty of storage for linen or other equipment. Two-in-one, what?"

Observing that the *malle-bain* did not strike my fancy either, he led me in desperation to another section of the store, displaying smaller items. He pointed to a bright-red piece of material which I recognized immediately: the famous red flannel waistband so highly recommended by old colonials in prevention and cure of all sorts of stomach and other intestinal troubles.

"Everyone wears it," he commented without much enthusiasm, "Very effective, you know." He sighed as I moved on.

"Now this you must buy," he urged—it sounded like an ultimatum—pointing at various styles of pith helmets, "if you want to survive in the tropics." (Barring an encounter with a rhino, I thought.)

I chose the light and least expensive one and he seemed relieved because the thing was obviously a style that went out of fashion after the first "Trader Horn" film.

"Now for the mosquito net," he smiled as if we had discussed the subject at length over the last couple of days, "what size do you want it? Single or double?"

"I can't take bulky or heavy equipment with me," I countered. "I am sure that I shall find one locally."

He let out an explosive snort.

"Nothing can be had locally, my dear sir," he chuckled, "absolutely nothing."

"For what government department are you signed up?" he queried at once suspicious.

"Not government, I am going for the Congo Red Cross," I apologized.

"Oh, in that case," he said his voice trailing off in an uncertain whisper.

"What about your uniform, sir," he coughed somewhat contemptuously, stressing the word "uniform."

"As a matter of fact," I answered a bit stiffly, "I need brass buttons with the emblem of the International Red Cross," underlining the "international" and adding, "that is if you carry such an item."

He rummaged in an obscure drawer and to my surprise came up with eleven brass red cross buttons, one short of the amount I needed.

"Will that be all, sir?" he asked, eyeing the purchase of one pith helmet and a dozen—minus one—brass buttons, with a deep sigh.

As I paid, he added; "Good luck, sir," underscoring every word.

Of course, this was by no means the end of our packing. Most of the chore fell to Dora many months later. Hoping to find passage to Africa easier from Britain, she had accepted an invitation to stay with friends in Barry Island, Wales. This did not work out as we had hoped and after six months she left for Antwerp. Transport of "stranded" wives was being arranged by the "Agence Maritime," but there was a long waiting list.

Together we had studied several publications of the type: "How to get there and come back." This resulted in a three-page list with general categories such as: wardrobe: formal, uniform, bush; headgear: bush and town; linen: personal, bed, bath, table, mosquito net; footwear: bush and town; toilet kit and supplies; sewing notions; writing materials; hunting equipment; kitchenware: pots, pans, crockery, china, lamps, stove; tools and accessories; miscellaneous: toys, Christmas gifts, flower, vegetable and herb seeds. "Miscellaneous" was a kind of safety valve where whimsical items could be added with impunity.

These days, such a list looks grossly extravagant, but the prewar "trousseau" was based upon the assumption, many times correct, that one would not have the opportunity to acquire any of the items listed locally, keeping in mind that "tours" were of three years' duration. We did pack some of our belongings and other items we could afford to buy before I left, starting, if I remember, with three trunks. By the time Dora and the children finally left for Africa, eleven months later, the number of trunks had risen to seven. At the end of a total of twenty-three years of overseas travel—twenty of them in Africa—the count was seventeen.

The word "trunk" needs perhaps a footnote. Essentially, it is a sheet-metal box with a hinged lid that can be locked by means of two padlocks. It is similar to what, in America, is called a footlocker. The trunk was as symbolic of colonial standing as the pith helmet; even more so because the latter slowly faded from fashion with the arrival of a new breed of colonials' most of whom fancied more elegant headgear. The trunk, of all shapes and sizes, remained a faithful travel companion till the end. Not only did trunks protect one's belongings against the rough transport practices in the colonies but, having survived perhaps the first tour, served as "temporary" furniture in the usually sparingly equipped colonial houses and were indispensable when staying in resthouses.

But as the years went by and the trunks had seen the worst of river-and-land transport, and had suffered many transoceanic crossings, their usefulness as a table or dresser became questionable as their normal rectangular shape was transformed into a mass of twisted steel, gouged dents, sheared corners and broken hinges, merchandise, in other words, even the most ambitious Colonial Outfitters & Merchandise clerk would loathe to recommend.

"Pawa," I was told, "lies in the Nepoko region of the District of Kibali-Ituri of the Province of Stanleyville, in the northeastern part of the Congo." That much I learned when I signed a three years' contract as Health Officer ("Agent Sanitaire") with the Congo Red Cross. Dr. Gerardi, also a new recruit, had left two weeks earlier. The role of the C.R.C. was, primarily, to assure medical care and assistance to the population of the Nepoko region; second, to contribute to research on leprosy and to seek means of control of the disease mainly through the organization of special villages for leper patients, where treatment of cases could be more efficiently achieved.

Now I stood completing the last forms before embarking from Brussels International Airport, seen off by Dora and my friend Hans, booked on one of the first planes carrying "relief" after the war to replace those who had been "stuck" in the Colony for five or more years without home leave. Because of the scarcity of transport at that time, 10 August 1945, my family could not accompany me. They would join me later when overseas transport would return to normal. The war with Japan was still on, although not expected to last much longer following the dropping of the first atom bomb.

This was to be my first flight. It certainly did not take place under ideal weather conditions. Low clouds and drizzle hid most of the airfield. A bus took the twelve passengers and disappeared in the gray morning, shortening considerably our painful goodbyes. The ride kept on going for such a long time that I was wondering whether my ticket was for a bus or an air fare. Finally we stopped in front of an absurdly small aircraft, a Lockheed "Lodestar" that had flown only a few months before on reconnaissance missions. We were ushered inside to take our seats which were arranged in a single row on each side of the cabin. The single seats were of the metal-canvas type, obviously a rapid conversion from a previous military type. With much shaking and backfiring, the two engines started. After a long taxiing and run, we took off in the gray nothingness. We were swallowed up in a world with no reference but for great masses of fog in which we seemed to float as an infinitesimal intruder. It got very cold. The cabin was not pressurized or insulated. Condensation water started running along the bare aluminum walls and I expected it to freeze at any moment. Frequent air pockets caused the plane to fall like a brick and rise like an elevator. For more than an hour we seemed to drift inside the same cloud and only the roar of the engines dispelled the illusion that this was indeed the case. And then, suddenly, through a large gap in the clouds I saw the earth from 10,000 feet. The visual impact was so strong that I wished we were back in a nice large cloud, closer to reality. But as it started clearing more and I got used to the new perspective, I also began enjoying the grandiose spectacle of seeing the world from above. I wrote in my diary:

Land at Migane airfield near Marseille in splendid sunny weather. We have lunch. Back in the air one hour and fifteen minutes later. Across the Mediterranean. . . Pass over the Balearic Islands. What a view! Perceive the African coastline one hour later and feel thrilled that this continent is to be my home for the next three years. Shortly thereafter land at Algiers, where we spend the night.

Day two: up at five. Breakfast at six and in the air at seven thirty. Cross high mountains—the Atlas. Vegetation dwindles to nil and we drift into a world with no sky, no horizon, no ground, no clouds: the Sahara. I fall asleep but wake when we are about to land on an undefined landing strip, part of an undefinable desert. This is Aouleff. It is 12:10. The heat as we step out is unbearable. We are herded into a lone white building and into a large room where the temperature is the same as outside except for the glare of the sun. The walls are bare but for two AIRFRANCE posters, and the picture of a pilot who killed himself landing here during a sandstorm. We are served a quick lunch composed obviously of ingredients that happened to be available in the pantry, while a small Arab boy keeps the air moving by pulling a punkah. There is a rumor that we might spend the rest of the day and the night here—something to do with fuel shortage—but an hour later we are allowed back on board. The interior of the aircraft has the temperature of an oven set for a medium rare roast. Glad to be back in the air, but gasoline fumes stay with us for a long time. Start noticing green vegetation and even scattered villages. Large cloud formations, some threateningly dark. After four long hours fly over a large river: the Niger, and land at the small airfield at Gao. Landing somewhat unusual, the aircraft approaching seemingly below the level of the landing strip and then has to rise so that instead of coming down to land, one could say that we came up to land! "It was the chief pilot trying his hand after the war years of inactivity," the radio told us when we commented upon this unorthodox manoeuvre. After a half-hour refueling stop we are off again and land at Niamey just as it gets dark. We did a "record" 1700 miles today!

Third day: up at 4 (GMT), in the air at 5:45. Follow the Niger for a while. First sight of the true rain forest from where

dense fog rises. More villages and towns and roads. Land at Lagos at 8:25. Lagos airport is just a couple of shacks, one marked "IMPERIAL AIRWAYS." Refuel and back in the air at 9:05. Immediately fly along the coast with occasional glimpses of tropical forest with dense canopy looking like broccoli. Land at Libreville at 12:12. Take off 25 minutes later. Fly over solid canopy for hours and finally land at Leopoldville at 15:43 (GMT). We have arrived in the Congo!
End of diary.

Leopoldville (now Kinshasa) was at that time, 1945, still a typical tropical colonial town with one-story buildings, bungalow-type houses, many of the "Sluismans" model, that is, made of prefabricated steel frames with room partitions of whatever material was available. It was hot and humid. As soon as we were given a room at the airport hotel—an assemblage of low cottages, everyone changed into what was assumed a proper tropical outfit. With pride and some apprehension, I donned my official Red Cross khaki uniform made of light material and the jacket could be worn without a shirt. It felt good. At the bar I noticed cigarettes, "Camel" I believe, prominently displayed in one of the showcases. First mistaken for some fake package of an old advertisement, they proved, upon close inspection, to be real, priced at five francs. I asked the bar boy if I could buy a package. He looked at me a bit puzzled and said: "Mais bien sur, Monsieur." I asked if, perhaps, I would be allowed to buy two packages. His astonishment deepened: "Voulez-vous un carton de vingt?" he proposed so as to cut short any more silly questions. I was flabbergasted. American cigarettes in occupied Europe had disappeared as soon as the Germans crossed the Rhine in 1940. I remember "sharing" the last "Camel" with my sister in 1941, smoking the last inch squeezed between the prongs of a fork. Many similar surprises would follow during the next few days: fresh oranges and other fruits, fresh meat, potatoes, cold cuts, and a whole array of other foods which for five long years had been only a memory.

A new member of the colonial medical staff, I made a courtesy visit to the "Médecin-en-Chef" (Chief Medical Officer). This first contact with a high official was rather informal and friendly because I brought news from his sister, whom I had known well at the Tropical Institute. It must be remembered that I was one of the first arrivals in the Congo after the end of the war and that direct, detailed, news from Europe was still very much sought after. When I left the chief's office, I felt like having cut the inaugural ribbon and on my way across the bridge. I had barely walked a hundred yards when I heard myself hailed from across the street. And there on the other side was Marcel Chardome, whom I had known at the Tropical Institute at the beginning of the war. One day he disappeared. That was the day when a detachment of Gestapo poured into the Institute in search of Marcel. They did not find him, nor was he at home. So the Germans took his parents instead. At the liberation of Antwerp, his parents had been set free.

Over a glass of beer Marcel told his story and I filled in parts which he had "missed." The reasons why the Gestapo had a particular desire to have a chat with him were numerous and well founded. You cannot blow up German Army transports and help repatriate downed Allied pilots and still be considered an advocate of the Third Reich. Some of us at the Institute knew that Marcel had something to do with the Resistance, but very few knew about his exploits. In 1943, Marcel and I had worked in the same laboratory complex of Professor vanden Berghe who would later become our boss again as director of the IRSAC Institute. I now learned that during all those years I had been working in one of the labs, that of tissue-cultures, "highly sensitive" documents were hidden. Among others, they included the detailed plans and maps of the sites where the Germans had placed explosive charges that would be detonated to destroy Antwerp's harbor facilities in case of an allied invasion and advance to Antwerp. (These documents helped the "secret army" prevent this destruction at the time of the liberation of the city by Montgomery's Second Army group.) At one time the tissue-culture room also hid a complete radio transmitter. Of all this I was innocently unaware.

Marcel continued his story. That night before the Gestapo searched the Institute, his group had held up a convoy of three army trucks loaded with supplies. There had been some shooting and then something went wrong altogether when a platoon of the Wehrmacht arrived on the scene and Marcel's group was forced to retreat in haste. Thanks to Marcel's skills as a leader, only one man was caught. Marcel himself thought it better not to sleep at home that night. The following day, however, he arrived at the Institute as if nothing had happened. At ten in the morning he left the building for the public library. This probably saved his life because ten minutes later two Gestapo men entered the doorkeeper's office.

"Yes," the man said, annoyed at being interrupted during his coffee break.

For his only answer, one of the Germans showed him his identification of the German Secret Police and asked to be taken to Marcel. The doorkeeper reached for the phone.

"No," said one of the G.S.P., "we know that trick. You just take us there."

They were taken to the laboratory where Marcel should have been busy inoculating rats or counting red blood cells. He was not there because at that very moment Marcel was studying the public library catalog. The Gestapo squad searched the building complex—not exactly an easy job with the great number of laboratories, darkrooms, storerooms, cellars, and the hospital itself. Their search was in vain and nobody seemed to know where Marcel could be. In fact, nobody remembered having seen him that morning. The Germans retreated in good order, leaving a rearguard to watch the building. Barely had the echo of their heavy boots died away when Marcel arrived, smiling, having found some good books. It is not clear how he missed the Germans coming out of the building. Of course, there are a great number of different entrances not all known by the public. Marcel's smile soon faded when we explained the somewhat strained situation. He decided it would be better to disappear before the Germans made another search. Of course, he didn't care to leave the building by one of the entrances. One cannot trust luck too many times. Marcel cleared the laboratory, leaving behind a smell of burned paper, got out in the courtyard and climbed the far east wall. He let himself drop into the narrow alley and at the end lost himself in the crowd. He dared not go home knowing that it would be under surveillance. He got a lift to the coast and, through his many contacts, a passage to England. A year later he was appointed to the Astrid Institute for Tropical Medicine in Leopoldville.

The day he hailed me, he was actually on his way to exchange books at the library.

"A sort of habit, you know," he said, "and it's so pleasant to go back to the lab without having to dodge the Gestapo," he added.

"I notice the walls are rather high to jump," I observed.

As we were not allowed more than a one night stopover at the airport hotel, the Congo Red Cross representative, who was also the OTRACO river transportation vice-president, made arrangements for me to stay a few nights in one of the cabins on board the riverboat *Berwin*, awaiting my flight to Stanleyville two days later. No sooner was I installed in my cabin when an African appeared asking if he could do some laundry for me. As this was long overdue, I gave him my khaki trousers and a shirt, stressing that I needed them back later in the day. I never saw him or my washing again. First lesson.

Two days later I boarded once again a twelve-passenger Lockheed "Lodestar" leaving Leopoldville for Stanleyville. We made the first landing at "Coq" (Coquilhatville, now Nbandaka) two hours later where I met a distant cousin whom I had cabled about my arrival. As had so many others, Koen Cuperus had been held up in the Colony without home leave during the war. We had not seen each other for eight years. After a total of eighteen years of colonial service he had reached the high rank of Provincial Chief of Agriculture. He was surprised that I too had chosen a career in Africa. Koen became my hero when he came back from the Congo in 1930 after his first three years' tour. I was fifteen then, thrilled and proud when he asked me to help him develop and print his photos. Soon I was working like a slave in the attic which he had transformed into a darkroom. I still remember the musty, hot (it was during school summer vacation) room in his uncle's century-old house in the ancient part of Antwerp on a street that bore his name: Cuperus Straat. At that time we used day-light (Ronex) paper for photo prints. I still have the two 5x7 enlargements I kept, showing Koen with two hippos he shot on the Congo River.

Our meeting was brief: my flight left half an hour later. I never saw Koen again.

Our plane followed the Congo River, providing a marvelous view of its meandering, multi-channeled course, midstream islands, and the enormous vastness of the rain forest extending in all directions. Two hours later we landed at Bangui, and another forty minutes at Libenge—like a commuter train. We finally arrived at Stanleyville (now Kisangani) in late afternoon.

I "took to" Stan immediately. It looked very tropical with its main avenue lined with tall palm trees, the nearby steaming

Congo rapids, the Wagenia fisheries, the exotic vegetation of the Tshopo Falls (now dammed), the colorful market, and the population dressed far less western-style than in Leopoldville.

Stanleyville is one of the oldest towns of the Congo. The first time the explorer Stanley saw the falls was in January 1877 when the area was virtually run by Arab traders. Arab occupation ended with the decisive victory of the Congo army in May 1893. In 1898, the present site of Stanleyville was marked out on the right bank of the river, a few miles below the last cataract. The oldest houses were built in 1909.

I learned that the next bus for Paulis (now Isoro) would leave in five days. In the meanwhile, I booked myself in the Hotel des Chutes and spent the following days in pleasant walks around the city and environs. I also paid a courtesy call on the Provincial Medical Officer, Dr. Liegois, who, in this capacity, was also the highest medical authority of the Nepoko region. As Stan would be the last big town before I would "disappear" in the confines of the forest, I shopped for a few things that might be in short supply elsewhere, such as toothpaste, soap, Dettol disinfectant, shoe polish, spare parts for lamps, thumbtacks and postage stamps.

The VICICONGO bus looked like a run-down school bus and provided the same kind of comfort. Its weekly schedule linked Stan to Paulis by a 370-mile-long dirt road, muddy at best, flooded and impassable many times, its entire length winding through the Ituri forest, where dry spells are rare. The road, a vivid red ribbon through a dark greenhouse, goes either up or down as it uncoils across the ridges of the intricate Congo Basin watershed with its hundreds of smaller and larger streams. At the bottom of each valley, a wooden bridge—trustfully—spanned the watercourse and as, with increasing momentum, the bus negotiated the descent and across the creaking planks shot up the other slope, the passengers were lifted from their seats, the luggage in the back was propelled between the aisles, and dense red dust would fill the air.

A reprieve from this ordeal came with the crossing of the Tshopo River. Here more than before we new colonials were rewarded with a scenery of the "real Congo" as the bus was forded across the stream on a platform built on top of eight large canoes pulled along a cable by half a dozen scantily-clad natives, their efforts coordinated by the chant of a rhythmic song. This was the real thing. It seemed to match what once had been only a boy's dream; my expectations had not been mistaken. And as we advanced farther into the forest, we must all have felt that we were leaving behind a familiar world and were now entering an alien environment: an environment some would embrace, others would tolerate and a few would loathe.

The journey inside the forest seemed endless. We stopped for a while at Bafwabalinga, better known as "Kilomètre deux cent vingt Neuf" (Km. 229), nearly the halfway point of the distance to Paulis. After 50 more miles we came to another large stream, the Lindi River, here about 300 to 400 yards wide—a charming spot revealing on the left bank a picturesque group of huts of the village Bafwasende, dwarfed by the majestic mass of the forest. A couple of dugout canoes glided silently along the bank. Layers of blue smoke drifted across the thatched roofs. A flock of small children were playing a soccer game with a paper ball. The ferry that took us across the river consisted of a wooden pontoon assembled on welded 50-gallon drums. In the following years I would come to realize the enormous dependency on empty 50-gallon drums to solve many logistics problems in Africa.

It was late afternoon when we reached another wide stream, the Ituri River. Across its wide waters, the massive church of the Catholic mission of Avakubi cut an immoderate silhouette against the stately background of the forest. While the previous two ferries were hand-operated, this time the crossing was assured by a ferry propelled by a small motorized launch. It seemed to have a hard time fighting the strong current. A few miles beyond the other bank we reached the hotel at Nia-Nia, our overnight stop. A large limousine was waiting near the entrance to the lobby for two of the bus passengers, both geologists, whom I had befriended during the journey. They proposed that I accompany them to Bayenga, the headquarters of a gold-mining company. The director of the company, they said, was a good friend of the director of the Red Cross, and they were certain that I would have no difficulties in getting transportation for the rest of the way to Pawa.

We were well received by the director of the mines and served a copious supper followed by equally generous drinks. It appeared that the mechanical shop of the mines was about to deliver a repaired generator to Dr. Zanetti the next day. The mine director ordered one of the drivers to load the thing on one of the pickup trucks and to take me to Pawa forthwith. It was then close to ten. All I remember of that very long trip was that we seemed to drive through an endless tunnel of vegetation along a shockingly bumpy road and that once I saw in a flash a spotted animal jump across the headlights. "Chui," the driver said. ("Chui," I later found out, means leopard—my first wild animal.)

I must have slept most of the time. Suddenly the vehicle stopped in front of a house. "Pawa," the driver informed me as he stepped out and disappeared into the night. It was one o'clock in the morning. I was alone with the whispering palm trees. My steps made a loud sound on the coarse gravel as I walked gropingly towards a house at one side of the road. I stumbled up some stairs to the front of a door, on which I began to pound. Uncertain steps sounded from inside and I could see a waving light approaching one of the side windows. The door opened wide. Inside stood Dr. Gerardi, clad in blue-and-white striped pajamas, a blinding flashlight in one hand and a 12-gauge shotgun in the other. "What the devil . . . ," he said, or words to that effect. My adventures in Pawa had begun.

Land of the Two Rivers

In the northeastern corner of the Congo rain forest lies a region known as Kibali-Ituri after the name of the two main rivers that drain the waters of their valleys. Here the northern savannas make deep inroads into the forest, carving a mosaic of forest relicts. In turn, the forest penetrates into savanna country over long distances along meandering rivers. It is a region of wide-ranging ecological diversity that gives rise to great faunal and floral variety. Attractive to migrating Sudanese and Bantu people, it led to recurrent struggles to secure choice territory and resulted in the unmerciful displacement of the sparsely dispersed hunter-gatherer Pygmies, the original inhabitants of the forest.

It is a rolling land of rounded hills and shallow valleys, well watered by numerous slow-flowing streams fed by a yearly rainfall of close to 80 inches. The rains fall mostly during the heavy and sudden thunderstorms characteristic of the equatorial tropics. The land is fertile. It is well stocked with both forest and savanna game and therefore the favorite hunting grounds of Pygmies and Bantu alike.

Perhaps 2,000 years ago, Mangbetu clusters of Sudanese people began to infiltrate this forest-edge country from the north, replacing both Pygmy and Bantu populations. Later, they in turn gave way to the Azande, known as the "Niam-Niam," notorious cannibals like the Mangbetu. Continuous wars resulted in a pattern of ill-defined and often contested tribal boundaries. These were finally settled by the control commission of the Belgian Colonial Government when the Congo Free State became the Belgian Congo in 1908.

At the time of their might, the Azande warrior tribes formed great and strong sultanates north of the Uele River, while the Mangbetu, to the south, established important culture centers where art, especially that of ivory carving, flourished.

The Mangbetu kings claimed power over life and death, but also raised art to extraordinarily high standards. In the heart of Africa, remote from major trade routes and isolated from prolonged direct foreign influence, their art remained one of the most authentic in the African continent. According to last century's travelers and explorers, the Mangbetu and the adjacent MaBudu tribe were among the most skillful African blacksmiths and apparently the only ones to use an anvil.

They were amazing architects. Georg Schweinfurth, who, in 1870, lived at King Munza's court, and later Miani (1872), Wilhelm Junker (1879–63) and Gaetano Casati (1879–83) were full of admiration for the artistic skills of these people and for their fantastic buildings made mainly from leafstalks of the wine palm, *Raphia vinifera*. Herbert Lang and James Chapin of the American Museum Expedition, who spent six years in this remote area (1909–15), witnessed the building of a gigantic palace near Medje, measuring 200 feet long, 80 feet wide and 35 feet high. These scientists, sent out to collect ethnographical as well as zoological material for the American Museum of Natural History, saw what was probably the last of the Mangbetu grandeur at the court of King Okondo. They were spared the gruesome sight, however, of human skulls and bones lying about on refuse heaps of the king's kitchen, as described by previous explorers. It is said that at the height of Mangbetu might, a dozen prisoners were slaughtered daily to furnish meat for the king's household of hundreds of queens.

The veneration by the people of their king was as overwhelming as their fear. Any object of beauty or value was to be offered immediately to him as a gift, for its possession when discovered might bring grave consequences to the holder.

It was by a stroke of luck that the American Museum Expedition secured a rich collection of objects just before King Okondo's death. Indeed, objects from past Mangbetu kings are extremely rare because custom demanded the immediate destruction of the residence at the death of a ruler, and the burning of all his possessions. Several of his many wives were butchered and served as the main course at the new king's inaugural feast. Others of the harem were buried alive with the dead king.

In the course of past struggles, the Mangbetu tried many times to overrun adjacent MaBudu territory. While they did not succeed in its complete occupation, they nevertheless gained large tracts of land, some rich in oil palm groves. The present MaBudu territory lies astride the middle course of the Nepoko River, roughly between 27°30′ and 28°30′ eastern longitude, and 1°40′ and 2°40′ northern latitude. The tribe is almost completely acculturated by the surrounding Mangbetu from whom they have inherited many customs including fashion and art, musical instruments and village organization.

Knowledge about the origin of the MaBudu is obscured by the mass migrations of Bantu people from the region of the Cameroon highlands around the first century, A.D. These migrations may have resulted from population increase and pressure when the introduction of iron implements from the north, especially the hoe, made it possible to grow more food.

Two main thrusts marked the Bantu migrations: one followed the Atlantic coast southwards; the other, skirting the Congo rain forest and highlands, arrived in the lake region of the western Rift Valley perhaps around A.D. 700. Other groups went farther south, eventually reaching southern Africa. MaBudu oral history and legends suggest that they come "from far away from where the sun rises," and that, one day, they had to cross a large body of water. It would seem that at the start of the sixteenth century, Budu-Nyari groups occupied areas south and east of Lake Albert, from which they started westwards, forcing a passage north of the Ruwenzori range and into the Semliki Valley. Here some of the tribal groups elected to remain in the valley: the Banawoma, the Bravomo and the Bapolomo. Their past affinity with the main body is found in their language, still closely related to Kibudu. The main body moved north until another group, the Nyari, decided to settle along the eastern bank of the upper Ituri River, in the region of present Kilo. The main Budu group pushed on, reaching the middle course of the Bomokandi River near present Rugu. Encountering strong opposition from other local tribes, they finally settled in a large area along both banks of the Nepoko River. This area was seriously reduced by Mangbetu pressure, but it failed to dislodge the Budu from the Nepoko region.

It is said that the general line of migration of the Budu-Nyari is well marked by extensive patches of palm trees. At one time, the MaBudu sought the help of the Arabs to repulse Mangbetu attacks, but this alliance ended in treachery when the Arabs, under pretext of help, were able to steal large quantities of ivory and also made off with most of the young women and men. At the beginning of the Belgian occupation, the MaBudu fought the colonial troups but later begged for their help in repulsing the Mangbetu.

The MaBudu are polygamous. They are mainly agriculturists. Hunting with bow and arrow is only a secondary pastime. Food crops are primarily bananas, oil palm nuts, manioc and beans. Women collect wild fruits and other natural products of the forest, such as mushrooms. Termites, collected during a few days at the start of the heavy rains, are an important seasonal additive to the diet of proteins and fats.

Close contact with the neighboring Mangbetu has clearly influenced all art forms of the MaBudu. Like their neighbors, they are excellent blacksmiths and even better woodcarvers. They are famous for their wooden drums, the "tom-tom" or "bush telegraph," widely used for sending messages from village to village.

The MaBudu are stocky; many are downright fat. They have round, jovial faces, disarming smiles and a great sense of humor. The men walk proudly, a short bow in the left hand, with no other load to worry about. Square-sided, box-shaped, woven straw hats, decorated with bright-red tail feathers of the gray parrot, adorn their heads. The lower parts of the body are covered with a piece of bark cloth worn between the legs and fastened around the waist with ropes or belts of antelope skin. Weaving as a traditional form of art was unknown among the MaBudu. Their material for clothing is obtained from the fig tree (*Ficus* spp.). The bark is stripped, placed on a flat wooden block and beaten to flexible softness. It is then buried in the mud on the bank of a stream for "maturation" and resilience. After washing, it is dyed with vegetable stains, deep black or brown or bleached with lime. The "breeches" are made from solid color bark cloth or from six-inch wide colored strips sewn together to the desired size.

The women, bare-breasted, walk behind the men with a straight-backed gait, rhythmically swinging their frontal grass or bark cloth skirts, their buttocks covered by oval-shaped shields made from colored raffia and strips of banana leaves woven in geometric designs, the *negbe*. A less sophisticated interpretation of the *negbe* is an apron made from strips of dried banana leaves. Complete grass skirts are mostly worn during certain ceremonies, such as funerals.

While traveling, the MaBudu woman carries an assortment of implements in perfect balance on top of her head, whatever the load. This may include the traditional small stool, a couple of pots, a mortar and pestle, and a bottle of palm oil stoppered with a wad of brown paper. Mothers carry babies on the hips.

MaBudu women love to decorate their bodies with patterns or lines, squares and triangles, using the black juice of the fruit of a kind of gardenia or with red from pulverized cam wood.

Chronicles of the previous century mention that the tattooing of body and face was universal. It certainly was still popular among the MaBudu while we were there in the late 1940s. Compared with certain other African tribes, the MaBudu's tattoo marks were usually discreet, however. Designs were made by small incisions to form a pattern of triangles, squares, stripes, Maltese crosses and so on. All MaBudu, however, showed thick ugly scars at the back of the necks, the result of deep cuts made immediately after birth "to let out the bad spirits from the body," as Mutima, our servant, explained.

A remarkable custom was the traditional elongation of the head achieved by tightly wrapping the cranium of a baby soon after birth and during the first years of its life. This distortion is also the cause of the sloping, almond-shaped eyes, already noticeable in young babies with wrapped heads. The filing to a fine point of the lower incisor teeth was still common among adolescent men and women, a leftover from cannibalistic days, we learned.

The women attach great importance to their hair styles. We saw them spending considerable time in doing and redoing their coiffures, even more so when preparing for festivities. They helped each other in braiding their hair in bunches or rolls which were later plaited to form various designs. These varied according to individual tastes and the popular fashion of the moment.

The traditional Mangbetu hair style is even more elaborate, requiring many hours of patient work. First, the hair from all parts of the head is divided into single tresses. These are then carefully stretched tightly over a hoop so that they stand up on top of the head like a kind of basket. A similar hair style was popular among Mangbetu men in the previous century.

We soon found out that MaBudu love to dance. Seldom did a period of full moon pass without a dance session in some quarter of the village. The music during these informal gatherings was provided by the singing of a monotonous strain accompanied by the clapping of hands or by the beat of a small slit-drum or an empty oil drum while men and women moved around a circle. The passionate beat was irresistibly enhanced by the rhythmic shuffling of feet of the dancers and by sudden outbursts of exultation from one of the dancers as he or she jumped into the center of the swaying circle of performers and with frantic body movements seemed to encourage the others to greater energy. We seldom stayed longer than a few hours at a dance, but were told that, although fairly orderly at the start, the party often grew wild and more erotic as the moon sank lower on the horizon.

During daytime festivities, action centered around a band consisting of kettle-, hide- and slit-drums, the latter often of unusual shape, the rhythm further marked by a few "rattlers" made from small, round, tightly woven baskets containing pebbles. A monotonous refrain was repeated over and over by the musicians as well as by the bystanders, accompanied by an occasional blare from a horn made from an elephant tusk.

On the occasion of certain ceremonies, the "armory" of the chief, represented by a number of spears and shields, is taken out. Although no longer in use in combat, these weapons are still symbolic of the chief's power and authority. When Katukunai, one of the MaBudu chiefs, traveled, his "armory" was always prominently displayed in front of his *tipoy* (carrying chair), the shields spun in half-circle gyrations.

Early visitors to Central Africa have described and commented on the extraordinary variety and shapes of a weapon called "trumbush" or "trumbash." It was apparently commonly used as a throwing knife during intertribal wars. It is probable that the more ornate ones depicted in some of the earlier books may have been knives intended for parade and as symbols of authority rather than as combat weapons. Gaetano Casati (1838–1902) in *Ten Years in Equatoria* mentions:

> This is a weapon of command and distinction. The king upon sitting down places it on a stool close by, and waves it when he is gesticulating during a long speech. It is astonishing to see how ambitious chiefs and warriors are to possess the elegant and glittering *trombask;* to be executed by such a weapon is considered an exceptional honour.

The blades of some of the old-style war knives I received from Chief Karume show one or more holes. In the past, each hole received a copper knob, the number of knobs corresponding with the rank of the bearer.

Less elaborate and with a wooden handle instead of the carved ivory handle of the parade knives were those carried by the ordinary villager. Their peacetime uses included all those expected from a bush knife. Also used for cutting grasses for roofing, weeding and other household chores, it was a tool for women as well as for men. When traveling, men carry the knife, together with the bow and arrows, as a sign of dignity— the umbrella of the London banker.

I found much beauty in an African village with its low huts thatched with weathered grasses, the red walls darkly shaded by the broad eaves and by the waving pattern of a nearby palm tree, the whole sharply contrasted against the mystical dark-green background of the forest and overarched by a silky sky grazed by lazy sheep-clouds.

MaBudu villages, small and large, are built along the same pattern of two parallel rows of huts separated by a wide avenue in between. The village grounds are well kept. In front of the chief's house two shadowy open sheds, flanked by a few palm trees occupy a kind of public square. Here elders meet and public hearings are held. One of the sheds houses the tom-tom or "talking drum," the "jungle telegraph" that relays messages from village to village at the speed of sound, for untold miles. MaBudu huts are rectangular, the largest side facing the central avenue. A typical hut has two rooms, one on each side of a central passage that leads to the backyard and to the kitchen. In the center of the kitchen floor four stones mark the hearth. A low fire smolders during most of the day, and is rekindled at night for preparing food and for warmth. The tar of burned wood coats the ceiling beams with a brown, sticky, sour-smelling patina. Ashes are used in the vegetable garden as fertilizer. Entrance doors are made from matting, planks or reeds. Custom demands that when the door is fastened, even if only by means of a string, no one is allowed to enter.

MaBudu homes are scantily furnished: a bed made of various parts of the raffia palm, a couple of low stools, a large wooden mortar and pestle, some baskets, a bow and arrows, a couple of calabashes, a few clay pots, a broom made of twigs, a couple of bottles with palm oil. While the furniture in some huts includes a table and chairs, others do not have a bedstead;

people sleep on a raffia mat spread on top of a layer of dried banana leaves. A small headrest, often artfully carved, is commonly used for resting and sleeping.

Among the pieces of furniture, a low, small carved stool is considered the personal possession of the housewife. When traveling, she will carry it on her head together with other paraphernalia. The stool is carved from a single piece of wood: a slightly concave seat, the single or double shaft and the base. Seat and base are round in shape, twelve to fifteen inches in diameter.

A completely different type of chair, mostly used by men, is made from five strong branches of equal length tied together in the center and then spread out. An animal skin is stretched across the top of each branch. By adjusting the lengths, a kind of reclining chair is obtained.

The thick-walls, the copiously thatched roof with just enough outside air inlets through the space between outer wall and roof make the Budu hut a comfortable shelter even in the hottest weather. Attempts to replace the traditional hut by modern concrete structures have met with little enthusiasm from villagers of rural areas who, among other things, complained of dampness that caused all kinds of pulmonary diseases.

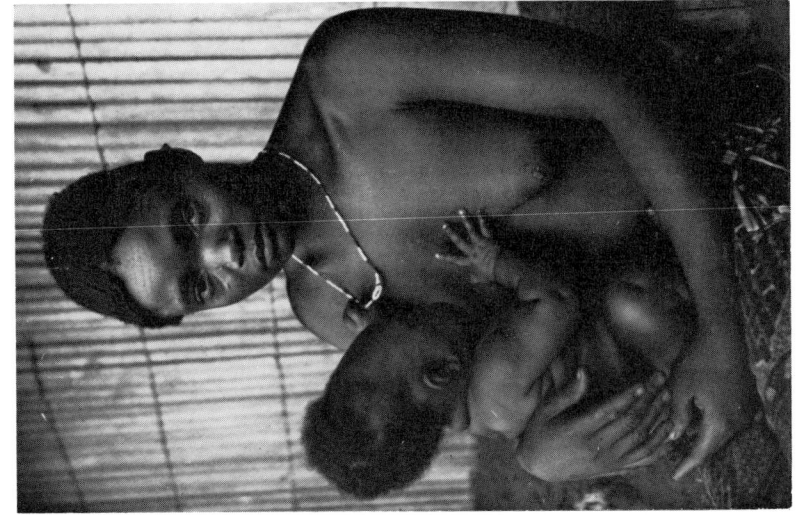

(Ma)Budu woman pounding manioc. Note stylish hairdo.

(Ma)Budu woman and baby showing elongated cranium achieved by binding the head from birth.

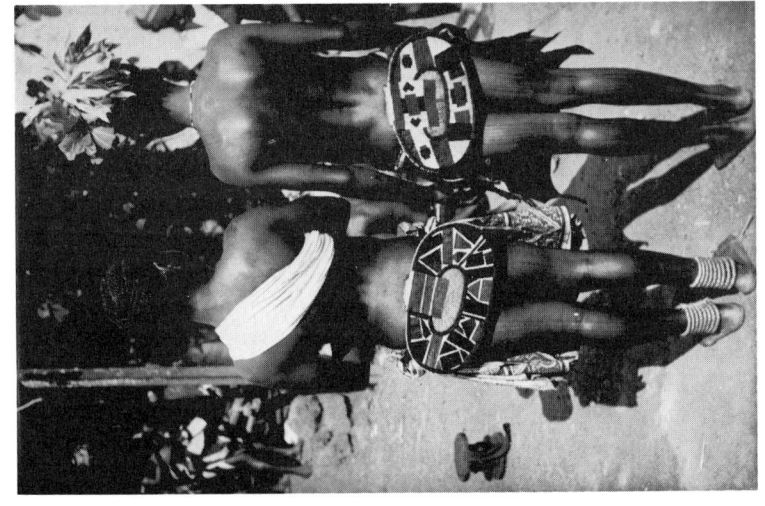

Mangbetu women wearing the traditional "negbe."

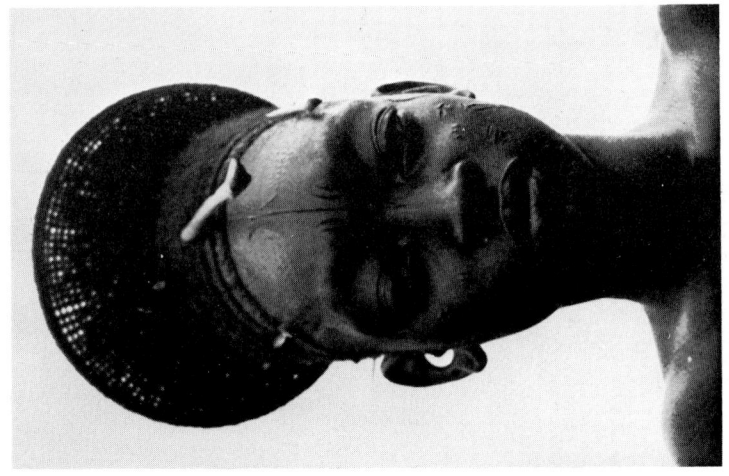

Mangbetu woman's hairdo in the shape of a basket and facial tattoo.

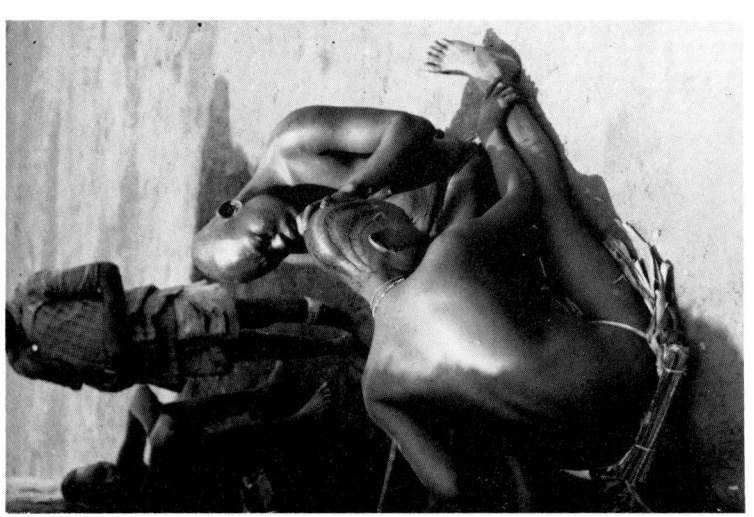

Hair-dressing (Ma)Budu style.

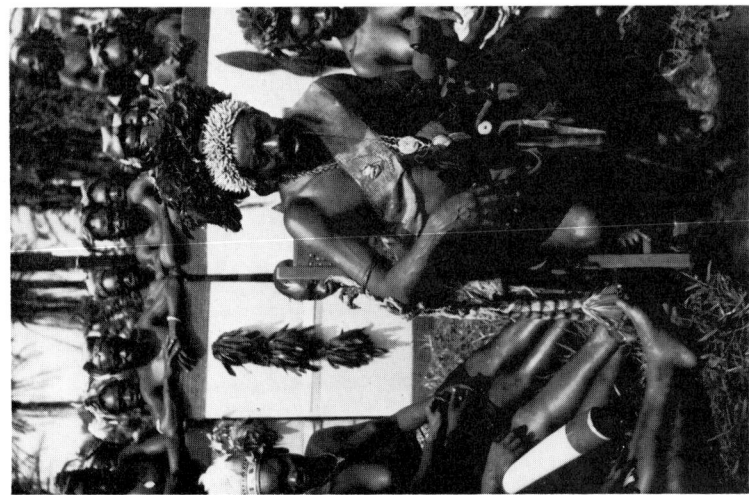

(Ma)Budu Chief Kotinai in full dress, surrounded by his preferred wives and his "army."

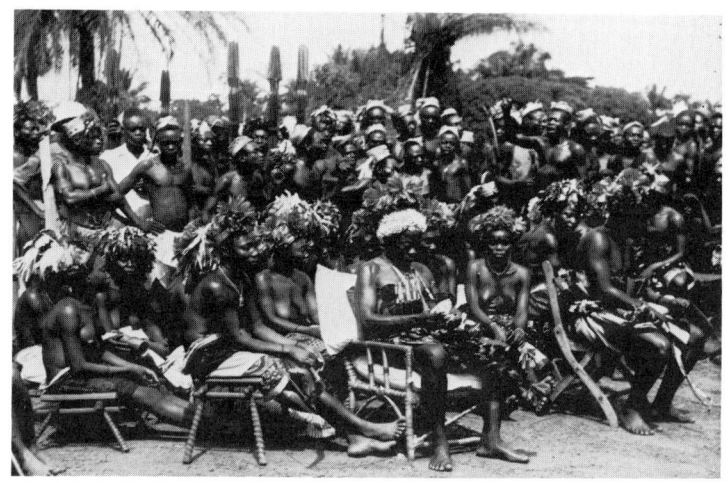
(Ma)Budu Chief Karume surrounded by his numerous wives.

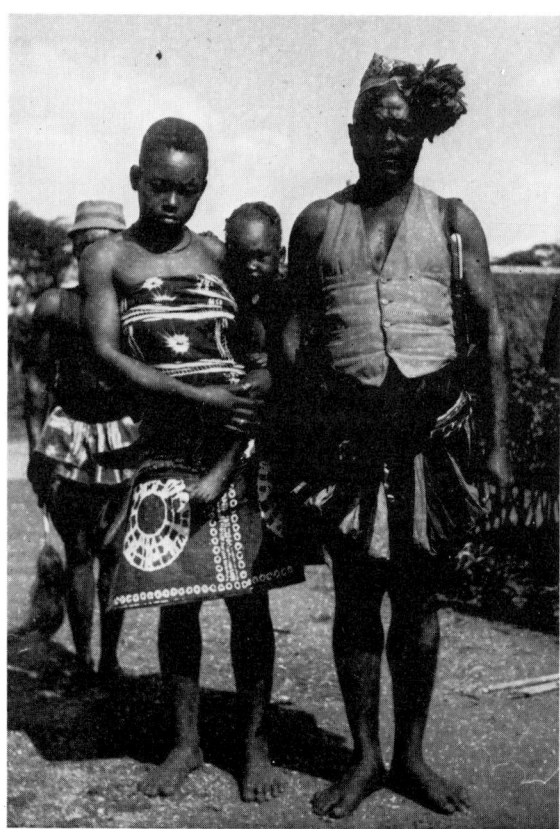
Capita Basiani and his youngest wife dressed in non-traditional but highly fashionable "kikembe" (cloth.) Basiani wears the traditional bark-cloth breeches, square rafia hat with chicken feathers and non-traditional vest—for dignity.

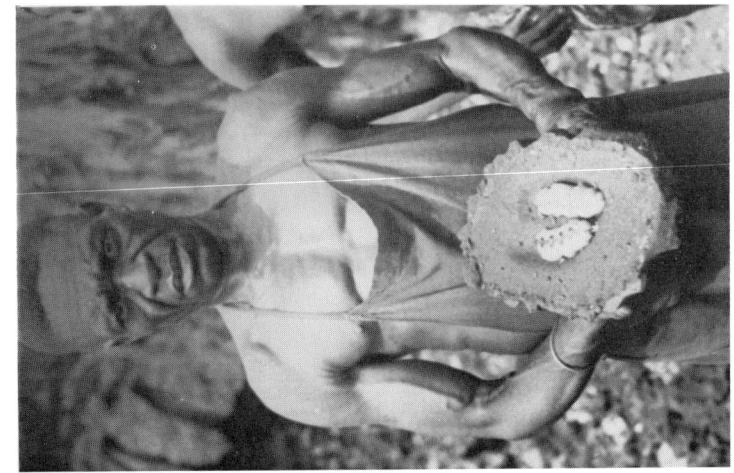

Makakaru, famous Pawa termite exterminator showing two termite queens in their nuptial chamber.

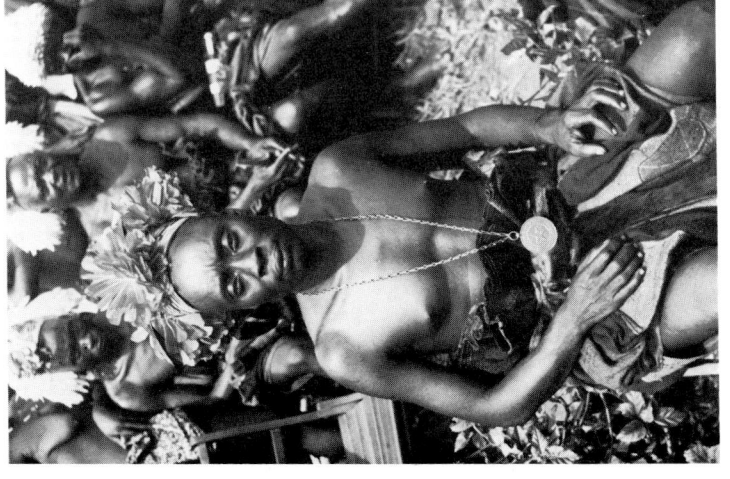

(Ma)Budu Chief Ndabani in traditional outfit (Basiani in middle background) and wearing the official government chief's medal.

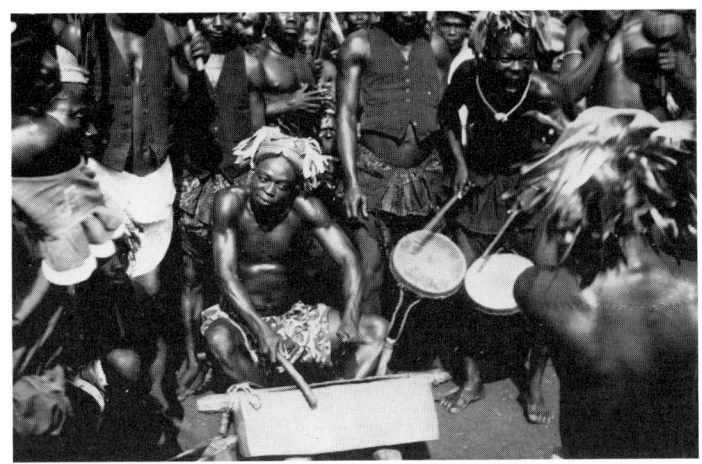
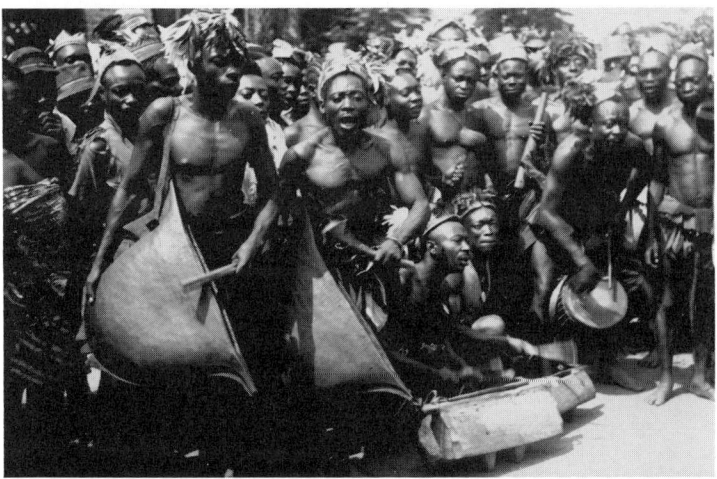

Budu orchestra in full swing. Note different types of drums: the beautifully shaped "gong" drums, slit-drums and hide-drums.

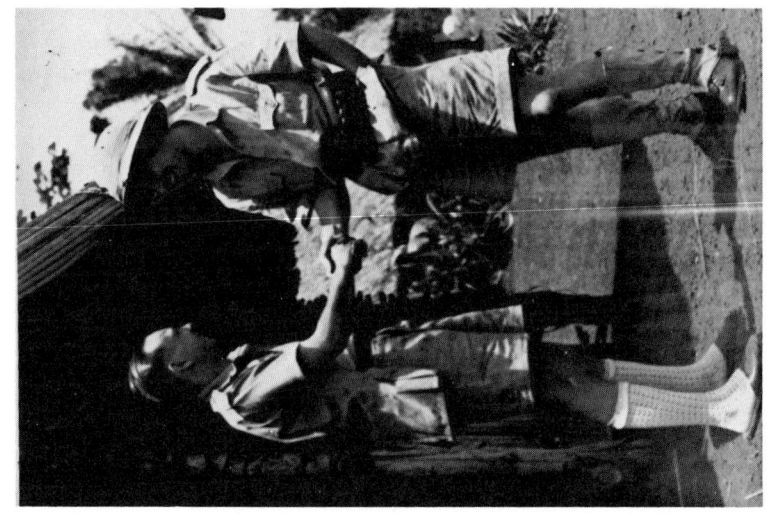

The author (at the right) meeting Freddie Wouters in one of his bush camps during a leprosy survey.

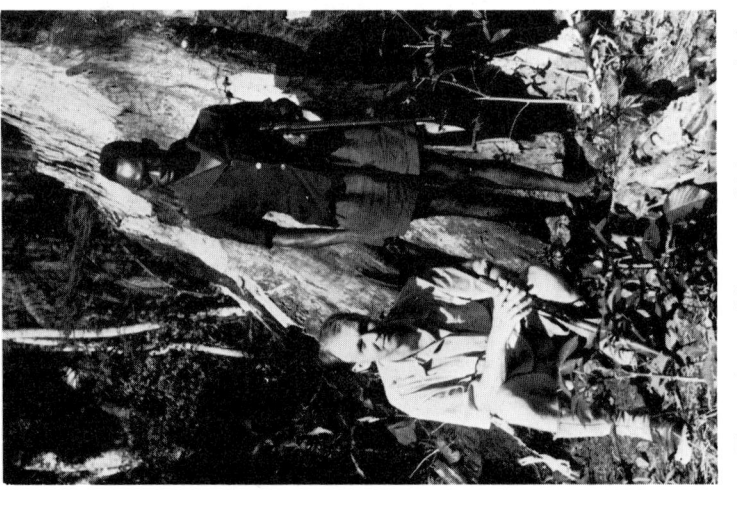

The author and his trusted Mutima ready for the hunt.

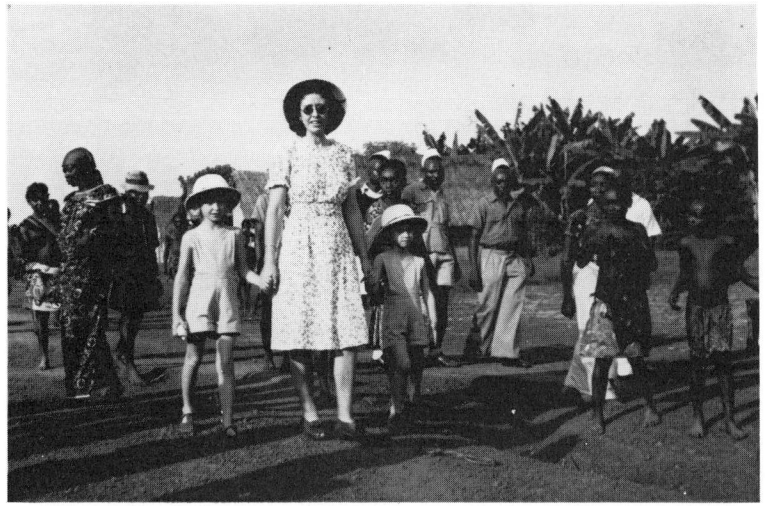

Dora with Winnie (six) at left. Jessie (five) at the right. during a stroll through Pawa's laborers' camp.

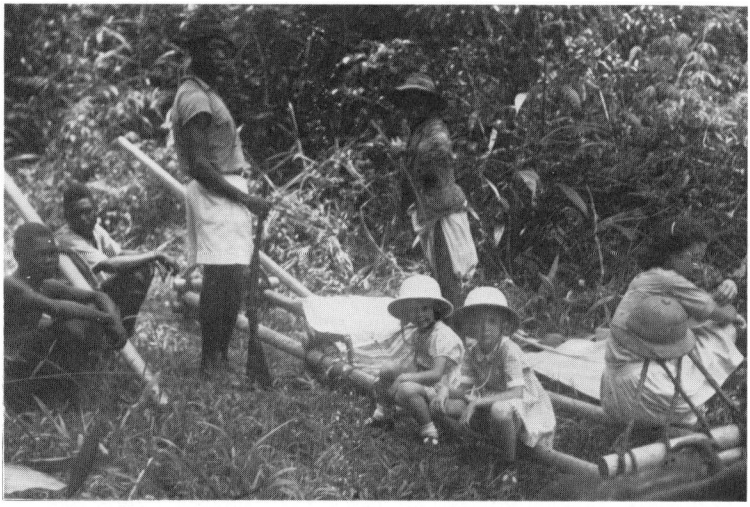

Tipoy (carrier chair) safari in the bush. From left to right: Mutima. Winnie, Jessie and Dora.

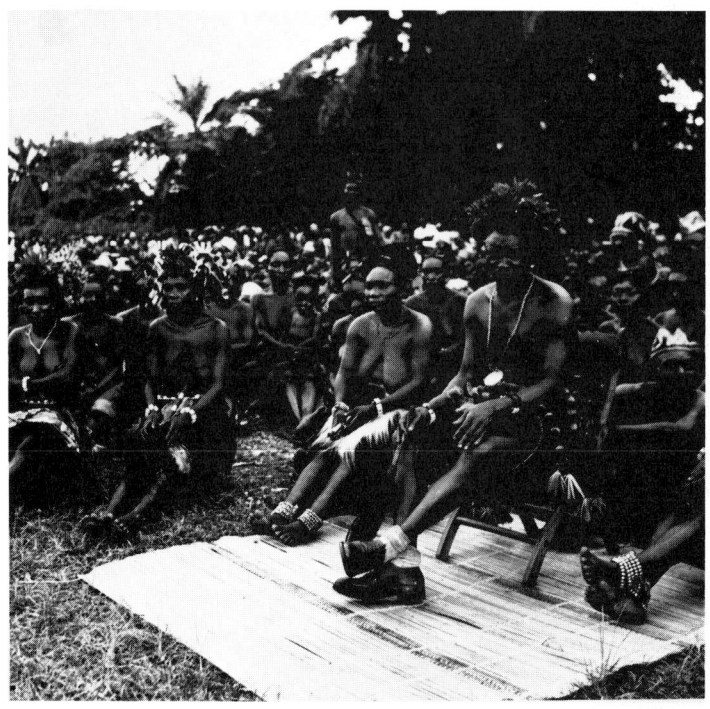

A Mangbetu Chief—traditionally outfitted (but for the walking shoes) and his harem.

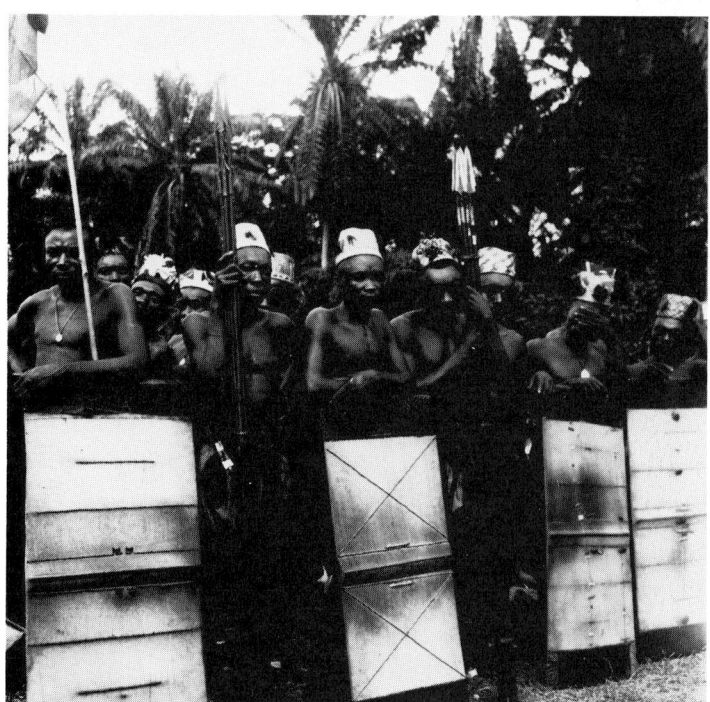

Budu army, tank division.

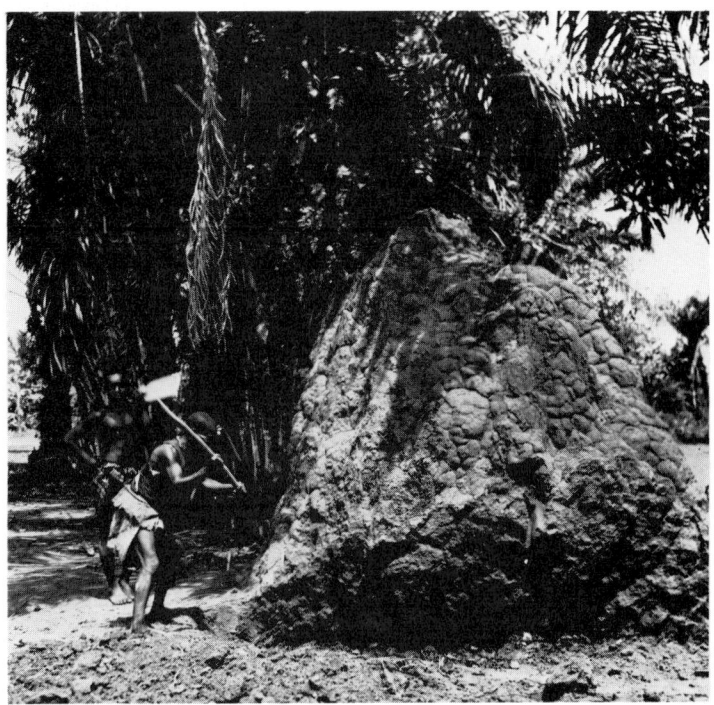
Assault on a termite mound in search of the queen's chamber. Her removal will cause extinction of the colony.

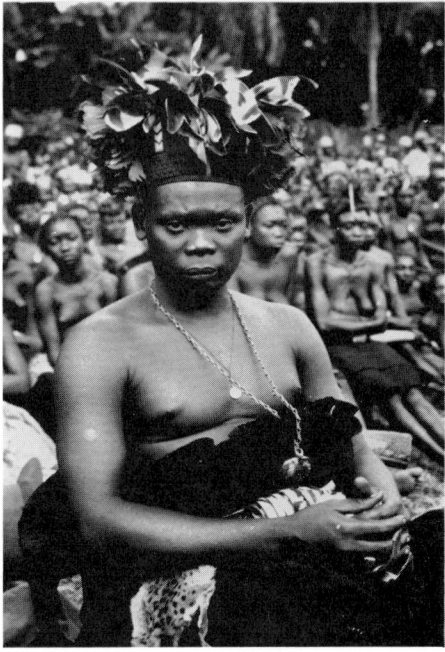
Mangbetu Chief Ebandrumbi.

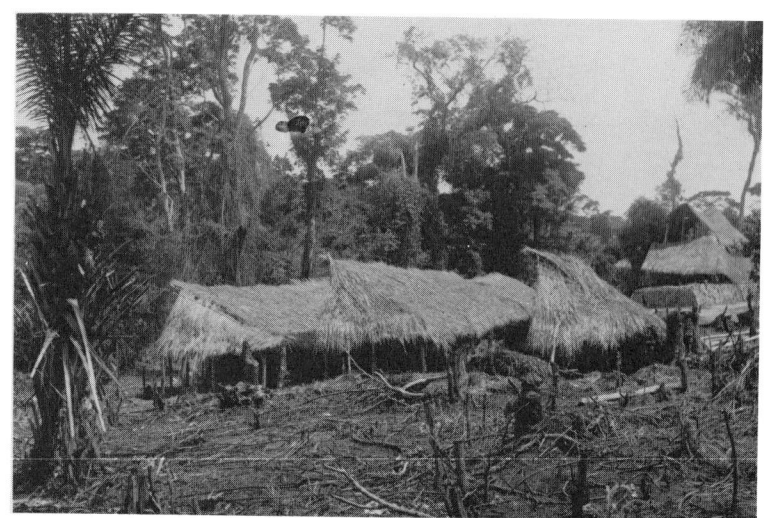

Brick-making works at Pawa, 1945.

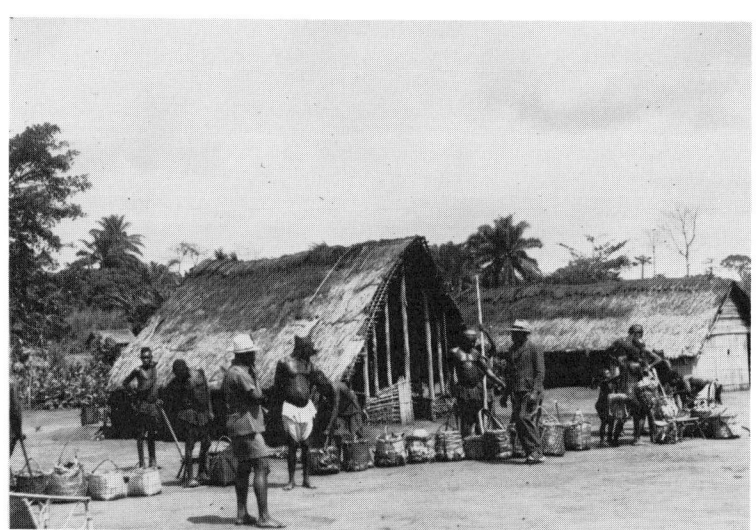

Leper camp at Pawa, 1946.

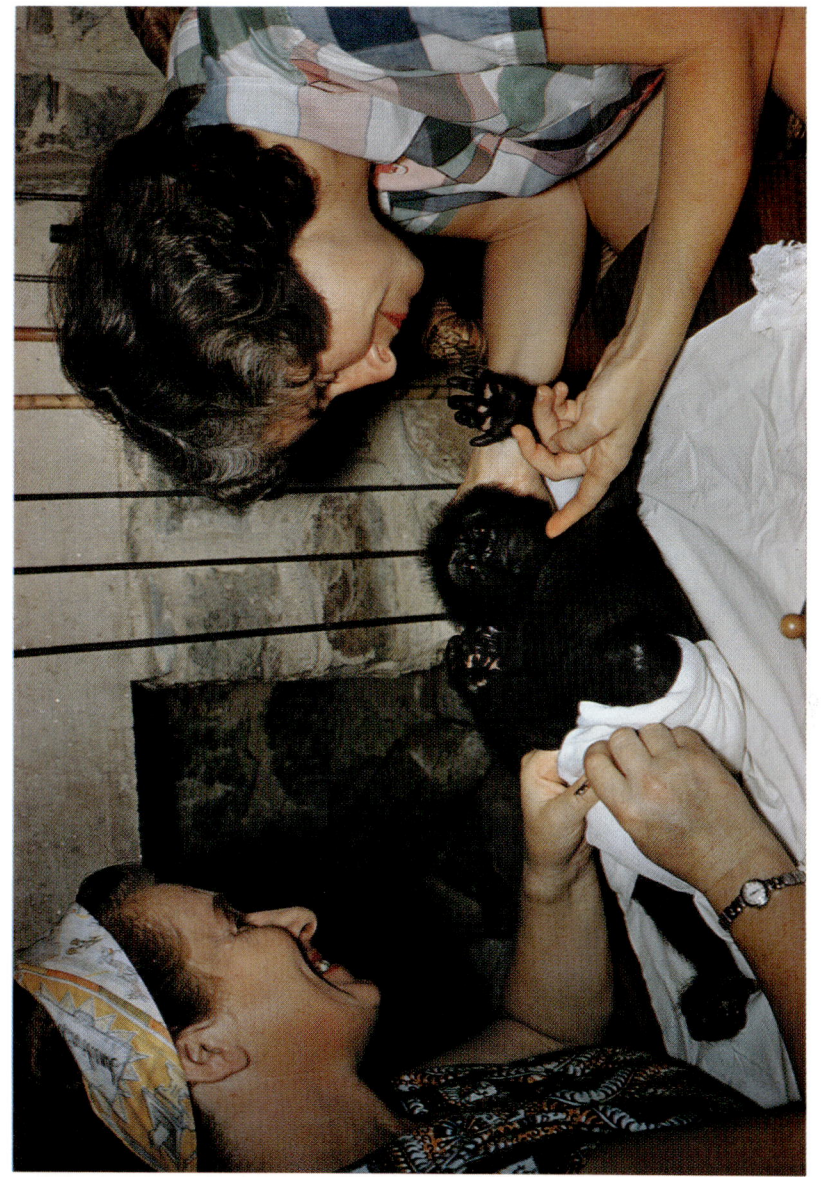

Dora Lambrecht, right, and Emy Cordier, left, admire an orphaned gorilla.

"See You at Pawa"

Those had been the words when I last saw Dr. Gerardi—henceforth called "Doc"—the day he left for the Congo, two weeks before my own departure. And here we met indeed, five thousand miles south and one month later.

Pawa is built on a slightly dome-shaped promontory. Its main and only road follows the central ridge like a backbone. On both sides, the rain forest spreads in all its splendor. Encroachment of the forest is kept in check over a width of 50 yards on either side of the road by continuous slashing of the elephant grass and other vegetation that would reach ten feet if not cut at least once a month. The road ends at the northern extreme of the promontory, its highest point. Here, the laboratory building and two houses face the downward slope leading to lush-green banana plantations of the Red Cross leper village. Beyond the leprosarium the land lies flat, marshy from moisture oozing from the surrounding forest. Then it rises gently, culminating in the sudden slopes of a series of red-brown hills. The hills are outcrops of extremely weathered latosols or laterite soils, characterisitic of most tropical regions of the world. They have a very high content of iron oxide and hydroxides that give these earths their red color. Under extreme conditions of weathering, the concentration of iron salts is such that large boulders and even mountain tops are composed of almost pure iron ore. Polished by wind, rain and blowing sand, they glitter in the sun with a metallic shine. During thunderstorms they are repeatedly struck by lightening—an awe-inspiring spectacle!

The turnoff track to Pawa lies about halfway along the road between Wamba—the territorial administrative post—and Paulis, end of the railroad to Aketi, a transport link to the Congo River. When grasses are short, one will find a sign reading: "Makoda—Pawa 1 Km." During the rains, it may be difficult to accept the overgrown tract as a motorable road. But at times when the recurrent stomach-aches of Brother Nicolas of the Catholic Mission have been particularly troublesome, Makoda and his men have been put to work and the road, now a sharp-edged slash in the banana and amnioc fields, instills some confidence that it may lead indeed to a place called "Pawa."

This is soon confirmed by the white-washed adobe walls of the houses of the Catholic mission and of the little church, partially visible through the secondary forest growth. Before reaching the hospital, a gap in the tall elephant grass to the left leads down to the brick kilns and a number of thatch-covered sheds where neatly stacked rows of pre-fired bricks are stored to dry. The depressions where the clay was removed are filled with milky water streaked with swirls of red earth, the home of a thousand frogs.

The hospital stands about 30 yards back at the other side of the road, 30 yards of relentless devotion by Sister Fidelia to grow some kind of lawn, but to little avail in this hard laterite soil. The hospital is a U-shaped, one-level brick building. The front is occupied by an office, two outpatient examination rooms, a room for surgery and an annex. Two long wards, each with an isolation room at the far end, form the two wings of the building, the left for male patients, the right for female—an arbitrary division because during hospitalization the men patients are joined by their wives, the women patients by their husbands. Kitchen, laundry and storerooms are located in outbuildings behind the main structure. Some distance farther back is a row of huts used by family members of the hospitalized, and a second row for pregnant women awaiting delivery.

Left of the hospital buildings are the main storerooms, including the pharmacy and garages, all new buildings. Behind are two sheds constructed from local materials for weathering and drying freshly cut timber. Pawa tries to be self-dependent as much as possible. Still certain basic supplies have to come by truck from Stanleyville, 370 miles away, or by train to the railway terminal at Paulis, 35 miles away.

Leaving the hospital area and proceeding along the main and only road, one comes to the next brick building on the right, the first house for the European Red Cross staff. It has a rather complicated floor plan because of the rooms that were later added as an afterthought. Like many colonial houses it features a verandah, called "barza," that extends all along the outside of the walls. The floor of the houses are at about two to three feet above ground level, isolating the building from ground temperatures, guarding it from possible flooding during heavy rainstorms while lending a feeling of security. Kitchen and annexes are located in a separate building in the back connected by a covered passage to the main part of the house. The back of this particular house directly faces the forest, only a stone's throw away. Doc, who lived here for a while, used to take pot shots at the monkeys who came to steal the bananas from the bunches hung from a nail under the barza.

The next house down the road, on the left, is ours. Following the classical colonial style, it has a central living room with bedrooms on each side. Again, the kitchen is a separate structure behind the living quarters. The house is long and low. Its clean, simple lines blend attractively with the uncluttered surroundings of a couple of palm trees and a few lean frangipani trees on short-kept grass. The barza is not fenced off, as in the other houses, making it look more spacious and enhancing its intimate relation with the garden. From the many houses we occupied during our fourteen years in the Congo, this was the one we preferred above all—maybe because it was the first house of our first tour in Africa and therefore of special sentimental importance. We became even more attached to the house when we had the opportunity to modify its floor plan after termites had sapped its structural strength by tunneling inside the main rafters and supporting beams and it became necessary to rebuild the house from the ground up.

Past our house, the road rises abruptly to end at the head of the promontory—a distance of about 300 yards—from where the country suddenly opens up to a panoramic view of an unexpected savanna with Mount Akunai in the hazy distance. This is the end of the road and of civilization, as far as visitors are concerned. Below lies the leprosarium with its 360 inmates and their families. If interested, visitors are conducted along an eroded path, forever invaded by stubborn elephant grass, to the village below. The first-time visitor braces himself for the worst, but the uninspiring, overgrown path belies the well-kept leper camp beyond.

After a pleasant hundred yards through the coolness of a banana plantation, the visitor is surprised to arrive at a wide, spotlessly kept village square. To the right is a series of light-colored brick buildings housing the dispensary and hospital rooms. Bright and airy, the structure leaves the impression of modern efficiency. To the left, the visitor is taken back to Central Africa by the very large communal shed built in typical local fashion, its dark, cool interior a great contrast with the bright brick building on the opposite side of the village square. An enormous drum stands at one end, its operator reclining in an easy chair, ready for any eventuality. The villagers like to keep in touch. Though they are free to travel, most patients prefer to stay in the village, some because they have difficulties walking, others because there is really no need to. This is precisely the aim of the Red Cross's effort: to create a pleasant village for those afflicted with the disease, one that is similar to other MaBudu communities, but with the difference that life is made easier for the patients: those too incapacitated by the disease are provided with basic foods such as palm oil, rice, dried fish and the like; others willing and capable till the community garden, plant crops such as bananas, manioc and maize. Inhabitants of the leper village are exempt from taxes and from cotton quotas. The village has its own chief and court and really functions as an independent community. While the CRC policy of maintaining leprosaria villages is a practical application of preventive medicine, the concentration of cases in one village facilitates control and care of the disease. In 1945, Pawa was only one of many leper villages thus organized by the Red Cross in the Nepoko region.

There is more to Pawa than meets the casual eye. To maintain as much as possible its self-reliance, the place hums with subsidiary activities, all vital to the main purpose of medical care and research, but largely unsuspected by the chance visitor. For instance, while the four houses, the laboratory complex and the hospital are the visible center of the community, its "suburb," housing 100 laborers and their families, lies unpretentiously at the prescribed 400 yards from the nearest European house, which happens to be ours. The "camp," as it is called, consists of two neat rows each of some 50 rectangular huts facing a wide central avenue. It is a pretty sight. A slight declivity near the middle lends a three-dimensional effect, the last huts rising to an outline against the cumulus-dotted sky. I took special pride in the camp because as "chef-de-poste" I was directly responsible for its upkeep, order and hygiene. One of the first jobs I had to perform soon after my arrival happened to be the complete reconstruction of the camp. I shall always remember my spurious confidence as I strode among the huts, feeling upon me all the seen and unseen eyes, hoping that I gave the impression of the personification of a "bwana," severe but just, friendly but strong, and wise to their tricks. The former qualities I can only hope to have fulfilled to a certain degree, the latter wisdom, I know, failed me many times. Throughout my association with African personnel I have had that uneasy feeling that things were not going as I was led to believe. Many times I found out, to my embarrassment but also with relief, that the truth had been told and that my suspicion had been unfounded. Involuntarily, I developed an attitude that made my personnel feel that I relied on their honesty and professional integrity and that I expected them to carry out their tasks to the best of their ability. Whether my almost instinctive adaptation to circumstances and responsibilities—I had never experienced before—was right or wrong, I do not know. In general, I seldom had trouble with my personnel and I do not believe that I was "taken in" by them more than average. I know of some colonials who spent hours investigating transgressions and who discovered some hair-raising facts. I may have been deceived many times, but I enjoyed the peace of not worrying excessively. However, I insisted upon absolute reliability and a sense of duty at all times from the hospital personnel and later from my laboratory of field assistants working under my direction. I always hated to apply any kind of punishment, but preferred the culprit to make up for his shortcomings by having him do extra work or be assigned unpopular chores. In the case of serious misconduct I preferred to fire the wrongdoer altogether without further admonishments.

All this was still far from my mind as I made my first lonely strolls through the Red Cross labor camp. I can still recall that sense of elation I felt during my first walk. Here I was, in the very heart of Africa, the dark continent of Stanley—in the very region where Georg Schweinfurth (1836–1925) and Gaetano Casati roamed, braving, as I made myself believe, the same dangers of those very surroundings and living among the same cannibalistic tribes. The shadows were still deep at eight in the morning. The women had already set about for their daily household chores. Fat babies were playing outside in the sun, looking strangely like chubby brown dolls. I felt terribly embarrassed when some of the babies uttered fearful cries when they saw me and scrambled to their mothers as quickly as their short legs permitted.

One of the early morning chores, it seemed, was the cleaning of the inside of the hut, a procedure during which all household objects were taken out. I remember how various groups of articles would make a wonderful subject for still-life photography. Among them were low carved stools, a wooden mortar and pestle, a bed made from mid-rib stalks of raffia palm and a few clay pots.

I entered one of the huts that had been emptied of its contents. In my capacity as chef-de-poste and as health officer, it was in my line of duty to look after the hygiene of the camp. I was taken aback by the hut's darkness and by the blend of odors which were to become familiar only much later: the mushy smell of damp earth, the sweet-sour scent of accumulated woodfire tar, and the emanations of fermenting palm wine. I stumbled over something that looked like a heap of hard red earth. "Makakaru" (termites) said Aponomanga, the capita (headman), who had accompanied me on this inspection tour. His other name was Ijuju and, being easier to remember, that was what I called him. I used the title "Capita," however, on occasions when something had gone wrong and I felt he had been responsible. He was short, stocky, a well-muscled man of about forty, with a serious face and worried eyes. When I met him that first day, he was sitting in the shade of a hut that was being thatched, ripping strips of bark from a branch held between his feet. "Kamba," he said, answering my inquiring eyes. "Kufunga miti," he added—a complementary explanation that was completely lost on me as I hadn't learned a word of Swahili yet. Then he got up and together we started our tour of inspection along the row of new huts.

A native hut may look like a heap of various materials haphazardly thrown together, but I was surprised at how methodically and well organized the actual building of a hut proceeded. At a new site, a couple of *mpagazis* (laborers) sat on the ground digging holes at given places by means of a *mpanga* (machete). Their prodding looked very laborious, almost futile because of the hard red soil, so solid with compact laterite pebbles. But they worked on steadily, unhurriedly, and soon the holes, a foot apart, had the required depth. A pole was lowered into each of the holes and anchored securely with earth and pebbles, pounded solid with the handle of the mpanga. The upper end of each pole had previously been cut in the form of a "V." The height of the poles was now adjusted so that the bottom of the V's were level with a rope fastened between the four corner posts. Long bundles of supple twigs were then tied by means of the fiber ropes Ijuju had prepared that morning, in horizontal rows one foot apart, inside and outside the row of poles. The spaces between the poles and the inner and outer lattice work were then filled with mud.

The manufacturing of *pot-o-pot*, a marvelously expressive word for mud, and its application onto the frame is a fascinating procedure. To make pot-o-pot, suitable earth is mixed with the right amount of water and then trodden with bare feet until it reaches the required consistency and smoothness. The surging noise and the slick of the glabrous red earth looks devilishly attractive and only the moral obligation of upholding the dignity of the white man kept me from taking off my shoes and socks and joining in the fun. While the tantalizing pot-o-pot–making is in progress, another man is patiently waiting for a grunt from the mud-making specialist. At this signal, he heaps some of the material onto the cut-out bottom of an oil drum, carefully adjusts a wreath of twisted grass on his head and, placing the load on top, walks off leisurely, balancing the burden with a corrective movement of the head. After the arrival of the mud-carrier, the most exciting part of the construction takes place when the stuff is slapped onto the framework in handfuls of juicy mud cakes. In most parts of the world, mud-slinging would not be looked upon favorably; in Africa it is an art.

The roof is an intricate affair, involving precisely shaped poles and the accurate adzing of support rafters. When the frame of the roof is ready, a one-foot-thick thatch is tied on. Spellbound, I watched the great dexterity of the thatcher in the way he placed, adjusted and tied the grass bundles that were thrown to him from below. The thatcher also applies the final trimming by cutting off the loose ends of the thatch. This is done with a mpanga and a wooden block held in the other hand. It looks amateurish, but after the man is through one can lay a ruler against the clean-cut edges. Inside, the newly finished hut smells sweetly of dry grasses and damp earth.

I thoroughly enjoyed my first days as chef-de-poste, but I was soon made to understand that my duties included more than just strolling in the morning sun. Gradually, almost imperceptibly, I was given more charges. When I reflect now on the amount of work I put away those days, I am surprised and wonder how it could all be done by a single person.

I feel peevish towards people who maintain that colonials had an easy life; interesting yes—easy by no means. Slowly but surely my list of activities grew to include: accounting and bookkeeping; making out the payroll and paying of African personnel; conducting morning roll call at 6:30; correspondence and mailing; keeper of storeroom and pharmaceuticals including preparation of prescriptions; general supervisor of all non-medical activities. After a few weeks, I had also to assume the duties and responsibilities of my true job as health officer with weekly visits to one or more field hospitals, taking laboratory diagnostic work in stride.

On Saturday afternoons, I "did" the *posho,* that is the market. Though interesting at first, the efforts of trying to keep some sort of discipline and order among a bunch of 200 natives, eager to buy bananas, rice and palm oil at cheap prices from about 150 forced sellers trying to get at least their merchandise's worth, became a nerve-racking way to spend a Saturday afternoon! The chore sometimes dragged on till sunset and even beyond when we had to finish by the light of the kerosene lamp. Wonderful memories, how I hated you at times! My role in the procedures was that of supreme commander of the posho. Certain neighboring villages of Pawa had been commissioned to supply an agreed quota of food weekly to native personnel of the Red Cross, an agreement worked out by the local chief, Ndabani, and by our own director. The capita of each of these villages had been instructed by Chief Ndabani to see that the required number of banana bunches and pots of palm oil arrived each Saturday at the Pawa marketplace. The capitas were hard-pressed trying to persuade their fellow villagers to deliver the weekly quotas and they often failed in this endeavor. When this happened too often or the shortage was too marked, I had, for the sake of my personnel's welfare, to report this to the chief. The unfortunate capita was then summoned to the chief's village to receive punishment, which was, by tradition, a number of strokes—usually from four to six—from the "fimbo," a four-ft. length of hippo hide, about one inch in diameter, tapering off at the far end.

The market activity started by weighing the bunches of bananas. A ticket with the weight and price was delivered to the owner. The ticket was often lost by the time of the sale and it fell to me, then, to estimate the weight. My estimation invariably brought two cries of protest: one from the seller proclaiming that the bananas were worth twice the price I quoted, and one from the buyer insisting that they were worth half my estimation. When, in spite of all protest, the buyer hastily paid the price I had quoted and when the seller accepted with a sheepish smile, I knew that my price had been close.

When the weighing was over, the head clerk of the Red Cross, a clever rascal named Masi, lined up the vendors in a single file. The buying proper then started. Each staff member or his wife formed a single file behind Masi and me and was allowed to buy one bunch each as we proceeded along the vendors' line. I allowed some leeway for large families, but soon the claim of numbers of children reached fantastic figures, denying all official reports of population trends. Protests were common; the bunch of bananas was too small, they were unripe, of poor quality or too expensive. I took a firm stand unless the issue developed into favoritism; I said that all should buy what came along at their turn or give up buying altogether. I was helped in this verdict by Masi, for whom the market chore was as boring a way to spend a pleasant Saturday as it was for me.

After the bananas came the palm oil. Here complaints were even more soul-stirring, the more so because the value of the oil offered was based entirely upon my estimate. I was surprised, however, that my price was usually accepted by both parties mainly, no doubt, because Masi had been a good teacher during the first weeks of posho. Masi, by the way, was one of the few CRC personnel who, besides his native Kibudu, spoke French, Kiswahili, Lingala and some other local dialects. When I quoted my price, he would put out his hand to receive the money from the buyer whenever the price was right. If the price was way off, he would look upward to Heaven as if seeking grace for a painful, though innocent, mistake. The trouble was that I did not always know in what direction I had erred.

When the posho was started early enough, that is around one o'clock, and there was not more than the usual palaver, it was possible to finish by five. With an immense relief and feeling of satisfaction, I would walk home, take a bath in hot if slightly cloudy water, don clean clothes and, reclining in an easy chair, see the sun set behind the forest at six. Fifteen minutes later it was dark. My boy Mutima would bring the Coleman pressure lamps, the S-shape-sprouted can with alcohol, and the matches. The blue flame of burning alcohol would dance erratically around the burner until, with a twist of the valve, the heated kerosene would burst into a strong white beam that turned uncertain shadows into sharply outlined objects. Even the palm fronds across the road would reflect the light and the forest would suddenly seem frightfully close. The loud hissing of the Coleman pressure lamps sometimes accompanied by faraway drumming and chanting was to be the background noise for the rest of that evening and for the next thousand Pawa evenings.

One Saturday, halfway through the posho, loud trumpeting and drumming made themselves heard above the clamor of the market. It announced the arrival of Chief Ndabani. His tipoy, borne by four chanting mpagazis, was brought in front of me, and lowered. Then out stepped the potentate, clad in traditional MaBudu outfit. His black-red-cream bark cloth, fastened around his waist in a broad sweep, gave the overall impression of the corolla of a huge exotic tulip. A classic MaBudu hat, adorned with red parrot feathers, finished his outfit but for one important item: his official chief's silver plaque that dangled on his bare chest. He was a man of medium height, heavily built, in his early thirties. His face bore a continuous obsequious smile. He had slit eyes with heavy, drooping eyelids that gave his face a rather sly expression. We shook hands native fashion: a handshake followed by holding each other's thumb. Ndabani stated that he wanted to make certain that his capitas were bringing the requested quotas of food, and asked if this were the case. Before I could answer, Masi start to complain bitterly about one capita who, indeed, had done very badly over the last weeks. He was immediately summoned and to my horror was ordered to lie down in order to receive six of the best lashes from the chief's favorite "polici," a combination constable-runner-law enforcer. This was the first time I was to witness a whipping, and I felt terribly embarrassed. But I couldn't stop the chief's order, nor could I turn away. With what I hoped was an impassive face, I watched the performance, outwardly unconcerned, inwardly sick. After the resounding six strokes, three on each buttock, the capita stood up, admittedly a bit painfully, rearranged his bark cloth he had lowered to receive the punishment, came to attention, saluted Ndabani and then me, and the thing was over without further ado while the posho proceeded as usual. The food supply from that capita was up to par for several subsequent weeks. I was to learn that these were normal proceedings and that certain capitas simply had to be reminded from time to time that the chief's law was still in force by the traditional method of "chicotte" (whip). The Belgian Colonial Government abolished this type of punishment in 1946, and government officials were no longer allowed to apply corporal punishment as it had been used for centuries in Africa as one of the milder sentences one could receive in African societies. Many chiefs, however, did not consider themselves bound to observe the revocation of their old customs, and it was said that the people themselves preferred to receive the "fimbo" rather than to serve imprisonment.

An administrative duty I hated more than any other was that of paymaster and keeper of the strong-box safe. I have always had a difficult time with money, either earning it or spending it wisely. However careful I thought I was, I was constantly short after checking the accounts at the end of each month. There were several sources of possible leakages. The most important one was, I believe, my own slovenliness in failing to mark unexpected on-the-spot expenditures; I was always in a rush. Another problem was that the paper money was so very old and greasy that many bills stuck together. Sometimes I noticed just in time that I was dishing out more bills than payment warranted. How often I didn't catch this error I shall never know. Another notorious source of shortages lay in the number of bills making up the money rolls received from the bank. Of course, one was supposed to count the money upon receipt, but who was going to count several hundreds of bills and a thousand coins while a long line of customers waited to be served before the bank closed at noon? Not able to account for money shortages, I had to make them up from my own salary. Luckily, the sums were never very large. Still, it was most annoying.

The payment of salaries at the end of the month was a source of endless arguments. Many times it would happen that no sooner had one of the men received his pay than he would be surrounded by creditors, eloped wives, greedy concubines, blackmailers, ransom collectors or unpaid fathers-in-law, to name only a few uncomplicated cases. Whatever the cause of the disturbance, I was usually brought in as an unbiased party. I soon learned to avoid involvement by all possible means.

To help me on payday and at roll calls, I had a clerk, a young chap called Otto. He seemed to be honest enough, but I don't know to this day how much he was implicated in my monthly losses, if at all (but I prefer to think that he was not). He had an almost sickly fear of our director. I know that he would take any amount of traditional punishment rather than explain irregularities to Dr. Zanetti. "That was what he was going to do," I told him after we had found a serious deficit once more. He immediately told me that he would rather forego a month's pay to make up for the shortage than face Dr. Zanetti.

Part of my administrative assignment was the hiring and firing of personnel. Requests for the dismissal of laborers came mainly from Brother Nicolas in charge of construction. Many times, the fired worker would complain that he had done nothing wrong. Often that had indeed been the reason for his dismissal: doing nothing at all. Out of principle, I seldom questioned the Father's decision, and so I prepared the worker's "kitabu" (book) by paying his due wages and marking the time and date of discharge. The "kitabu," soiled and greasy as it may have looked, was an official document, a sort of identity paper which all Congolese adults were supposed to possess and presumably keep up to date whenever the owner changed address, or job or traveled outside his or her district. It helped in keeping track of population movements and in census-taking. Inhabitants wishing to travel were required to have their "kitabu" signed by an administrative or medical authority. Travel could be refused if, for instance, the person was involved in a court case or as a preventive measure against the spread of communicable diseases.

As for hiring personnel, the "kitabu" provided information about the applicant. For instance, a frequent change of jobs would not speak well for the applicant. In the case of household personnel, there was an unwritten agreement among the housewives, the ones who usually did the hiring and firing of servants, of how to report in hidden terms eventual shortcomings of personnel dismissed from their service. A quotation: "departure for home leave" or "departure for relocation" not followed by other comments would generally be considered a favorable reference. Unfavorable references were handled in various, sometimes witty, ways: "clever magician" (thief); "loves the sun" (lazy); "great traveler" (often absent); "collects empty bottles" (drunk) and so on. Another method of reporting negative references was by exaggerated qualifications, such as "extremely careful" (a slob) or "extraordinarily pleasant" (unpalatable character). The reason for these hidden messages was that it was unlawful to give references that would be prejudicial to the owner of the "kitabu."

One of my more pleasant duties, alas often too time-consuming, was to check on various outside activities. Among these: brickmaking, felling of timber, the processing of chaulmoogra oil, termite control, and the manufacturing of soap. Then there were the occasional trips outside Pawa, such as hauling supplies with the lorry (or truck) from the Paulis railway station or taking the medical requisitions to the other Red Cross stations at Ibambi, Medje and Babonde.

One of my occasional inspection tours included the various workshops. I was most fascinated by the blacksmith and his helper. I regretted that I could not spend more time in the dark, mysterious sanctuary of his isolated shed at one end of the village. The smithy was enshrouded in a sort of enigmatic cloak that even Brother Nicolas's wrath didn't seem able to penetrate. In African societies, smithery is one of the oldest of arts, and smiths are considered a highly respected, elite group within the community. It was perhaps this traditional rank that made our blacksmith a bit standoffish. It made the Brother suspicious, and I too felt that more was going on in the smithy's abode than met the eye. The dark workshop did not promote enlightenment. Nothing, however, justified Brother Nicolas's suspicion. The smith was given pieces of sheet metal to make into various objects for buildings or equipment, and smithy made them, to exact specifications, and on time. Neither he nor his helper ever caused any trouble at work or at the posho, their wives never escaped, they were never wanted in court, their skill was beyond reproach, and they could make everything that could be made from iron. They were so unobtrusive that I don't even recall their names, or their faces. Though we had a lingering suspicion that some of the raw material was turned into more potent things than door hinges, we could never prove a single case. We made occasional surprise visits to the shed only to find door hinges and other innocent implements. Perhaps the smithy was guiltless.

One of my favorite inspection tours was a visit to the brick kilns. They were located near a low-lying marsh where gray clay was found. The clay was kneaded into soft consistency by two men treading the glutinous mass with their bare feet until proper uniformity was reached. The clay was then shaped by hand into cakes slightly larger than the size of a brick. These were pressed into their final form in a hand-operated press. The dark-gray molded cakes were then stacked underneath low-flung sheds to dry, leaving spaces between the rows so that air could circulate freely and insure even desiccation, which would take several weeks, depending upon the season. The great moment came when the Brother decided that everything was ready to fire in the kiln. The dried brick cakes were assembled on top of three tunnels made of baked bricks of previous vintage; the whole was protected from rain by a thatched roof on high poles. Again, the bricks were stacked in such a way as to leave sufficient gaps between each to allow free circulation of hot air throughout the mass. The finished kiln looked somewhat like a miniature replica of the pyramid of Sakkarah. The tunnels were now loaded with logs and the fire started. The secret of success was that once the fire was started, it had to be kept going steadily day and night for a week or more, depending upon the number of bricks.

Going out to look for the lumber team was always an adventure. On an assignment, the team was sent out for many days at a time. To find them in the forest took the cooperation of willing guides and long marches. This made the Brother very cross. He claimed that the lumbermen went deep inside the forest on purpose to avoid surveillance. This meant that we had to send another team to haul the timber long distances to the road where it could be loaded onto our lorry. Working deep inside the forest gave the lumber team plenty of time to loaf around to visit relatives or markets as the Brother, not unreasonably, suspected. They were easily informed well in advance in case of a surprise visit, many times by a village "gudu-gudu" (tom-tom).

They were safe. Then, one day, the Brother had a brilliant idea: instead of sending laborers to bring the timber out to the road, he had it carried all the way to Pawa by the lumber gang itself. They didn't like that at all. First, it so happened that they worked a long distance from Pawa; second, it was rather degrading for a "scieur-de-long" to haul timber. On their next assignments, they found good trees quite close to the road and everything was put right again, at least for the time being.

The task of the "scieur-de-long" teams, once the suitable tree was selected and felled, was to cut the bole and the larger branches into sections of convenient lengths. Each of the sections was then cut lengthwise into boards one inch thick or into timber of current sizes. The timber was then carried to the side of the road where it would be picked up and transported by our lorry. The cutting of the sections was done by means of a "long saw," roughly seven feet in length provided with a wooden handle at each end. The bole section was secured horizontally across a crude scaffold and cut by two men, one standing on top of the section, the other below. At Pawa, the wood was left to "season" under large, well-aired sheds. Because well-cured wood may take years, the stock was replenished regularly as the seasoned wood was consumed.

The forests of the northeastern Congo contain a large variety of valuable woods. The one most commonly used at Pawa for general construction of beams, rafters and door- and window-frames is commercially known as African mahogany *(Khaya anthotheca)*, locally known by the name "Makamba"; it has nothing to do with American mahogany, except for its red color. It is a big tree, reaching 100 feet when full-grown, found mostly in the peripheral zones of the rain forest. When freshly cut, the wood is pinkish, turning dark red-brown on contact with the air. Another beautiful tree is the "Limba" *(Terminalia superba)*, often 100 feet tall with a diameter of up to seven feet. In the gloom of the forest, the tree stands straight and white, its trunk supported by buttresses of tall, support roots. Its lovely wood has the color of light oak, works easily and is perfect for furniture and cabinet work. Another beautiful wood in use at Pawa is "Kasa-kasa" *(Erythopleus guineensis)*. Unfortunately, it is very dense and hard and difficult to cut with hand tools. The wood is resistant to insects, and so tough that it can be used for making wheels. The tree has a close, well-developed crown of dark green, conspicious among the other forest species. The young tree grows tall and straight until its crown reaches the upper canopy. It then rests and develops some branches and leaves as it competes for sunlight.

In 1945, the Congo forests covered approximately 50 percent of the country's surface or about 300 million acres. As in other tropical forest regions of the world, the Congo forests are slowly being reduced through commercial exploitation and the encroachment of an expanding population. Pawa's tree-logging, although minimal in scope, was part of an overall destructive process that, one day, may become irreversible.

One other activity was specific and unique among Pawa's industries: the collection and processing of the fruits of the chaulmoogra trees. About 100 trees had been planted in the cleared strip that separated the edge of the forest from the road. During the time I was at Pawa, chaulmoogra oil was still in use as the treatment of leprosy. The oil derives from a tree (*Hydnocarpus wightiana*) that grows into a thickset bush about ten to twelve feet high, resembling somewhat a coffee tree in general appearance, and visitors often mistake it for such. The fruit, the size of a small orange, and the color of dull-green velvet, contains forty black, shiny seeds. The outer shell is rather brittle and can easily be crushed by hand. The fruits drop when ripe. They were collected twice a week by Sukari (sugar), who was also responsible for their processing in addition to his other duties of beating the gudu-gudu. On most days, one would find Sukari balanced on an old packing crate under a shed, patiently removing the slimy black seeds from their shells to spread out to dry for several days. The shed was shared with the CRC planton (messenger) who whiled the time away by rolling tufts of raffia fibers on his thigh into homemade string. When thoroughly dry, the chaulmoogra seeds were ground in a meat grinder. The resulting gray-colored paste was then pressed in a hand-press from which a clear, slightly yellowish oil dripped into a jar, each drop languidly forming long crystal-clear teardrops that sparkled in the sun. The dried seeds yielded about 15 percent clear oil. The oil was heated and filtered several times. The final preparation was an admixture with sodium gynocardate or creosote in various concentrations, according to whether it would be used for intravenous, intradermal or intramuscular injections. The bottles were then carefully sterilized, labeled and stored in the dark.

Trees yielding volatile oils containing chaulmoogra acid and closely related fatty acids and derivates belong to the family Placoutiacea. The genus *Hydnocarpus* is found in tropical Asia. The trees that were planted in Pawa belong to the Indian variety, *Hydnocarpus wightiana*, said to give the best yield of oil. The tree is endemic in the tropical forests of the Western Ghats of East India, up to an altitude of 2,000 feet. The flowers are greenish-white and unisexual, so that both male and female plants are needed for seed production.

Although chaulmoogra seeds were mentioned as treatment for leprosy in the oldest Chinese and Indian records, it was only in 1853 that the oil was introduced to Western medicine by a Dr. Mouat of the Indian Medical Service. A legend tells of how a certain King Rama developed leprosy and fled deep into the country. He subsisted on herbs and berries, among them the seeds of the *kalaw* tree, and found that the disease soon subsided. He went back to reign. Then one day he found a once-lovely young princess in a cave, completely disfigured by the disease. He told her about the *kalaw* berries, and he himself went to collect them for her until her health was restored. They were married, raised sixteen sets of twins and lived happily ever after, so the story goes.

After the rediscovery of chaulmoogra oil as a cure for leprosy, perhaps not so radically effective as the Hindu legend wants us to believe, it still remained the only available effective drug for many years. It was estimated that in 1963 there were still some 13 million leprosy victims in the world, 80 percent of them in Africa and in Asia. A shortage of available chaulmoogra oil was felt long before that time. In 1920, Dr. Joseph F. Rock of the United States Department of Agriculture was assigned to locate important natural habitats of the tree, to study the organization of regular supply and to determine whether it would be possible to establish nurseries in other parts of the world. He sailed to Singapore. From there his travels in search of the rare plant brought him through the steaming jungles, high mountains and swift rivers of Siam (Thailand), Burma and India. He collected and shipped to Hawaii a number of closely related species in the hope that at least some would produce seeds containing the useful drug. Most were failures. With great courage, he resumed his search and after a gruesome two-day march to a mountain pass, he found the slope on the other side covered with *Hydnocarpus kurzii*. Collecting as many seeds as he could, he sailed back to Hawaii where they were grown successfully on a 100-acre plot. By 1921, thousands of seedlings from the three species Dr. Rock had collected were flourishing and bearing fruit, among them *H. wightiana,* which proved to be one of the better species. Dr. Rock died in Honolulu in 1962, at age seventy-nine.

Much About Soap and Termites

One could say that Sukari was the chemist expert of Pawa because besides the processing and mixing of chaulmoogra oil he also made soap. While I never followed the process closely—it was messy and smelly—I know that it involved the saponification of crude palm oil by the alkali obtained from ashes of banana leaves. I doubt that the soap was of high refined quality, but that didn't matter much. It was used mainly for boiling slightly soiled bandages from the hospital, after which they were thoroughly rinsed and dried for many hours in the fierce, sterilizing sunrays. They were then used in the leprosarium. With our tight budget we tried to cut expenses wherever possible. Sister Cypriana, in charge of the welfare of the various leprosaria, was a particularly tough economist and the soap-making business was one of her ideas.

Sukari, bless his soul, was also the man who announced the end of the working hours, at noon and at five, by beating the gudu-gudu. I had never known him to be late. His signal started with spaced beats that picked up speed and ended in a prolonged roll. His popularity was on the low side, however, when at six in the morning and at two in the afternoon, he had also to call the men to work. Our working hours were typical of colonial times: reveille at six; roll call at six-thirty; breakfast between eight and eight-thirty; lunch between noon and two; end of the workday at five.

Makakaru was another classic Pawa character. Whatever his true name might have been, no one knew or used it. 'Makakaru' is Kibudu for 'termite'. The name stuck to him because as long as human memory could recall, he had been officially engaged in the endless fight against these troublesome insects. Makakaru had dedicated his whole life to this noble enterprise. And while chances of promotion were slim, so were the chances of running out of work. As a matter of fact, many times it looked as if the termites could build their mounds faster then Makakaru was able to tear them down. However, a few barked remarks from the director usually restimulated Makakaru's energy and shook him into action to check the termites' advance into the chaulmoogra plantation and their attempts to undermine the road. Makakaru's philosophy was quite simple and therefore profound: the only thing he asked from life was that the termites would keep their activity at par with his passion for work. He also knew, however, that this was asking too much and that he would have to face the director's wrath whenever the equation was markedly out of balance. At one time I won his temporary blessing when I had detailed a gang of mpagazis to help Makakaru collect large amounts of earth from termite mounds, after I had found that this smooth, compact material was ideal to surface the tennis court I was then building.

Makakaru's attack on termite mounds, leading to their ultimate destruction, was simple and straightforward, as one would expect from someone in the business for several decades. Over the years he had gathered strange but, no doubt, properly adapted instruments to carry out his trade in an efficient and comfortable way. His equipment included a crowbar, a hand-spray–gun, a bottle of creosote, an old trowel, a storm lantern and the usual mpanga. He would walk along one side of the road with a rather firm step and an intense expression on his face. His once-blue uniform was faded and in rags. One might be excused from believing that this was due to the hazards of his job. Not at all. All CRC personnel received a new uniform at the beginning of the year. Makakaru sold his as soon as it was issued. Arriving at the termite hill of his ruthless choice, he would carefully deposit his instruments and study the nest for a while. A long while. Then the crowbar would be put to work. By the time Sukari's gudu-gudu announced high noon, Makakaru would have located and removed the fat, ugly huge termite queen. Once the queen was removed, the colony was doomed to die and its population scattered. That strong monarch is the termites' dynastic link with its millions of subjects. The queen is easily one of the most repulsive objects I have ever seen. Her head and thorax are of nearly normal termite size, but her abdomen is a wriggling huge, fat, creamy sausage six, seven or more inches long, two inches wide. The queen is confined in a thick-walled chamber made of the finest, smoothest red earth precisely shaped to the size of her bloated body. It is from here that she mass-produces a daily output of thousands of eggs. Overpopulation is unknown because the worker-termites simply keep on building a larger mound. Only the death of the queen will terminate a colony.

If asked, Makakaru also performed his task indoors. He was, however, clearly a field-man; more at ease at heaving the crowbar than working the scapel, one might say; uncomfortable and rather destructive when working in confined quarters behind delicate furniture, for instance. The mess he usually made during his house visits was appalling. After he was thrown out of the director's house, followed by verbal abuses he hadn't heard for a long time, either in Lingala or Kibudu, it became clear that his inside duties were over forever. Makakaru returned to his outdoor operations and their many possibilities of resting in the shade of a chaulmoogra well away from the "wazungu's" (white men's) whims.

My own battles with termites started soon after I occupied the house. One morning, after Sukari's gudu-gudu fantasy had scattered my dreams that this might be Sunday, I became aware of something unusual in the room. Looking down on the floor I saw to my utter amazement a mound of red earth about one foot high, close to my bed, and looking suspiciously like a termite hill. It was. It looked so unassuming, so natural and casual that I hesitated to tell anyone, afraid that it would be known that "the new boy complained about a mere termite hill in his bedroom, the other day. What is Africa coming to!?" When I did tell the director a week or so later, he was quite concerned, however, and asked the Brother to investigate the matter. It did not stop the relentless, insidious termite demolition work. A year later the house had to be taken down and rebuilt when the roof threatened to fall on our heads, major beams having been reduced to pulp.

This first open attack was followed by more subtle but equally destructive ambushes. First the back of my shirt was tunneled through over a length of ten inches the very first time I hung it on a peg against the wall. A couple of days later my pajama followed suit. I hung my clothes on a chair. I organized the defense of my belongings by injecting creosote into the holes in the walls that were indications of tunneling activity, this after consultation with Makakaru. I doubted the effectiveness of this measure, but it was symbolic of a declaration of war; I was ready to man the barricades. The reality of how fast I was losing the war came to me abruptly when, one day, I leaned against a doorpost and my hand went right through the wood or rather through the thin layer of paint that had once covered the wood. I began to work on the wood as well. Pretty soon the house smelled so strongly of creosote that I had to sleep outside. And still it was a losing battle. Taking out one of my notebooks from a bookcase, one day, I found it pierced by long tunnels that went through all its pages. Another day, the termites got into my food cabinet and, besides the cheese—replaceable—ate the frame from the wire mesh—which wasn't. Anything left undisturbed for any length of time and containing cellulose in one form or another, was subject to often unnoticed, internal destruction. Termites hate to work in the open. When I lifted a demijohn of precious wine, stored away for special occasions, the handle of the basket came off and the bottle crashed on to the cement floor, spilling my hoard. Not only was this an endless war, but victories were a bit too one-sided as far as I was concerned.

This was the situation when my family finally joined me at Pawa. For some reason, the battlefield remained quiet, void of any military operations, truce seemed in the air. But I was ill at ease and apprehensive that the enemy might be regrouping its forces and shaping up for a breakthrough. This happened one night when a noise like a deep sigh came from the ceiling as if someone had given up holding a heavy weight and was about to throw in the towel. Next morning we discovered a definite concavity at the left side of the roof. And while this rather improved drainage, we also knew that the termites had won a major battle, if not the war, and that they now were merely considering mopping up operations. We lived for another four months in the house and then we had to move out in a hurry. While our house was taken down and being rebuilt, we went to live in the house of the director on leave in Europe. Our new house was built on the same spot and according to my own floor plan. This time, the supporting walls were well isolated from the foundations by a solid slab of concrete. It was a lovely house.

While termites are undeniably a scourge in many tropical and subtropical regions causing staggering losses in stores and buildings, for some African populations there is one compensation during a part of the insect's life cycle. With the first heavy rains, winged termites start leaving their mound by the millions to swarm about the surrounding country. Their awkward flapping flight is of short duration. They land in an uncoordinated fashion within a short distance from their escape hole, lose their wings and each starts crawling around in search of a mate. But before many can fly away, African children are fast to build a crude, small basket of twigs and banana leaves over the escape holes to collect this most appreciated food supplement. Even those that land outside the traps are quickly seized and eaten *in vivo* and *in toto*, wings and all, a few termite wings getting stuck around their greedy mouths. Slightly roasted in their own abundant fat, swarm-termites are considered a dish of unparalleled savor and are of great nutritional value. The taste is oily-nutty according to my daughters, who once participated in a catch.

At the time of the swarming, Pawa, with its numerous termite mounds, was literally covered with flying termites. They were to be found in every crack and nook, covered all surfaces and flew inside the houses at night, where they burned themselves inside the pressure lamps, leaving a stench of charred bodies and destroying the lamp mantle in the process. It was a curious sight on the morning following their nuptial flight when thousands of crawling termites covered the parade grounds in front of the roll-call office, each female closely followed by a male—or vice versa, I never knew—moving in pairs for some unknown destination with the inborn instinct of starting a new colony.

Besides the activities mentioned before, my other duties included: surveillance of sanitation and general upkeep of the station; supervision of rolling stock and spare parts; control of fuel and oil; dispatch of transportation; inventory and purchase of domestic, laboratory and hospital supplies; checking teams of carriers responsible for the delivery of adequate amounts of water and firewood to the three senior staff houses. To these duties was added the supervision of an African elephant hunter after we had received a government permit to kill one elephant per month to supplement the diet of the lepers. I soon found out that, in this case, supervision was a rather symbolic function for after the hunter, an old army sergeant, was issued a gun and five rounds of ammunition, he disappeared in the forest for the following two weeks. The next thing I heard from him was by way of a CRC runner who dashed into my office with the tail end of an elephant and rather vague information of the whereabouts of the shot animal. A party of mpagazis, at last enthusiastic, was sent out to cut up the animal so that the pieces could be transported to the nearest road where the truck would load what was left. I had no illusions that all that meat had been left undisturbed. When the very smelly vehicle pulled in, I had the greatest difficulty in containing the crowd, so eager were they for meat. The trunk, the choice piece, went to the hunter. On another occasion, the hunter would return after many days without elephant tail but with spent empty shells and a hair-raising tale of how a couple of elephants had refused to die and had nearly killed him. If only he could have had five or possibly ten more rounds. There was little chance for me to verify his stories, but I had the strongest suspicion that the hunter had shot and sold some animals for his own profit. However, as long as he kept the leper camp supplied with meat I was willing to forego investigation, for which I could ill spare the time.

As if I had not had enough work already, one day I proposed to start a class in simple parasitology and microscopy for our young male nurses working at the hospital hoping that some might become interested in pursuing a more advanced medical career. I had six students and we held class one day a week in one of the school rooms at the mission. None of them spoke another language than Swahili or Kibudu. Teaching parasitology in Swahili was quite an experience. We had much fun trying to find the right Swahili word for various objects and verbs that did not exist in their language. But by means of drawings and demonstrations under the microscope, I managed, I believe, to explain some of the basic principles of the transmission of diseases and the involvement of certain insects in the process and how, in many instances, transmission could be avoided by simple rules of personal hygiene and sanitation.

And then, one day about halfway through my tour, a new man arrived fresh from Belgium to take over my administrative responsibilities. I was finally free to devote my time to medical work. This still included running the medical laboratory, pharmacy, dispensing drugs and supplies to other Red Cross centers, blood tests of lepers who were under experimental drugs and, finally, the weekly visits to three field hospitals. It was still a lot of work, but then it was the kind of work for which I had come to Africa. Pawa provided me with a solid background of experience, a lasting love for Africa, and a taste for learning and exploring that would eventually lead to a joyful career of research in insect-borne parasitic diseases, a term as broad as I can make it.

The Hippocratic Oath

During his speech before the graduating class of 1943 (Diploma in Tropical Medicine and Hygiene), the director of the Tropical Institute, Professor Jerome Rodhain, vigorously stressed his determination to see any one of us severely punished were we to be found guilty of dishonoring our profession or found liable of malpractice. This was 1943! The language, along with the cutting edge of his voice, made a deep impression on all of us. It was still fresh in my mind when I started my health officer's career in Pawa, two years later.

The Congo Red Cross's main obligation in the Nepoko region was to assure the delivery of medical care to the population, replacing that usually provided by the government medical services. In addition, Pawa was also designated as a center for the study and control of leprosy. The Nepoko was, indeed, a region of very high leprosy incidence.

Leprosy is an ancient disease. While the medieval populations in Europe were devastated by sudden and tenacious epidemics of smallpox and plague, a sly and more hideous disease crippled the inhabitants in a slow, unrepentant grip: leprosy. It is not so much the number of victims that strikes the imagination of recorders of medieval history as the mystery that always seemed to surround the disease and the latency by which the victims underwent slow decay, limb by limb. If plague, the Black Death had swept the land indiscriminately, the stumbling walk of the emaciated, crippled leper would have somehow been more horrifying than the mercifully quick death of a plague victim. Forcing the isolation of the lepers into specially provided houses, the citizens gave way to feelings of mystic horror rather than reasoned quarantine, whose principles were only discovered centuries later. The image of the leprosy victim, swaying clappers and uttering the hoarse cry: "I am a leper, I am a leper," is as much part of the imagery of the Dark Ages as the coffin-laden flat wagons that carried the plague victims.

Leprosy was already known well before that time, however. Certain skin diseases described in Egyptian records of 1350 B.C. during the reign of Ramses II are held to be typical of leprosy lesions. Leprosy was known in China some 5,000 years ago. The disease is described by Aristotle, around 345 B.C. on the

Greek coast and in Asia Minor. Its spread was precipitated after the conquest of Egypt by Cambyses in 525 B.C. and Xerxes in 480 B.C., and the later maritime colonization of the Mediterranean. Both the Hebrew scriptures and the New Testament report its presence. Spot dates show the advance of the disease in the European hinterland as recorded in: Italy (62 B.C.); Germany (in 180); Spain (fifth century); France (sixth century); England (in 625); Ireland (in 869); Wales (in 950). By the tenth century, leprosy was recognized in most European countries. It seems that the disease became even more widespread during the twelfth and thirteenth centuries through Crusaders returning from their eastern campaigns.

A most remarkable event in the epidemiology of leprosy was its rapid decline in Europe, for no apparent reason, during the fourteenth and fifteenth centuries. By the end of the eighteenth century, leper houses, no longer required, were shut down in most countries. In the nineteenth century, the disease had disappeared from Europe except for small pockets in Sweden, in the Pyrenees and Maritime Alps and in a few areas of the Baltic coast. General improved hygiene and better diet may account for this decline, at least partially, while perhaps the isolation in leper houses had the desired, if unsuspected, effect of interrupting the transmission of the responsible disease agent. There is little doubt that leprosy was carried into the New World by African slaves. Exploration and travel account for the rather recent introduction of leprosy in Oceania and Australia.

At the present time, the highest incidence of leprosy occurs in humid tropics. As these are often areas of low living standards and poor sanitation, climate alone cannot be taken as the sole factor of predilection. Moreover, the occurrence of the disease and its spread in Europe for so many centuries in the past tends to refute the theory that a tropical climate is a prerequisite for its transmission.

In 1940, the infection rates per 1,000 inhabitants in Africa were as follows: Belgian Congo, 20; French Equatorial Africa, 16; Nigeria, 10; Sierra Leone, 10; Uganda, 5.4; Rhodesia, 5; Gold Coast and Cameroons, 5; Mozambique, Angola and Zanzibar, 3 to 5. In the Belgian Congo, the highest incidence occurred in the Nepoko region.

Gerhard Hansen was the first to identify the acid-resistant bacillus, *Mycobacterium leprae*, (Hansen 1871) as the agent of the disease. Acid-fast bacteria are those that retain the original red color when stained with the Ziehl method, whereas bacteria not belonging to this group, lose the red color as a result of the dilute acid treatment and absorb a blue counterstain instead. Among the many acid-fast bacteria, two are infective to humans: the Hansen bacillus of leprosy and the Koch bacillus of tuberculosis. Both bacteria are zoologically closely related, but are individually indistinguishable. In biological specimens, however, the Hansen bacilli are found in little bundles like match sticks, usually of more than ten, while the Koch bacilli are found in smaller groups of three or four bacilli at the most, and often single. The two bacteria can be differentiated biologically, if the live bacilli are inoculated in laboratory animals. The regular failure to introduce lepra infections in laboratory animals is the reason why relatively little is known about the physiology of this bacillus and its action in the tissues. This excludes the possibility of experimental therapy. (In 1974 it was experimentally proven that *Mycobacterium leprae* can be inoculated directly from human lepromatous lesions into the armadillo, *Dasypus* spp.) Of Dr. Hansen himself, little is known besides his discovery of *Mycobacterium leprae* in 1871 as the cause of "Hansen's disease," a term often used because it is thought to sound less pernicious. Hansen was a Norwegian physician born in Bergen in 1841; he died there in 1912.

Leprosy is one of the most frustrating diseases to treat and to study. Nothing is known exactly about how the infection is transmitted, except that prolonged contact with a leper will almost certainly result in contamination. Acid-fast bacteria have been found in several insect groups and even in leeches. As experimental work is practically impossible because only humans and armadillos are susceptible to the infection, and as the bacilli cannot be cultured in any known culture media, these findings of other occurrences of the organism have not been followed up much, and the implication that an insect might be a vector has been disregarded. The bacilli are found in almost every tissue of the body of an infected person, but more manifest and conspicuous lesions are seen in the skin and peripheral nerves. The disease symptoms have been classified according to the site(s) of the main pathological manifestations, with numerous intermediate and substages. When subcutaneous it is cataloged as "L" (lepromatous); when found in the nerves as "N" (neural). According to the type and stage of advancement, a leper may look like a normal person, but still be a carrier of the bacillus and contagious to healthy people, or may look like a decaying body with ulcers and dwindling nerves that have reduced legs and arms to necrotic stumps. The disease can last several decades, even a lifetime, or cause death in a few years, according to how the infection evolves and how much care is taken of the patient.

The basic principle of the CRC antileper campaign was the segregation of patients in villages that were run and administered insofar as possible like any other traditional African village. Serious cases, who could not help raise their own crops, had their diets supplemented with staple foods such as dried fish, palm oil, rice, ground nuts and bananas. The villages were designated by the abbreviation "V.A.I.L." (Village Agricole d'Isolement de Lepreux). It was a successful experiment mainly because the patients did not feel confined, but lived an almost normal village life. The segregation of lepers was not officially compulsory, though strongly encouraged. The lepers were allowed to bring their immediate family members to the V.A.I.L. village, on condition that it made their voluntary isolation less difficult to bear. Family members willing to share this existence had to face the reality, however, that by accepting cohabitation they exposed themselves to continuous risks of contamination.

There is little doubt that the lepers had a far better life in the V.A.I.L. villages than they would have had in their home villages. They were given help and advice for raising food crops, were free from taxation, received medical care on the spot and were given food supplements. Another step in the CRC program towards reducing the natural incidence of the disease was aimed at protecting babies born of infected parents. It was proposed, and again this was entirely free choice, to take care of these infants in a nursery school. This was free of charge or obligation. The parents could visit their child any time they wanted or, indeed, could ask that it rejoin the parental home, where, however, it would face almost certain infection with the disease. Indeed, the following statistics show probability of contamination: with a leper father 10 percent of children become infected; 16 percent with a leper mother; and 40 percent when both parents are infected. What is more, the first sign of infection in the child may not be seen for as many as ten years after contamination.

Whereas a male patient joining a V.A.I.L. village is often accompanied by his wife and children, such marriages often do not last long; the wife, or wives, return to their parents. This denouement is commonly followed by long court sessions and quarrels, as the husband is entitled by native custom to the return of the dowry. As can be imagined, that is a very lengthy procedure involving many passionate squabbles.

The chaulmoogra treatment of leprosy was of doubtful efficacy in most of our cases. Of equal or perhaps of greater value during the course of the weekly chaulmoogra injection sessions was the general improvement in health through routine medical care. We believed that the treatment of secondary diseases such as malaria and intestinal parasites—together with a proper diet—would shore up the immune system and give the patient a better chance to resist the Hansen bacillus. The general well-being of the patient was also greatly improved by the cleaning and systematic treatment of necrotic ulcers, so common in leprous patients.

New hope was born when, towards the end of 1946, we received the first samples and information of a new drug "Promizole," a derivative of the sulfanilic acid group. Early trials looked very promising indeed. Administration of the drug in the prescribed doses was often followed by a rapid response: skin lesions disappeared, lepromatous swellings subsided, and patients gained weight and felt better. Results, however, were not constant and when I left Pawa in 1949, the new drug had given as much disappointment as it had hope. Nevertheless, we were grateful that a general improvement had been seen in almost all patients under Promizole treatment; in some, the progress had been halted; in a few, an apparently complete cure had been achieved. In all instances, the results had been far better than with chaulmoogra treatment. Anemia, however, was a serious side effect of the sulfa drugs in patients under prolonged therapy. A strict monitoring of the patient's blood's hemoglobin and red cell count was therefore necessary. It fell upon me to carry out these weekly blood tests of the first ten lepers under experimental sulfa treatment. As they had been chosen from among the most contagious, I fully realized my own risks of exposure to the infection. My hands were none too steady as I handled my first patients. In the procedure, I had to puncture the skin of one of their fingers with a needle, draw blood—swarming with Hansen's bacilli—into three different mouth-operated pipettes, and further manipulate the potent stuff in subsequent tests, including the counting of red cells, white cells and hemoglobin content. After a time I gained greater skill, and no doubt became more efficient in handling more safely the risky assays that soon became a part of the routine of a colonial health officer.

My greatest satisfaction, however, lay in my weekly visits to three "dispensaries" (field hospitals). After 40 years, impressions have lost the keenness of novelty, others have gained in importance and passion, many have been forgotten. It would be difficult to describe in detail those moments when I attended to my Budu and Pygmy patients in the primitive structures grandiosely called "field hospitals"—the warmth of the red earth floor, the coolness of the mud walls, the dancing sunlight through the raffia shades, the smell of leprosy, disinfectant, tropical ulcers and the smoke-permeated bark cloth of my patients as they filed past the examination table.

After a month's internship at the Pawa hospital I was given the responsibility of running the dispensary at Abiengama, some ten miles north of Pawa. During this apprentice period I had watched "Doc" and Sister Fidelia in their work and acquainted myself with the organization of the medical care for some hundred, or more, outpatients. I had also watched the head doctor perform surgery on a hernia case. After five minutes I had to leave the room to avoid crowding the operation table: the sight and the sound of the scalpel cutting live human tissue was too much to bear so early in my medical profession.

The dispensary at Abiengama consisted of a rectangular mud-walled structure divided into three parts. I held my weekly consultations in the middle part, behind a large table. In the wall behind me, a square opening provided a draft of cool air that helped disperse the putrid odors of the more severe cases with tropical ulcer. On my left, a room separated by a bamboo curtain, was used for more private consultations, such as syphilis cases, and for giving injections. To my right was a room reserved to store drugs and medical equipment and which, for a short while, I used as a dentist's cabinet. If I had time, I would examine stool samples under the microscope for intestinal parasites or would leave them with Madianga to examine during the week so that I could have the results on my next visit. My weekly visits were planned for Wednesdays so they would coincide with the passage of the weekly Stanleyville—Paulis mail truck at the junction with the main road, about ten miles north of Abiengama.

My consultations started with the lining up of the patients in front of the building by Benjamin, the African assistant who accompanied me from Pawa.

Madianga, in charge of the dispensary during the other days of the week, handed out the identification and treatment cards that I had made out for each patient during an earlier visit. They showed their names, serial number, date, a short history of their ailments and the recommended treatment, which was then administered by Madianga during the week. On following visits I would indicate any changes in treatment, if necessary, or note end of treatment when the cure was achieved. At the end of each month I took all the cards home and from the data compiled my monthly reports. Weekly attendance varied from about 50 to 150 patients. On rainy days there were as few as ten. I suspected that visits to the dispensary were also made occasions for social gatherings, a place to visit to hear the latest information about distant relatives and friends. And while there, why not take a pill or two, to make the journey worthwhile in more than one respect?

The clamor made by the patients while they waited their turn outside was often so loud that I had to exert my imperialistic authority and have them pipe down a bit. This was usually replaced by the wailing of the babies awakened by the sudden silence. As order was restored, the line advanced once more. Patients presented themselves to my right, the women giggling and bashful; the men with grave determination. Many did not speak Swahili but only the local Kibudu tongue, so that my assistant had to translate. Medical complaints were mostly minor ones, ranging from rheumatism, or a headache to a common cold. Cases of chest ailments with heavy coughing increased abruptly one week after I began administering a self-prepared cough mixture that was flavored with mint. This sudden increase had me baffled for a while, the more so since it occurred in the dry season when everybody should be bouncing around in good health and spirits. Then I saw the light. In the next batch of cough mixture I replaced the aromatic ingredient by a strong-tasting disinfectant. The epidemic disappeared as quickly as it had begun.

Most of the time diagnosis was not too complicated and there was always malaria, if confirmed by blood smears, or intestinal worms if found in stool samples, to fall back on in case I was at a loss. About 90 percent of the children between the ages of two and five showed malaria parasites in their blood. Rates decreased gradually to around 30 percent in adults. All, young and old, male or female, had one or both of the common intestinal worms: *Ascaris* (roundworm) or *Ancylostoma* (hookworm), accompanied at times by the rarer *Trichurus* (whipworm) or *Taenia* (tapeworm). Most had microfilariae in their blood, mainly *Depetelonema persistans, Dipetelonema streptocera* or *Loa loa*. There was no sleeping sickness in the Nepoko region. We saw large numbers of frightful tropical ulcers, the moist environment and high temperatures, no doubt, contributing to the process of ulceration of even slight wounds, which occur mostly on the lower limbs. The most serious diseases, however, were leprosy, pneumonia and the sexually transmitted diseases, syphilis and gonorrhea, the result of the great promiscuity of the population. Yaws, a kind of ulceration of the skin called framboesia, is caused by an organism, *Treponema*, closely related to that causing syphilis, and was seen especially in Pygmies. It is nonsexually transmitted by body contact with the open ulcers of an infected person.

The number of syphilis cases in treatment at the Abiengama dispensary reached the 100 mark at one time. Diagnosis of syphilis was not always easy in older cases. When there was doubt, a sample of venous blood was drawn and later tested serologically at the Pawa lab. The trouble with the syphilis test was that yaws infections, old or new, would also cause positive reactions. In new yaws or syphilis cases, diagnosis was not difficult because ulcers caused by yaws are quite distinct from syphilitic lesions.

I was rather pleased to have Pygmies among my regular patients, as they were usually reluctant to have anything to do with a white "witch doctor." I tried to encourage their attendance by showing that they were no different from my other patients and by giving them all possible care. Though they were sometimes ridiculed by others, including my own assistants, I never batted an eyelid. I liked their shy but independent style of behavior. They were very amused, and so were the other patients, when I tried a few Kibudu sentences I believed I had mastered by listening to the same questions my assistant asked the non-Swahili-speaking clients: "Do you sleep well?"; "Do you have a temperature?"; "Are your stools hard or soft?"; "Do you have pain when you urinate?"; "Are you married and are you living with your wife (or husband)?"; and so on. My attempts may have been terribly confusing especially when, as I have reasons to believe, certain words were incorrectly used. The hilarious outcry some of my efforts provoked left me with no illusions that my Kibudu was somewhat outlandish at times, to say the least, but the good spirit it created contributed perhaps to the Pygmies' willingness to come for treatment.

One day I took along a series of dentist's forceps. They came in all shapes and sizes, some of fascinating design. An old woman had begged me for many weeks to extract a painful molar. Encouraged by stories of successful extractions performed by another health officer, I decided to try my own hand. When the woman arrived, I led her to the private consultation room, had the bamboo drawn and tentatively applied the appropriate forceps to the offending tooth. I still do not understand what happened in the next seconds, but suddenly the forceps were slack in my hand and between them was a bluish tooth, repulsive with age, but otherwise the result of a perfect extraction. Instead of the wailing patient I had expected, covered with blood, there was the wrinkled face of a beaming old lady, an expression of gratitude in her eyes I long remembered. My reputation as a tooth extractor spread fast and wide and the following week the length of the waiting line in front of my dental cabinet would have been a warming sight to any professional practitioner. I made some more successful extractions, most of them easily performed as many teeth were so decayed that they came out at the first attempt. But as I was spending more and more time on this sideline practice, it began to interfere with more orthodox medical activities. On the advice of the director who feared also that my dental avocation would not conform to my official duties as health officer, I had to declare my dentist cabinet closed (without much regret) and referred all new toothache sufferers to the Pawa hospital.

As in other countries of the world, the symbol of my profession was the stethoscope. Doc had showed me how to use it and how to distinguish between a pretender and an acute case of pneumonia. Equally important to me was the precious time it gave me to think and make up my mind about what was wrong with a patient while I applied the instrument to various parts of the chest and back.

One day the director decided that the future of the Nepoko resided with the children and that a special effort should be made to see that their health was monitored from the day of birth. I was instructed to hold a special session at each of my visits and to examine *all* babies from newborns to one year olds, weigh them, take their temperature, treat infections, give the mothers a measure of milk powder, and keep a record of data on a special postnatal card, with a copy for the mother and one for our own files. Contrary to what I expected, the measuring of the anal temperature was less cumbersome than weighing a baby. The babies started howling the moment they had to leave their mothers and be put onto the scale, swaying their arms and legs, which made accurate weighing a bit of a joke. The second week I brought small pieces of chocolate that seemed to calm them down somewhat. But when, several weeks later I ran out of my stock of chocolate, it started a near riot, the mothers accusing me of meanness, even malice. After that, attendance to the "goutte de lait" fell sharply and as chocolate remained a rare commodity for a long time, only free milk and a piece of soap kept it going.

Abiengama was the village of residence of Chief Ndabani. It was named after his father, the previous chief who died in 1942. Like many MaBudu villages of some importance, it was composed of two rows of huts neatly aligned, leaving a broad open space in-between. The chief's house was at the entrance to the village, to the left, and was the only brick house. It was huge and contained many rooms, most of them empty. Here, reclining in his lounge chair, Ndabani spent most of his leisure hours and they were many—under the barza, listening to the stories or complaints of his subjects. His favorite wives would sit around him on the typical low stool and share the "malafu" (native alcoholic drink) or the cigarettes he contemptuously accepted from the members of his entourage or from visitors. A native policeman, uniformed in blue "kaniki" (a kind of denim) was always standing by. Besides his uniform that at times included a red fez, the mark of his profession was a pair of handcuffs dangling from his leather belt and, symbol of law and order, his "fimbo" ominously stuck in the same belt. Punishment applied with a new, straight fimbo was bad enough, I would imagine, but when it was applied with a flexible whip or one with a twisted end in the hands of a fiendish policeman, it could easily take the skin and flesh from the offender's quarters. Wisely, the offenders never complained about this traditional flogging, but rather cursed their bad luck when the executor happened to be one using a crooked fimbo or applied strokes with a twist. Victims of the fimbo came to our dispensary for treatment of lacerations. They usually healed well with daily applications of mercurochrome to prevent infection.

The dispensary was only a few hundred yards away from Ndabani's village, but I seldom went to visit him, except for strictly official and urgent matters. Personally, I did not especially like the chief's sly manners and I had the feeling that he did not like me, nor any other white man, for that matter. Moreover, a visit would not be considered polite if I had to make it short and I certainly would have hated to waste time just sitting under Ndabani's barza with no common ground for conversation. I sometimes regret that I did not use this opportunity to learn more about local history.

At the suggestion of the director, I did visit Ndabani the day I took charge of the Abiengama dispensary. I found the chief sipping malafu in the shade of the barza. Someone produced an empty beer glass and Ndabani poured what remained in the calabash. The glass filled with a milky liquid in which all sorts of unidentifiable matter floated. Looking politely unconcerned, I drank the stuff. It had a sweet-sour taste with a definite alcoholic twang, not unlike a "Tom Collins," as a matter of fact. It was rather potent and after a couple of drinks it seemed only normal to accept Ndabani's invitation to accompany some of his men who would show me where and how the malafu was collected. The afternoon that had started with an innocent courtesy visit ended near sunset with my return in rather ragged clothes after a long journey through deep forest and quaggy marshes. True, we had reached the raffia trees in full malafu production. I had climbed the rough step-rope to see for myself the fermentation process. Briefly, this process develops as follows: rain water collects in the hollow part inside the crown formed by the upper fronds of certain raffia palms. If all goes well, the level of the liquid is maintained naturally through the compensation of water input from rain or dew, and evaporation. In the meantime, certain starch and sugar compounds derived from flowering buds and tree sap are dissolving and when they reach the correct concentration, trigger the fermentation process. Malafu-producing trees are easily spotted by the swarms of bees attracted by the sweet-smelling liquid. They may play an important role perhaps in transporting certain essential yeasts from fermenting trees to nonfermenting ones. As soon as an active malafu-producing tree is spotted, a claim is made by the discoverer(s), who have from then onwards a legal right to the output. The brew is sampled from time to time until judged to have reached the required degree of maturity. This may depend upon the owner's thirst and upon the pressure from his relatives or friends. The liquid is then drawn out into gourds and kept in a dark, cool place for mellowing and consumption. After I had seen the whole process I suddenly realized that the organic material I had tried to fish unostentatiously out of my drink had not been vegetation but rather dead bees or parts thereof. An illegal treatment of malafu was its crude distillation, producing a concentration of the alcoholic fraction called "arak."

Abiengama was also the site of a COTONEPO station, a company that brought the raw cotton from the natives to be processed for sale on the world markets. Here, the cotton pickings underwent their first mechanical treatment, after which the crude fibers were packed into bales to be shipped abroad. The station was run by a European supervisor. It was only civil to pay him a visit occasionally on the days I was attending the Abiengama dispensary, 200 yards away. I confess that I did not make those visits without reluctance—not that the company agent and his wife were unpleasant people, far from it. But it made me late to pick up the mailbag at Basiani. It was here that, accompanied by numerous whiskeys, I heard a good many stories of the "old days," and again I wish I had made notes, for this region had been famous for the exploits and pranks of a bunch of embattled bachelors, stories told and retold over many a Kibali-Ituri campfire. The hospitable couple's house was the frequent stopover for passing travelers and one of them was the cause of a fearsome adventure. It happened on the occasion of my first visit when, together with Doc on our way back from our walk to Akunani Hill, we had been invited for a drink. We had spent several hours gossiping and storytelling and I felt relieved that after only three whiskeys we were about to leave when the noise of screeching brakes announced the arrival of another visitor. It was an old-timer, an ex-COTONEPO agent, known to everyone as "the Baron," now running his own transport company. There was no escape. We had to stay for another drink, the Baron guaranteeing our safe return in his truck carrying a load of gasoline to Wamba. The party gained even greater momentum when two friends of the Baron also stopped by. They had a supply of fresh meat bought at Paulis and said that it would be damn silly to let it spoil during the trip to Wamba. So a great repast was prepared, in which everyone participated in the cooking and in the consuming. All quite jolly!

Night fell and by the time all news had been exchanged, every worthwhile story had been told and the second whiskey bottle showed signs of depletion, it was close to midnight. When Doc and I strongly opposed the suggestion that we should all stay for the night, the Baron grudgingly agreed to take us to Pawa. With great misgivings, Doc and I squeezed in the front seat next to the Baron at the wheel, adjusting ourselves to avoid the sharp edges of transgressing seat springs. I felt somewhat reassured when the truck kept pretty well to the middle of the road. Then all of the sudden the floorboards caught fire. It seemed quite unfair that Doc and I should end our lives in Africa, so soon after they had started, in the wake of an inglorious drinking spree. But the Baron was not an old-timer for nothing: he managed to stop the truck before our feet caught fire, bailed out into a ditch, began scooping up handfuls of sand which he tossed skillfully on the flames, swearing and blaming the bl . . . hand brakes. After a frantic struggle with the latch, Doc managed to get the door open and we too abandoned ship. The fire put out, we spent some time gathering the Baron's team of African helpers who had disappeared into the bush as soon as the lorry had swayed to a stop. They could hardly be blamed, perched as they had been on top of 600 gallons of gasoline.

We resumed our journey to Pawa, minus hand brakes.

Basiani and Beyond

Living in Pawa, one could hope to receive food and other supplies usually associated with civilization from two sources: Stanleyville, 370 miles away, or Paulis, only 35 miles from Pawa. Without one's having a personal vehicle, the shops might as well have been on the moon.

During the rare occasions when Dora managed a ride with one of the Red Cross cars to Paulis, she returned with luxuries such as butter, mantles for the Coleman lamps, matches, batteries, and more rarely, biscuits and chocolates. Or a piece of meat which, as during World War II in Europe, one wondered "whether to stuff it or eat it." Ninety-five percent of the year our animal proteins derived from chickens provided by the local villagers and those from our own chicken coop.

Vegetables could be ordered from a farmer in the Haut-Ituri, a mountain region where climate and volcanic soil allowed farming of temperate crops, and transported by "car-courier" (mail-car) traveling weekly between that region and Stanleyville. The state of freshness depended upon factors such as road conditions, the soundness of bridges, bushfires, the state of repairs of the vehicle, the number of friends the driver had along the road and whether he remembered stopping at the Pawa road junction. The arrival of goods from Stanleyville, at about equal distance from Pawa as the Haut-Ituri, and subject to the same vicissitudes of road hazards in addition to four major river crossings, was equally unpredictable. Goods for Pawa, from either direction, were deposited at the road junction 20 miles north of Pawa, near the village of capita Basiani. My weekly visits to the dispensary at Abiengama, about half-way between Pawa and the junction, were scheduled on Wednesdays when the "car-courier" passed the spot, so that I could either meet the lorry or collect the goods and the mail which the driver would leave with Basiani.

Basiani was a stocky, overweight Budu with a broad, round face that switched in a second from a splitting smile to an expression of deep gloom. He had the features of a well-to-do, successful, non-dieting businessman, a picture that would have been complete with the replacement of his bark cloth breeches for a pin-stripe formal suit, a shirt and a flashy tie, and the exchange of the stump of sugar cane for a cigar.

The entire population of the village was directly related to him, understandably as he had twenty wives and many times that number of children. We suspected that a good deal of smuggling and other shady transactions took place during the Basiani stop-overs but I certainly did not wish to make it my concern. The running of C.V.C. (Compagnie Vici-Congo) trucks was none of my business.

I came to know Basiani well. Passing many hours waiting in the village for the mail, I grew to like him in a way. He must have guessed that I could not fail to observe certain unusual activities when the "car-courrier" stopped at the village. It is possible that my presence inhibited a certain amount of irregularities. I always thought that Basiani looked rather uneasy when I arrived at the junction *before* the mail did. I never questioned the activities during the unloading and loading of the C.V.C. vehicle. In return, Basiani and his men helped us in every way by looking after our mail and packages—or keeping it overnight when the lorry was late—for me to pick up the next day.

Basiani often visited the Abiengama dispensary to chat or for treatment of arthritis, the result of an old syphilitic infection. He had a quiet sense of humor. One day, while I was sitting at my table examining patients, a man, obviously a mental case, walked in and started sniffing all parts of the walls as he toured the room. Basiani, sitting as usual in the corner on my left, followed with his eyes every movement of the madman with a studious, spellbound interest. A complete silence had fallen on the audience as if time stood still. After the lunatic had inspected all the walls in his fashion, he gave a last, departing snort at the doorpost and left without further ado. Without uttering a word, Basiani turned towards me, an expression on his face that seemed to say,: "A bit peculiar in my opinion. What is the world coming to?"

It was Basiani, I suspect, who coined a nickname for me, a custom applied to all newly arrived Europeans. Oddly enough, the name was later interpreted in a way, I am sure, he had not intended. I believe the origin of the nickname was as follows: Basiani was a born beggar. Routinely, when we met he would ask for cigarettes or other small favors. I didn't feel obliged to form the habit of giving him something each time we met. I felt that this would spoil our noncommittal relationship. Basiani, however, translated this as stinginess and so began to refer to me as "mekono ngufu," meaning "hard-fisted." Unfortunately for Basiani, and luckily for me, "mekono ngufu" was interpreted by others as meaning "strong hand" and as such accepted because it was thought rather well to fit my obstinacy for granting, or accepting, any favors. And so, thanks to Basiani, bless his soul, my passage among the MaBudu will be remembered by the flattering name of "mekono ngufu," the "man with the strong hand."

How many hours I squandered at the Basiani junction waiting for the mail and food baskets! I usually reached Basiani at about four in the afternoon, but very rarely found the mail and food baskets waiting for me. With luck, the lorry would arrive around five; many times it was nearer six, and all too often it failed to appear altogether. My return on Wednesday was, of course, anxiously awaited by the Pawa inhabitants. How popular was I when I returned with both the mail and the baskets, but how humiliating when I arrived empty-handed! First, the mail was delivered at the laboratory, where the director would open the sealed bag and start sorting. I was then free to go home, leaving instructions to the driver for the delivery of the food baskets. By that time it was dark and I would sink gratefully in an easy chair and start opening my mail, if any.

While the dispensary of Abiengama served a large population mostly concentrated along the motorable road and the COTONEPO center of Abiengama itself, the inhabitants of areas farther inland started complaining about the lack of easily accessible medical care for their villages. As they were cotton-producing populations, the directors of COTONEPO, who financially supported the Red Cross, approved the demand for increased medical care inland. Budubudu was the place chosen as being the most central and when the new CRC administrative agent arrived at Pawa to take over my nonmedical responsibilities, I was directed to organize the new dispensary. Its construction was organized by the district officer. The ground plan was identical to that of Abiengama, but instead of mud walls, the new structure was made of a double layer of elephant grass, called "matete." It looked very romantic, very "South-Sea-Islandish," so I thought. A table and a chair were the only furniture I could lay my hands on. Shelves and other storage facilities were made out of matete mats supported by Y-shaped poles. It was all very primitive. Perhaps because of this I began to prefer Budubudu to Abiengama, feeling that I was working under real jungle conditions comparable to early colonial times. Budubudu was pleasant in more than one way. The people were friendly, clad in traditional bark cloth and, if the amount of clothing is to be taken as a criterion, less civilized than the Abiengama crowd. Well away from the main road, attendance at the Budubudu dispensary was certainly below that of Abiengama and I often found time to walk around and even hunt monkeys, which were numerous in the surrounding forest. It was at about that time that I had acquired an Italian Brecchia 7mm rifle, sold very cheaply as army surplus. It was a one-time deal. The price of the weapon included 100 rounds of ammunition, but no more ammunition for the rifle would be available thereafter so that the rifle would be useless after the last round was fired. Moreover, many rounds misfired and I would not have recommended it for hunting lion or buffalo. But the price was so low that many bought the rifle, if only for target practice. Because of its unreliability for larger game, I practiced my hunting skills using the Brecchia on monkeys in the Budubudu forest. Hitting a small animal, such as a red-tail monkey high up in the trees with a single bullet from an uncertain rifle is arduous, to say the least, a fact which the monkeys found out to their great satisfaction. Only the noise seemed to bother them.

Budubudu—what a nice ring the name has—was twice the distance from Pawa as Abiengama. From the main road, an overgrown track led inland until the GadaGada swamps stopped further nonsense. The only reason for the road at all was that it led to a cotton collecting point where, once a year, COTONEPO agents bought the crop from surrounding fields. The track started out in the savanna, but soon wound its way into the forest. Near the edge of the forest was a large solitary fig tree. From the bare patch at its base I guessed it was some kind of meeting place. I was told that the tree was the place where goods were exchanged between a small group of Pygmies and MaBudu, with neither group ever meeting face to face. After a successful hunt, the Pygmies would deposit chunks of meat and leave. Once out of sight, the villagers would arrive with rice, manioc, maize, bananas or the like and place them next to the meat. They would then retreat in turn. The Pygmies would reappear and examine the vegetables. If they decided that the exchange was fair, they would take the vegetables and disappear, leaving the meat. If not satisfied, the Pygmies would retreat without removing the vegetables. The villagers now had a choice of either removing their merchandise or, if they were anxious enough for meat, adding some bananas or whatever else they had to offer. Agreement was reached only after one of the parties had removed the other's proffered merchandise.

It was during one of the first Budubudu trips that I experienced my earliest encounter with elephants. One day, for reasons I don't recall but probably due to a breakdown of the pickup truck I normally used, I traveled in the three-ton lorry driven by Adomana, a former army driver who had participated in the 1940-45 Abyssinian campaign and still showed remnant army behavior and discipline. He was a quiet, pleasant chap, if somewhat stubborn and droll. On our way back from Budubudu, which we had left rather late in the afternoon, and driving peacefully along the forest tract, we suddenly came upon a group of five elephants. Adomana slammed the brakes and managed to stop not more than 30 yards away. As this was my first encounter with a herd of elephants, I was thrilled to the core. At this distance the animals completely filled the frame of the windshield—a dark gray mass of leathery skin upon which the soft pink light of the setting sun brought out every detail. We waited patiently, rather amazed that the elephants had not been scared away by our sudden appearance. Perhaps the wind was blowing away from us because it took more than fifteen minutes before some of the animals finally decided to move away from the road towards the forest edge—except for the largest one, which remained obstinately in the middle of the road, balancing its trunk rhythmically as if in deep meditation. The animal seemed oblivious to us and we wondered how long this would last. Adomana, wisely, said he did not dare to use the horn, afraid that the elephant would panic and stampede in our direction. It grew darker and while I personally enjoyed the free entertainment, Adomana, it seemed, had made other plans for spending the night. He grew sullen and quite angry at times, calling the elephant all kinds of names not necessarily appearing in the zoological nomenclature. At last he could bear it no longer. Without explaining to me, he grabbed a stick that happened to lie on the cabin floor, opened the door, slipped from behind the steering wheel and walked slowly towards the elephant that seemed to have fallen into a deep sleep. I was so surprised that I didn't dare to move, but looked on with great fascination. Adomana manipulated the stick as he would handle a rifle during parade and went through the movements of presenting arms, while confronting the animal with a speech delivered with the seriousness of a private addressing an officer: "Salamu bwana mkuba. Sisi taka kwenda mungini sababu nzala saidi. Bwana yango, muganga kabisa, vilevile nzala saidi. Bibi yake ngoya saa mingi. Akisanti, nitaka kupita nzia sasa hevi. . . ." ("Greetings, big master; we wish to go home because we are hungry. My master, a real doctor, also is hungry. His spouse has been waiting many hours. Please, we should like to take the road . . .").

The speech went on for quite a while. Then Adomana, now quite disgusted, again presented arms, turned around army style and returned to the lorry. Slowly, the elephant seemed to come to its senses and hesitatingly joined the group at the edge of the forest. Adomana did not waste time. He gunned the engine, crashed the gears and the lorry shot forwards before the elephants could change their minds.

"Unaona" ("You see"), said Adomana with great satisfaction.
I nodded and replied:
"Wewe yua tembo kabisa." ("You really know elephants")
"Ndiyo" ("Indeed") was his nonchalant answer.
And so ended my first elephant adventure.

Of Hunting

I knew that once in Africa I would go hunting one day. It seemed as natural as having a drink in a pub. And that's how it went. My first weapon was a very old 12-gauge shotgun with an external hammer, acquired cheaply from Doc after he had bought a more sophisticated shotgun himself. As far as I can judge, it worked fine although the hammer fell off a couple of times. All the shots I missed with the gun I have to blame on myself. Not that I was a novice in the handling and care of firearms. My days in the army had given me ample opportunity to get acquainted with a 7.6mm Mauser, a rifle I have carried for 545 days and nights, cleaned and rubbed so that it shone like a knight's sword, and which cost me two weekend passes. But a shotgun is something else still. Here the choice of "shot," that is the gauge of the pellets, is as important as aiming. Although it had a double barrel, it seemed to hold always the wrong size of shot or, as I preferred to think, it was always the wrong kind of animal that crossed my path.

My first hunt was in the company of a genuine earl who had hunting experience from home, "on his lands, you know." He downed a pigeon (*Streptotelia* sp.) at his first shot. After two clean misses, I was surprised that I, too, got a bird. His next victim was a hornbill. We had the three birds prepared for supper and ate all three in spite of the pishi's (cook's) misgivings. He warned us that the hornbill would be too coriaceous to eat, and furthermore, taboo for Europeans.

My greatest triumph came many months later, and I have to acknowledge the active participation of my faithful servant Mutima in this experience. I have to tell about Mutima later because if I start now I shall never finish my hunting stories. Let me give a quick snapshot of him, however. Mutima was an unusual MaBudu in that he was tall and slender but no one could mistake his watermelon-shaped head for anything but a typical member of the MaBudu tribe. His eyes were like slanted slits. He was intelligent and witty, demure when circumstances required it, spirited and lively on all other occasions, a good dancer, a splendid marksman with bow and arrow, silent and dependable, full of humor, but in the home serving me and my family with the supercilious air of a purebred butler. If I hadn't liked the name of Mutima (meaning "heart") I would have called him Jeeves. I engaged Mutima the day of my arrival in Pawa, when he was perhaps 18 years old. He stayed with us for the next 14 years we spent in the Congo. We saw him get married and raise a family. I delivered one of his sons one dark night on the slope of a hill. But, back to the hunting.

The countryside around Pawa is essentially solid rain forest. The savanna, to the north, is too populated and cultivated to carry any large numbers of game. So most of the animals were to be found in the forest. The use of the verb "to find" is a bit misleading here. Finding game in the forest is not an easy matter, nor is hunting there. But Mutima and I had set our hearts on getting ourselves a wild pig. There are three genera of wild pigs in Africa: *Phacochoerus* in the savanna; *Potamochoerus* in dense vegetation communities, and *Hylochoerus* in deep forest areas. The latter two can attain proportions comparable to good-sized European wild boars. All can be quite dangerous when cornered. For many months Mutima and I rose at four on Sunday mornings: "kuku ya kwanza" in Swahili language, meaning literally "first cry of the rooster" (five o'clock being "kuku ya mbili": "rooster's second cry"). After the classical fumblings and overturning of furniture, clatter of falling pans and pots, we would finally make off, full of hope but frozen to the bone. I have been embarrassed, when replying to people's questions about the climate, that during my years in Africa I have suffered as much from the cold as from the heat. An extreme example of this fact was in the Kalahari Desert where, many years later, we suffered 110 degrees during the day while the water in our jerrycan froze solid overnight.

Stepping out into the garden by the back door, we would cross the sleeping labor camp vaguely outlined against the steel blue sky in which the stars were silently alive. An icy wind swept between the two rows of huts piercing our light clothes, a contrast to the hot dampness that would follow in a few hours. We were glad to arrive among the protection of the close trees. Here another problem faced *me*, however. While Mutima, with his MaBudu eyes that could see in the dark, trotted along at a good pace, I became subject to unfair, vicious attacks from aerial roots, slanting vines, spiny creepers, fallen boughs and mudholes. Mutima sailed through the forest serene and effortless like the midnight breeze. I followed emitting sounds not unlike a laboring steam engine. The branches I did not snap underfoot were those still on the trees. I suspect that Mutima was very much annoyed with my forest manners. He stopped from time to time, no doubt to let the clamor die down and enjoy the silence of the forest for a while and to allow him to listen for the sound of a prowling animal. I have little doubt that my unethical behavior was responsible for our negative results of the first months. Mutima never openly commented on my clumsiness, but his attitude, when he stopped after I made an even more than usual blunder, wrote whole chapters on the subject "how to hunt with a white man and survive the ordeal." But Mutima was a good teacher and I began to learn the finer points of moving among the trees and undergrowth according to the etiquette of the forest hunter.

Leaving so early in the morning on those hunting trips, we found that all bushes and grasses were still loaded to capacity with dew; it took only a few minutes of walking through the stuff to become completely soaked. With the icy wind it made a good combination. One never quite knew when the sun came up in the forest. One moment it was night and the next one a ray of sunlight would pierce the canopy, making the dew sparkle. An hour later we would miss the cold wind we had cursed so bitterly before. But the hunt was now nearing its climax and weather and winds were no longer important. The forest came alive, not so much with sound and motion as with an unseen and silent presence that was felt more than revealed.

One day, some time after the first sunlight had broken through the canopy, Mutima had stopped and stood listening with deep intent. He pursed his thick Bantu lips in a pensive way and finally declared: "ngulube" (pig). He signaled me to follow him, and I tried to move as silently as I could, more to please Mutima than to avoid disturbing a wild pig which, after so many weeks of unsuccessful search, I had stopped believing existed in these regions. But suddenly, after another halt, I could hear faint nibbling sounds and grunts and my heart began to beat quicker with the expectation that makes every hunter prone to cardiac arrest. We crept forward and arrived at the rim of a kind of depression in the forest floor. Here undergrowth was dense and I could not make out what was going on. Mutima, of course, read the situation like an open book and was making all sorts of signs that would have been the delight of Sitting Bull. I could feel that he was inwardly cursing all white people and me in particular. But suddenly I grasped the layout. I guessed, more than I saw, the movement of something below me at the bottom of a bomb-craterlike hole. Inserting a buckshot in the old shotgun, I crept as silently as I could forward to get a better view. In the gloom I discerned a dark object from which grunting noises escaped and I assumed that was the target. I took a good grip of the gun, leaned forward, lined up and let go. In addition to the explosion that rent the fresh morning air, many other things happened simultaneously. Upset by the recoil of the gun, I felt myself sliding over the rim and would have fallen on top of the stricken, but according to the shrieks, very much alive animal had not Mutima grabbed me by the arm, preventing what would have been a most embarrassing tête-à-tête with my victim. In my attempt at keeping myself from sliding down into the hole, the gun had fallen from my hands. Mutima, once more, saved the day by retrieving it before it fell down into the pit. I wondered what the next move would be, but here too Mutima had the solution. He said that the pig was mortally wounded—and I was grateful for his recognition of my marksmanship—but not dead and he asked whether he could use the gun to finish it off. I felt that I had had enough thrills for the day and so, with another buckshot in the barrel, Mutima crept into a favorable position and another explosion shook the forest, finishing in style what I had begun in a fumbling way. The joy of Mutima was reward enough for the many weeks of effort. The animal was a huge *Potamochoerus* (bush pig). It took only a short while for Mutima to run to the nearest group of huts and to recruit a couple of men only too willing to tie the animal by its four legs to a sturdy bough and to carry it to Pawa. News of our triumph had preceded us and when we arrived at the camp, lip-smacking people were waiting along the path from the forest. Photographs and the preparation of bloodsmears were only a temporary delay to the feast that followed and of which, fairly enough, Mutima was the hero.

The bush pig was the only large animal I was to shoot in Pawa. Weeks of fruitless attempts to duplicate our exploit went by. Around this time, I became increasingly interested in monkey malaria parasites. I must confess that monkey hunting was quite exciting. Here at least we were almost certain to see the animals although, often, the monkeys managed to keep at a distance too great for my shotgun, and they were too small and quick for using a rifle. I am glad to report that my hunting was not done purely for the sake of "sport," but included an element of scientific interest. No hunter can deny, however, whatever the excuse he puts forward, that deep inside himself he does feel the ancestral sense of satisfaction when finally the quarry is brought down with a successful shot, a thrill that comes down undiluted from our earliest ancestors. My monkey hunting was done in the name of science, an attempt to investigate the deep-tissue cycle, called exo-erythrocytic cycle, of malaria parasites in the mammalian host of which, at that time, only the blood forms were known. In birds, the development and multiplication of malaria parasites outside the bloodstream were known to occur in the liver and it was assumed, but so far unproven, that a similar tissue cycle existed in mammals. And as malaria parasites in monkeys are closely related to those of man and as monkeys were available in great numbers in the forest just across the road, I had to admit that both my hunter's instincts and scientific interests were too powerful a temptation to resist. Besides, the animals I shot had another practical value in that the meat was not wasted. The MaBudu consider monkey meat a great delicacy and Mutima, his family and his friends were the main beneficiaries of my scientific interest. Let it be known at this point that, to my great regret, my endeavor did not result in a scientific breakthrough. The exo-erythrocytic malaria cycle in monkeys was duly discovered in the liver, but not by me and not in the forest. It was found through experimental infection in the laboratory a couple of months after I had started my monkey hunting trips. Anyway, it was an exciting period, both the hunting and scientific expectations, especially after I had found that the blood samples of most of my monkeys showed malaria-like parasites (actually *Hepatocystis kochi*) and that the liver showed abnormal white areas. Pieces of liver, preserved in formalin, were sent to Professor Rodhain of the Institute of Tropical Medicine in Antwerp for sectioning and examination but, as said above, someone got the answer sooner than we did.

Cercopithecus ascanius is the species name of the monkeys commonly found in the forest around Pawa. The red-tail monkey, as it is called, is seen throughout the Congo basin. Mostly all *Cercopithecus* monkeys are deep forest dwellers. Two species make the exception: *Cercopithecus aethiops* lives in woodland savannas; certain subspecies of *Cercopithecus mitis* seem to be equally at home in the forest as well as in woodlands. The genus *Cercopithecus* is generally divided into twelve species, eleven of which are represented in the area of the former Belgian Congo. Many species have a number of geographical races differing from the type mainly in color patterns, but sometimes also in behavior. Five *C.ascanius* subspecies or races have been described from the Congo. The red-tail found around Pawa belongs to the subspecies *schmidti*. It is widely distributed in the forested areas of the northern and eastern Congo basin, southern Uganda and western Kenya. This monkey was studied extensively in connection with yellow fever research. The finding of 60 percent positives for yellow fever antibodies out of 118 *C.ascanius* tested from the Bwamba forest, Uganda, indicates the active transmission of the virus in the forest canopy. From information like this, and similar observations in monkeys of the Amazon basin, it has been concluded that yellow fever is primarily a canopy-transmitted disease through mosquitoes living in that same ecological niche. Occasional "spill-overs" into the human environment occur, resulting in the further transmission of the virus by ground-dwelling mosquitoes, causing temporary epidemics in human populations.

Besides the crowned eagle, *Stephanoaetus coronatus*, man is the red-tail's worst enemy. Monkeys are trapped and shot for food, but also in defense of food crops which they raid systematically throughout the year. The fur of certain monkey species is sought for ceremonial and ritual purposes in certain tribes. *Colobus polykomos* fur is especially appreciated for hairdress as exemplified by those worn at certain ceremonial dances in Ruanda. The MaBudu, and many other tribes of the forest, including Pygmies, use the *C.ascanius* rufus tail to encase the terminal ends of their short hunting bows. As soon as the monkey is killed, the tail is cut off and its skin removed in a single piece by pulling it away from the central vertebrae, like the skinning of a sausage. Still supple and soft, it is then stretched around the bow's end. In drying, it encases the wood so tightly that it can't be removed, except by soaking.

It is with nostalgia that I look at the bow in front of me, received from capita Makoda 45 years ago.

Perhaps the best way to "read" the rain forest is by hunting. It is then that one is alert to all movement, to all sounds, to all smells. One learns to distinguish between the swaying of the upper branches caused by wind or by a monkey; between the rustling of leaves made by the passage of a snake or by that of a mongoose; whether the sudden fall of dewdrops from the canopy was due to a bird or from their own weight. Broken twigs on the ground indicate the passage of a large animal, a sharply cut vine the passage of man. And, of course, the soft sandy ford across a river is an open book for someone like Mutima, who could tell you how long ago a python slid by, how many monkeys came to drink and whether the tracks of a leopard were made before or after the monkeys crossed.

During early morning hunting trips I had many opportunities to witness the awakening of the forest. Dense fog would delay sunrise by more than an hour, until the heat of the sun would suddenly burn away the moisture and reveal the massive, high canopy. At that moment a single cry of a bird would be heard, followed by a second cry, half a scale higher. Then a hornbill would cackle, expressing its displeasure at being awakened before the sun had a chance to dry its feathers. All at once, the rest of the orchestra would fall in with flute, tuba, piccolo and cello. The hornbill would try its wings and with a loud gaggle, glide with sporadic wing beats to a higher spot in the canopy, closer to the sun. Frolicsome young monkeys would practice a few jumps until called to order by the leader and the whole troop would move off in orderly fashion, in search of fruits.

Unlike sunrise, sunset comes subtly, the transition from the natural gloom to nightfall imperceptible until one realizes that darkness has fallen. The approach of nightfall is recognized by animal behavior. Bird cries are subdued, often confined to one or two species. Monkeys are moving back to their sleeping quarters, desultorily picking a fruit here and there, the young ones urged on by their mothers. The last group rustles the leaves as they settle for sleep, a few complaints and then everything is quiet. A bird's last tweet-TWEET, tweet-TWEET is heard, and night covers all.

Spending long hours in the forest, I became quite fascinated by it and its denizens. I watched monkeys for long periods with rapture as they moved nonchalantly high up in the canopy, swinging from tree to tree with precision and matter-of-factness. I recognized two peaks of activity: one in mid-morning after the sun had burned away most of the heavy dew, and one during late afternoon. Time of activity may change from locality to locality depending upon the time of year and local conditions. For instance, fruit trees such as certain *Ficus* species, become attractive during their short fruit-bearing period, not only to monkeys, but also to all kinds of birds. The noise and bustling activity in the trees at that time were considerable and delightful to watch. The territorial imperative was temporarily forgotten and everyone snatched what was available in as short a time as possible. Monkeys, their pouches full of figs, would still try to prevent hornbills from getting their fill. Smaller birds darted unchallenged to the edges of the smaller branches. The forest echoed with cries of frustration and grunts of satisfaction.

Observations about the travel behavior of monkey bands gave us information on how best to hunt them. At first, Mutima and I would roam the forest at random. After a while it became clear that large bands of monkeys traveled according to a certain pattern, reaching the same general areas at the same time of the day. All we had to do was to take up a position in that area at the estimated time and, by listening carefully, determine the line of travel of the band. These were exciting moments of hope, but also of frustration. A loud rustling of leaves would make our hearts beat faster, but this was often followed by prolonged periods of silence when the band decided to stop to investigate a fruit tree or in a moment of indecision or sensing danger. Ants would crawl on my neck and my body would start itching all over. But I didn't dare to bat an eyelid, well aware that Mutima's intent gaze included my behavior as well as that of the monkeys. And then suddenly, and even while we watched carefully, the monkeys, to our great surprise, would be right on top of us. If we were spotted, the monkeys would express their wrathful indignation with exciting and angry clicking sounds and flee in all directions, disappearing in a wink, the distant waving of branches and leaves appearing like so many joyful farewells. Mutima would pick up our equipment with a disgusted expression on his face, turn around and without a word trot back to Pawa. Whatever the reason the monkeys fled before I had a chance to have a shot at them, I would feel the guilty party. But Mutima, when asked by Dora how the hunting had gone, would turn into a diplomat and a faithful servant by replying: "Makako iko nyama ya mayele" ("Monkeys are intelligent animals"). As we became more familiar with the habits of the monkeys, so did our hunting improve. I also convinced myself that by now I could walk as fast and as noiselessly in the forest as a MaBudu. At any rate, after the first few weeks of rather unpretentious hunting, we started returning home with one or more monkeys on each of our trips. I had learned to wait patiently for a good shot rather than shoot at the first monkey that came in sight. By that time I had also acquired a new long-barreled repeating shotgun and I used number two shot instead of the larger but small patterned buckshot. As every hunter knows, it is the approach and the positioning for the shot that is important. The shot itself takes only a fraction of a second, and then it's all over. The greatest sustained excitement was to determine the direction of approach and hear the monkeys swing from tree to tree, nearing our hiding place. I confess that I never managed to match Mutima's sense of observation nor his keen eyesight. He could hear the monkeys from far away and spot them among the foliage well before I could. In exciting whispers he would direct me to gaze at a likely opening for a shot, but often I failed to see the animal before it moved and then it was often too late for a good shot. I soon learned that shooting animals from beneath a tree poses certain problems. For one, the gloom of the forest, especially during late afternoon, made it difficult to see dark objects against the glare of the sky. Another drawback was that many times thick branches would be in the line of fire and form a protective screen between me and the target. This I realized after a while, puzzled by misses of apparently easy shots. From then onwards, and whenever possible, I tried to shoot from an angle and this produced better results. If I was quick enough, I could get another shot off before the band dispersed and, with luck, got myself another monkey. On one occasion I shot three under circumstances I have now forgotten.

The height of the excitement came when after a successful shot, which echoed like a bomb in a cathedral, we would see the victim stagger, lose its grip and, crashing through the lower branches, fall with an ominous thud onto the forest floor. Sometimes it took a while before Mutima could locate the dead animal in the entangled undergrowth. Perspiring with excitement and from the humid forest air, I would unpack my army sack and take out the accessories for making blood smears. The dampness of the forest floor was such that the blood smears did not dry quickly and I had to move the slides back and forth to speed up the drying. It sometimes happened that shot animals got stuck in the higher branches. Those were lost to science because most forest trees lack lower branches by which one might reach a higher level and remove a stuck animal. Mutima showed me the way to carry a dead monkey: the long tail was tied over the back onto the neck and the animal was carried by the middle of the tail. A monkey weighed no more than 10 to 15 pounds, so one could carry two animals if necessary. We usually arrived home just after sunset. Mutima would disappear with the dead monkey(s) into his quarters behind the house to return some time later with the liver and the spleen of each animal. I put small pieces from each organ into fixing fluid, carefully labeling each bottle with a serial number I kept in a small notebook into which I entered all relevant details. One day, out of curiosity we asked Kiberiti, the cook, to prepare some choice pieces of monkey meat for us to eat. He said it was bad for white people to eat monkey meat. Obstinately, we insisted that we wanted to try it anyway. The macabre touch of Kiberiti in presenting the dish together with two little hairy hands decidedly cooled off our eagerness. However, we did taste the meat and found it rather insipid and sweetish. With a masterly psychological trick Kiberiti had cured our curiosity and even if we had liked the meat, I doubt that we would ever forget the imploring little monkey hands. The monkey meat was all theirs the next time.

Although I claimed scientific justification for hunting monkeys, I still felt self-conscious and guilty about it at times. I started wondering about life in the trees and how monkey bands reacted when one of their members was shot.

"And why are you so keen on hunting monkeys?", the old colonial asked me, sipping his third whiskey.

"Do you know of anything else to hunt in these parts?" I countered.

The old colonial, who had spent the best part of his fifty years in the forest of the Congo basin, and I, freshly out in Africa, sat on the barza of his house. It was the end of another hot, damp day and we were enjoying, as colonial customs prescribe, a "sundowner."

"I'm getting tired of bush pig hunting," I proceeded, "I get up at four on Sunday mornings to be in the poli (forest) at five, cutting and wading my way through undergrowth and swamp. My only success has been one bush pig, three months ago. The novelty of wading through muddy rivers and having my skin torn to pieces has worn off. But we see plenty of monkeys."

"I always found monkeys difficult to hunt," said the old colonial glancing meaningfully at his well-rounded waist, "they see like radar; they hear as if equipped with amplifiers, and they travel as fast as lightning."

I laughed indulgently.

"I know that was my first experience too, but since then I have worked out a special technique," was my reply.

"There are not many things you can teach an old colonial," said the old colonial, a bit piqued.

"There's where you are wrong," I teased. "Old colonials are so very sure that they know everything about Africa that they overlook the most obvious things."

"I shall be glad to hear about your new technique," the old colonial said coldly.

"Oh, I wouldn't say it is a new technique," I assured him hastily. "As a matter of fact it's merely the application of a very old method, probably the first form of hunting used by man, namely ambush."

"Elementary, Watson," said the old colonial, reaching for the bottle.

"Right," I replied, "but effective. I have noticed that bands of monkeys come to sleep in the tall trees not far behind our storeroom complex. During early morning they retreat into the depths of the woods on the other side of the river. In the evening they return to their sleeping quarters. All I have to do is position myself near the river about five in the afternoon and listen for the direction from which they will cross the stream. By the time they arrive, I am well prepared to shoot at least one from my hiding place in the underbrush."

"Indeed, elementary," confessed the old colonial, "but why shoot monkeys at all? Do you like the meat?"

"Not really," I said, "My men are the ones to profit from this hunting. The reason I shoot monkeys is to make blood smears and to take pieces of organs for the study of malaria parasites."

"Don't tell me monkeys have malaria the same as we do," asked the old colonial, incredulously.

"Yes, they do—although not the same kind as human malaria parasites," I replied.

"If you know, why are you still interested in taking and examining blood?", the old colonial wanted to know.

"Well," I lectured, "it has been found that in bird malaria, because they, too, carry malarial parasites, there is a secondary development cycle of the parasite in the liver, known as the exo-erythrocytic cycle. So far, this was never investigated in mammals. It is logical to assume that such a cycle occurs also in primates, that is monkeys and man, hence my interest."

"Have another whiskey," the old colonial yawned.

"No, thanks, I'm off."

"Well, it's rather late. I wish you every success in your monkey business and those exo . . . , what'd'you call them?"

* * * * *

After I had learned that the exo-erythrocytic malaria cycle had been discovered in the liver, as we had suspected, and had been fully described officially in one of the scientific journals, I lost interest in monkey hunting, and as wild pig hunting was mostly an unrewarding affair, my wanderings in the forest became less frequent. It was, however, during one of those aimless strolls that Mutima saved my life. We were on our way back from an early morning trip and, arriving at a particularly dense part of the forest, we both stopped short at the sound of a sudden snort. My first thought was: bush pig, and this was confirmed by Mutima. He seemed, however, perplexed for reasons I could not fathom. He moved more cautiously than ever in the direction of the sound. The forest was so dense and dark that only instinct could have told him that something was not right. We moved still closer. The sound was now so distinct that I prepared myself and my gun to shoot at a split second, intensely watching the dark foliage in front of me. Suddenly, Mutima whirled around and, almost brutally, pushed me back several paces. From his stone-serious face I guessed something was terribly wrong. Without questioning, I let him lead me away from the place until we reached more open ground, but we could still hear the faint grunts. I asked what was wrong. "Chui," he said. He explained that at the point where he had suddenly turned back he had seen a leopard crouching on a branch above us, ready to jump. His theory was that the leopard had wounded the bush pig, but had been disturbed by our approach—from the leopard's point of view—most untimely. And it certainly was not going to let its meat be taken away—perhaps it would even add to it! Mutima's awareness of danger had saved us both from a very unpleasant adventure. On the other hand, I told Mutima, with an assurance I was far from feeling, that I could have shot the leopard had he told me, and shot the pig afterwards. Mutima said that the leopard was about to jump and that a hasty retreat was the only chance of making the best of a rather compromising situation. Thank you, Mutima.

Perhaps Mutima did not have too much faith in my shooting and I don't blame him. My reputation as a good shot, which I did not deserve I confess, was well established, however—a reputation I earned in the following way. Doc, Fred, a newly arrived health officer, and I decided one day to make a foot safari to a mountain near Zatwa about ten miles south of Ibambi, Doc's residence, from where we would start. An old colonial, whose name I forget but who was known by the natives and us all as Paipai (pawpaw), gave us a sketch map and some historical notes about the area. According to Paipai, the mountain Asonga had not been climbed since the day he and Pole Pole (slow), the name the natives gave to Dr. Butler, the famous ornithologist, had made the trip to the top in 1920. Not that the mountain was difficult to climb, simply that there was no reason for anyone to do so. One Sunday morning we set out, late as usual when it involved Doc. Ours was an impressive caravan of our house personnel turned into porters, their brothers and uncles, and volunteers who added themselves along the way at the sight of Doc's array of guns. The climb was easy, a slowly rising path over laterite stony soil through alternating patches of short grass and secondary forest. At one time, as we were walking through one of the forested parts, a tumult at the head of the column signaled that something was afoot. Approaching the group in front, they pointed to a spot inside the forest and with restrained excitement repeated "Ndeke, ndeke mkubwa" ("a bird, a big bird"). After a long while we could make out at a distance of maybe 60 yards a large hornbill—nothing very unusual, really, but we hadn't seen anything larger, so far, and our people said it was good enough to eat. My two companions did not seem anxious to risk spoiling their reputation, flimsy as it may have been, trying to hit a bird with a 22-caliber rifle in half-darkness at a distance of 60 yards—too far for a shotgun. They looked at me and Doc gave me the 22-rifle, the expression on his face trying to imply great sacrificial friendship and sportsmanship. With no reputation to lose and wanting to try the 22-rifle which I had never handled before, I jokingly took the gun, sighted briefly so as to get it over with and squeezed the trigger. No one was more surprised than I to hear the cries of joy, amazement and admiration from the large crowd as the bird fell, shot through the head! My protest that this was sheer luck was taken for false modesty. I wonder if Doc ever forgave me that shot. My servants shared the triumph of their master and they were ever so happy and proud. I don't remember much about the rest of the trip, which was uneventful and uninspiring even after we reached the top, a bare laterite rock. I remember mostly the warm feeling of having gained the respect of a bunch of "savages." Getting a bit brazen myself, I told Doc and Fred that I usually shot birds in the eye so as not to mess up their plumage.

The Bachelors of the Nepoko

Within the short period between the two World Wars, most of primitive Africa was exposed to a western technology a thousand years more advanced. The reaction came in the late 1950s when the former pupils eager to prove to themselves and the world that they too were citizens of the twentieth century with the rights to govern their own destiny, discarded, many times arrogantly, the guiding hand of their western masters. In the Congo, the influence of western ideas upon the way of life of both the indigenous and European populations was unequal, depending upon regional characteristics, topography, history and trade routes. Places of great commercial, industrial or administrative interest had known only short periods of what is known as the "old Congo." World War II was followed by an explosive development of cities such as Leopoldville, Stanleyville and Elisabethville, and so were areas with potential agricultural expansion of cash crops as in the Kivu Province or with ore deposits such as uranium and copper in the Katanga Province. At the time of my first visit to Leopoldville, in 1945, the city looked and felt like an exotic place with a colorful "colonial atmosphere," especially in the eyes of a new arrival as I then was. When, in 1952, I passed Leopoldville again, it had lost its tropical easy-going ways to become a busy modern complex of tall buildings, efficient no doubt, but sadly intimidating, alien and impersonal. Africa seemed far away even though one could be mauled by a crocodile one mile upstream as surely as in the Nepoko River.

The Nepoko region, lying well outside the slipstream of the lively Congo River trade and equally isolated from the brisk business activities in the eastern provinces, was during our time relatively untouched by the frenzy of "development," in spite of some inroads made by increasing demands for palm oil, cotton and coffee. In 1945, the traditional relationship between whites and the indigenous population, the former the authority, the latter the servant, remained unchallenged. Except for abuses, contingent with all rules and societies, the relationship between master and servant seemed an unquestioned and accepted social standard at that time. Some colonials, especially the resident planter, enervated by a harsh climate and alien environment, among a potentially hostile population, estranged from his own traditional culture and customs and tempted by his position of authority, applied strict disciplinary rules and occasional violence. In defense of some of the planters it must be said that often they saw their plans, investments and hopes ruined by an indifferent labor force and overseers, too late realizing the absence of responsibility in casual labor and differences in values. Many of these arguments are being swept aside and replaced by the term "imperialism." In the Congo, some traders made a fortune and got away in time before the wave of independence obliterated their gains; some lost all their money and their health in some forsaken corner of the forest; still others were on their way to "making it," but lost their lives under the avenging knives of hysterical fanatics.

There was little integration—no more or less than in many other parts of the world where class differences or caste systems exist even between people of the same country. In the Congo, fear of exposure to tropical diseases enhanced the motive for segregation between the potential indigenous disease carriers and the susceptible European residents. Congolese public health regulations required a minimum of 200 yards between native and European quarters. All grasses and other vegetation had to be kept short in a perimeter of a minimum of 20 yards around houses to reduce contact with mosquitoes outside resting sites. In large cities, the "buffer zone" between the native and European quarters was usually much wider than the prescribed 200 yards. Exception was made when lodging personal servants, many of whom had living quarters in the back of the resident's house. Such an arrangement was more prevalent in smaller towns and isolated settlements than in the big cities.

In Pawa, both Mutima and Kiberiti had their separate brick houses in the back of the garden. We tried to discourage the living-in of relatives except, of course, their immediate families. Kiberiti had two wives. Mutima was a bachelor when he first came to work for us—until he married Nyama-na-poli (literally "animal of the forest") and had a child every three years. MaBudu tradition banned intercourse between man and wife as long as the baby is breast-fed. The proximity of the servant's quarters was advantageous for everyone. For the servants, the living quarters and conditions, including health, were generally far superior to those they would be able to find and pay for outside the settlement. For us, it was agreeable to know that Mutima was only a shout away. During the slack hours of the afternoon, Mutima would arrive to "put the house in order," but most of the time we had long conversations, he doing most of the talking. He was a marvelous storyteller. He knew dozens of traditional tales about animals and I wish we had had a sound recorder and camera because the stories he told could only be fully appreciated through sound and movement to catch his intonations according to whether the leopard, the hornbill or the cricket spoke, and his gestures and the rolling of his slanted MaBudu eyes. He also talked about life in "the old days" and how his father, in turn, had told him stories of tribal wars when each side devoured the slain enemy . . . "zamani," he added (long time ago) to put us at ease.

Every region has its own flavor and the Nepoko was certainly no exception. The "decor" was the dreamy tropical forest, interlaced with rolling savanna and pockmarked with clearing around groups of huts made of red mud, thatched with coarse grasses, through which the smoke from wood fires dispersed in an endless cloud. In this "decor," the actors revolved in their proper social echelons: the traditionally dressed MaBudu, his or her well-formed dark-brown body glittering in the sun or rain; the olive-skinned Portuguese businessman out to make a fast buck in palm oil, in the meanwhile living in the back quarters of his crammed store; the sallow-faced Greek, importer of canned foods and sundries; the pale "official" ridiculously attired in the classic colonial gear of the 1940s.

As was customary in the "old Congo," most of the old-timers" were bachelors. One of the colorful Nepoko characters was the Baron (our lifesaver in an earlier chapter). Retired after a career with one of the gold mines, he now lived on a small coffee plantation tucked away along one of the small back roads. Traffic along that road was extremely rare and as he could not afford a car himself, it was sometimes months before the Baron received any news from the outside world. Understandably, the Baron made sure that the ever-so-rare traveler along the road would not be "wasted." As soon as he heard the approach of a car, he would run outside and blow a whistle until the car stopped and the driver stepped out to investigate what was causing all the excitement. By doing so, the excitement merely started. He would be dragged inside, even in face of the strongest protest, and be served whiskey-and-soda as long as he or the Baron could hold it. No one escaped, as I found out personally one day. To ignore the whistle would be an offense with grave social consequences, a chance to be taken only if the offender was sure never to return to the area. Everyone knew the Baron, who was considered, by white and black alike, as a kind of spiritual father of all "Nepokonians." He was the mainstay of colonial traditions, the representative of that generation which had made the Congo possible and which was now reluctant and with much misgiving to hand it over to the younger generation. Granted, not all those early colonials developed a high spirit of idealism. The Baron certainly belonged to those who truly loved Africa and its people and although their conduct might not always have been above reproach, they nevertheless had been the main contributors to the development of the country.

Of the newcomers, the so-called "after-war relief," young Doc was certainly one of the most colorful. In contrast to many of the new arrivals, he was a bachelor. Perhaps because of this, his adaptation to life in the colony followed that of the old-timers, almost invariably bachelors. Whatever the reason, Doc fell right into the pattern, including the acquisition of what was commonly called a "ménagère," a native girl who supposedly ran the household but whose services were expected to extend beyond the call of such duty. Considered immoral by the Church and the "landlubbers" back home, the custom was an institution as old as colonialism, and served in many instances the purpose of providing a kind of stable household, probably better managed than if passion and impulses had run unchecked. Anyway, the custom was there; and it was followed with great enthusiasm by most bachelors. As with everything else he undertook, Doc's arrangements for setting up his household were complicated. His medical specialty was dermatology, in particular skin lesions caused by syphilis, so an ad hoc screening was applied to all his household personnel. Knowing the medical history and statistics of the MaBudu population, it will be appreciated that it took a lot of screening before finding a servant that pleased and was at the same time above all free of suspicion of being a carrier of *Treponema pallidum*. By the time Doc had subjected a suitable female candidate to a meticulous, and I mean meticulous, examination of all body parts and drawn blood for every conceivable serological test, most applicants had lost interest in the job. Apprehensive of what exactly to expect after a first week of testing, the aspirant usually went home, bewildered and confused. But one day, Doc's pishi (cook) arrived with a girl who not only passed all the tests but was even willing to stay. It became clear, after a while, that there were some strings attached to the deal. Not long afterwards, Doc, when calling Abati, his lady-in-waiting, found himself surrounded by three girls. Abati explained that her widowed mother had suddenly died, leaving her two sisters familyless and that the girls had agreed to help in Doc's household chores until they found a more permanent occupation. As both girls were quite good-looking, and preliminary tests showed them free from the "white scourge," Doc made no further objections. One week later the count was four girls, and then five, three weeks later, the pishi having come up with a passably credible story for the fourth addition, but one less satisfactory for number five, who she explained would be staying only temporarily. The quality of the fifth girl failing to meet Doc's high standards, he put his foot down and said that he positively did not want to run a kind of girls' finishing school for the whole of the Nepoko and that recruiting should be stopped immediately and even reduced. Faced with the obligation of making a selection, he did not have the heart to send any of the girls away. So when visiting Doc, one would find at least three girls attending to the whiskey and sodas and seeing that the guests were provided with comfortable chairs placed in a way to catch the evening breeze.

But Doc was very demanding. His personnel had to be constantly at his side, at his beck and call. He would shout for Abati, who remained his number one girl, for the slightest excuse. Often he forgot why he called and would dismiss her to call her back a moment later as he remembered. He would even call her to light his cigarette, the matches being only a step away. I felt very sorry for his personnel, but there must have been some hidden advantages for his servants remained faithful and seemed resigned to follow Doc's whims, however bizarre they were.

It was as if Doc had a premonition of an early death and that he did not want to miss anything, however daring or unorthodox. This attitude brought him no mean amount of trouble and was the source of many colorful adventures. Some, no doubt, will remain classics of the Nepoko and it is to be hoped that they will be remembered by the Budu habitants and retold as part of their own oral tradition.

One of the stories was about a wild party that presumably took place at the Baron's house, during which Doc disappeared with a Budu girl in the direction of the cotton shed. Those who had observed the maneuver guessed what was going on. They were somewhat surprised when a moment later a servant came running, asking the host for a lantern requested, he said, by the muganga (doctor). Willing hands prepared a storm lamp, but also followed the servant to observe, through the gaps in the reed walls, what Doc's game was. It was really quite simple and, knowing Doc, to be expected: before committing himself to acts of ardent love, Doc wanted to make sure that no VD risks were involved. What he was doing, while his amazed friends looked on clandestinely, was to submit the girl to a detailed medical examination, by the light of the lantern. The whole scene must have been highly grotesque and, no doubt, extremely annoying and offensive to the girl. The Peeping Toms were discreet enough to retire from the scene after their first curiosity was satisfied, and Doc's diagnosis was never revealed.

Doc acquired a car in a somewhat roundabout way. Having spent a lively evening in the company of the Baron and his friends, he drove back from Paulis in the panel pickup borrowed from the Red Cross. First, he had to take the Baron home. The Baron was soon asleep; and halfway, Doc also fell asleep. The car jumped the road on a downhill stretch, skidded across the ditch and landed, upright, in a patch of elephant grass. As the car came to a sudden halt, Doc awoke with a start. Feeling the limp Baron across the seat and fearing the worst, he began to examine the "body." At this the Baron woke and demanded politely but firmly that Doc keep his hands on the steering wheel and carry on with the driving. Doc told him what had happened. At this, the Baron screamed with laughter, repeating over and over that this was the best part of the whole evening. Doc was not so sure of this when, the next day, he faced the director who gave him the choice of buying the car "as is" or paying for the repairs. Doc chose the first alternative and he didn't come out too badly on the deal. Except for the somewhat battered exterior, the car had sustained surprisingly little mechanical damage. Doc kept the car in reasonable working condition and used it for the rest of his three years' contract. On one occasion, I borrowed the car to spend a vacation with my family—not without some breakdowns, as I shall relate later.

Doc was one of the most unemotional persons I have ever met. Time had little meaning for him when he became absorbed in some problem. He would ignore everyone and everything around him, including time. He was always late for appointments, not by a few minutes, but by hours. He would spend half a day examining a patient with an ailment of particular interest, especially skin infections, questioning him repeatedly on the same subject, sometimes drifting away from those relevant to the disease. He thought nothing of continuing consultations at field dispensaries long after sunset, by the light of a pressure lamp. He was a most nerve-racking person to work with, but he was a brilliant doctor, a determined organizer, a splendid neighbor and a man absolutely devoted to the call of duty whatever time of day.

He spent his weekends in the most eccentric ways, leading sometimes to extraordinary events. His most commonplace outings seemed to generate adventurous flavor, for example, the day he was traveling peacefully in a native dugout on the Nepoko River, and was attacked by a wild bee colony and forced to jump into the water. The river was in flood and he and the boatsmen barely made it to the banks. He would think nothing of spending a night in one of the villages, a practice rarely followed by other Europeans, except when the village was provided with a government rest house.

Before taking over the responsibilities of the CRC medical post at Ibambi, Doc had to spend a couple of obligatory months at Pawa. I came to like him, but was relieved when he left: at last I could keep regular hours and go to bed at the time I felt like it without being awakened in the middle of the night to see "an interesting case." It was during his stay in Pawa, however, that I learned to apply what I had studied at the Institute of Tropical Medicine. Doc was a patient teacher and I was still a novice at that time. Even in his practice of medicine Doc would somehow become involved in unusual situations. One I shall never forget: an autopsy Doc and I carried out on a syphilitic woman who had died suddenly, pregnant with an eight-month baby. Doc wanted to find out how the disease had affected the fetus and if so, in what way. It was a Saturday afternoon, of course, and we had to hunt for Benjamin, the head hospital attendant, for the keys to the different cupboards, select the surgical instruments, prepare fixation fluids and, finally, locate the autopsy room known to exist somewhere in a patch of forest behind the hospital. The room had not been in use for several years, and the clearing in which it once stood was completely overgrown. Benjamin even had difficulty finding the path leading to it and we had to cut our way to the entrance with a mpanga (bush knife). When the small structure was finally exposed, I stood aghast: it looked more like an adobe ruin of uncertain age. Resolutely, Doc tugged at the door and the whole structure, including the posts, came tumbling down on him in a cloud of dust, amid the loud, sizzling, noisy protests of termites disturbed in their uncounted years of unchallenged privacy. The inside was as dark as an underground cave. When we opened the shutters, surprisingly holding fast, we were able to discern a concrete slab in the middle, ominous in its size, and a bench along one of the walls which crumbled when I touched it. Benjamin had some of the mess cleared up by an unfortunate "pagazi" (occasional laborer) who happened to pass by. Then the body was brought in. At that moment, a loud wailing went up from the outside. In order to avoid social complications, we had hoped to perform the autopsy without the knowledge of the family. Unfortunately, they had seen the removal of the body from the hospital. This was rather disturbing for we knew that native tradition would not allow us to tamper with the body. Benjamin found some kind of excuse for why we would have to perform certain tests behind closed doors, a rather symbolic expression under the circumstances. He advised us to work as fast as possible while he would try to assuage the relatives waiting outside in the bushes. Gingerly we set to work. I wonder if anyone can appreciate what it felt like being with a corpse in a hot, stuffy, crumbling room, dark except for a faint circle of yellow light from a hurricane lamp that threw weird, oversized shadows of scalpels and forceps on the opposite wall; the musty smell of decaying wood masked by the stronger smell of decaying tissues; the crisp sound of a scalpel cutting through human flesh accompanied by the vibrating noise of nervous termites; the occasional loud laments from the outside that seemed to increase in volume. Big drops of sweat dripped from my forehead as I watched Doc and helped him with the instruments. Doc operated slowly and methodically, as always, intent on the business at hand, apparently unconcerned and unaware of the hostile environment and noises. The stench of kerosene and the open body became overwhelming and even Doc blanched. We finally had to open the shutters a wee bit. It increased the volume of the wailing, but it certainly improved the "breathability" of the air. Finally we got the fetus out, a male. After a preliminary examination it was stored in a large jar with fixing fluid, for later study. After taking samples from several organs of the mother, her abdomen was sewn up and all traces of surgery cleaned away as much as possible. We covered the body with a white cloth and allowed the waiting relatives to take it away—under a renewed outburst of lamentations.

In spite of a hot bath, clean clothes and a couple of stiff whiskeys, the smell of the room remained anchored in my brain for hours.

Fate was very unkind to the Pawa medical profession. Doc, having left the Red Cross for a government appointment in the Kasai region, met with an accidental death in 1950; our director, Dr. Zanetti, died in the SABENA airplane crash at Libenge in 1948. Young Dr. Swerts, who later came to replace him, was killed by the Congo rebels during the independence revolution in 1960.

First Letters Home

Dora kept all the letters I wrote her during the many months I was alone in Pawa while she was with friends in Wales, hoping that British shipping lines would resume calling at African ports sooner than other lines. This proved to be a wrong assumption as we found out later. Some of those letters are a great help to knit together fragments of memories and to rekindle vague recollections. Abstracts of some of them provide insight to my feelings during a period of adaptation to colonial life.

My first letter from Pawa was dated 28 August 1945, a fortnight after I left Brussels airport:

Finally arrived at Pawa. I have been given a house which is undergoing repairs and will, eventually, be rebuilt, so the Catholic Brother in charge of construction, told me. As it is, the house is very attractive with a simple, typical colonial floor plan: a central large living room with a bedroom on each side, one with a bathroom, the other with a large storeroom. The bathtub is made of concrete. The hot water arrives through a pipe in the wall connected on the outside to a 50-gallon drum heated underneath by a wood fire. Behind and separated from the house is the kitchen, connected to the living-dining room by a passage—a sort of bridge—the whole being built about two feet above ground. In the back of the kitchen is another storeroom, the pantry. At the far end of the back garden are two small houses for servants. All Pawa permanent structures are made from our self-made bricks, not red, but of a warm creamy color. Facing the main and only road is a front garden and a central driveway (see sketch). Of course, everything is new to me. I have to look after the house, rations, wages, laundry, furniture, lamps, water and wood supply, supervise and give orders to the "boys," supervise the "garden boy," and so on. All this is made more difficult because I do not speak the language, Kisahili, commonly used in all of East Africa and the eastern parts of the Congo bordering British Territories. I have taken on a houseboy—name: Mutima—and a cook—name: Kiberiti. The garden boy is, at present, still being provided by the Red Cross. Our house is located midway between the hospital at one end of the "central avenue" and the laboratory, at the other end, a half-mile stretch. Along that "avenue" are the house of the director, Dr. Zanetti—across from the laboratory—our house, Dr. Gerardy's house, the garages and workshops, the storerooms and pharmacy, and finally the hospital. A short distance beyond are the church and other buildings of the Catholic mission, and the village of Makoda, the capita (headman).

For the moment, I still have my meals at Dr. Gerardy's. This morning, however, Mrs. Zanetti sent me four chickens and some vegetables. In the meanwhile I also received some more furniture, all locally made in our own workshops.

Wednesday, August 29, 1945.

From this morning onwards I am really on my own. Kiberiti, the cook, prepared a breakfast of porridge, eggs, bread, cheese and coffee. The evening menu was: vegetable soup, broiled chicken, cabbage, fried potatoes, and delicious pancakes for desert. Mutima, the houseboy, served it in great style. "Dinner at the Ritz" comes to one's mind. The lonelier did I feel afterwards, the blackness of the forest staring back at me from beyond the open double front door. The bright circle of light projected by the Coleman lamp across the barza and part of the driveway is the only visible outside world. The weather is very pleasant, not too warm at the moment because of a constant breeze. The air is wonderfully clear because we are in the rainy season. Most of the rain comes down during the almost daily thunderstorms that usually develop just after sunset. At this moment a storm is brewing in the distance, the vanguard wind rustling the palm leaves. The nights are cool. In fact, I sleep under two blankets.

This morning I made a tour of the Red Cross territory and installations with Brother Nicolas, from whom I am going to take over to become officially "chef-de-poste" (station manager). These administrative functions will be additional to my medical and laboratory work.

Tuesday, September 4, 1945.

"In the gloaming, by the fireside, with you I'll be content . . ."

It's a fact, I am sitting by the open fire, a glowing wood fire that throws sudden light beams into the room. Mutima pushes the logs further inside with his bare foot, and adds another—log, that is. I feel cozy. Outside a retreating thunderstorm rattles the window panes. A steady rain drips from the roof of the barza. I am reading Priestley's *Daylight on Saturday*, a novel about life, love and death in an aircraft factory during the war. Mutima puts the teapot and cup on the little table next to my armchair. Having run out of sugar, he places a cup with sweet condensed milk next to the cup. "Sukari nakuisha," he says (the sugar is finished). A minor disaster. The armchair is low, wide and comfortable. I've donned my slippers and if I had tobacco, I would light a pipe. The rumbling thunder, the drumming rain, the hissing lamp bring charm to the room that otherwise would feel lonely.

I tell Mutima about winter in Europe, using the few Swahili words I have learned. That, for instance, rain (mvua) isn't water (maji) anymore, but solid like that he has seen in the freeze compartment of the fridge in the laboratory. By way of illustration, I show him the photo of Edwards in the snow taken in Antwerp last January. He says something like "Ena weye," meaning, I suppose, something like "holy smoke," and claps his hands.

Wednesday, September 5, 1945.

This afternoon went with Dr. Zanetti to the Protestant Mission at Nebobongo, not far from the Red Cross hospital at Ibambi, to be an interpreter for Mr. Scott, the English reverend. It was a very pleasant trip during which I saw more of the country. We came back by a different road and stopped at two places of Dr. Zanetti's friends. It is an ingrained, rigid tradition in the colony that you do not pass a white man's house without stopping. In the old days it was a measure of security to see if everything was all right, as it still is of course, but having become a rule for good manners. Breaking the rule would be an extreme social discourtesy.

Today, I discovered another streak of "butlerism" in Mutima. With both pairs of long stockings in the laundry, I had donned ordinary white socks held up with an elastic band. Mutima caught me as I was leaving the house and said that I could not go out like this. "Hapana mzuri," he said, which I interpreted as "Not proper." I had to rush to early morning roll call, however. By the time when, after breakfast, I prepared to go out again, he had washed and dried my long stockings, over the kitchen fire I suppose, and said that I had to change. I have been chided on other occasions for an unbuttoned coat, rumpled trousers and a dirty sun helmet.

Sunday, September 9, 1945.

As it was a lovely morning, Dr. Gerardy (called "Doc" from now onwards) and I proposed to have a long walk and decided to visit the mountain that dominates the panorama in front of the laboratory. Our boys did not allow us to go on our own, but insisted that they come along to carry our food and water. This proved excellent advice! As we left, the askari from the nearby village (usually an ex-soldier turned into policeman) joined us, carrying an umbrella—in case of rain. How he learned about the expedition, we don't know. We took the main road to Abiengama, which runs parallel with the direction to the mountain. A fresh breeze made walking pleasant in spite of the warm air temperature. At one point, we had to jump across a huge, meandering army ant column in the process, so it seemed, of moving their eggs to another spot. What an interesting sight! Thousands of ants, each carrying an egg underneath its body, scurrying frantically onwards in close ranks. The sheer numbers of insects that had already passed had hollowed out a narrow trench in the laterite earth of the road. The "trench" was manned, or should I say "anted," over the whole length by a tight row of large "soldier ants," standing up, it seemed, guarding the migrating column. As Doc stepped near, a score of "guards" immediately attacked his shoes. Two hours later, that is at one o'clock, we arrived at Abiengama. Here the real safari started when we left the road and followed a narrow path to the left that plunged into a deep valley. We crossed a stream over a tricky bridge made of two slippery tree trunks. After a while, the path went up again through eight-feet-high elephant grass. We climbed steadily, the elephant grass giving way to short turf and then to bare hardened laterite rock that also covered the ridge of a prominent hill. From here we had a wide overlook of the surrounding country including the tiled roofs of Pawa, shimmering in the far distance. Here we met the capita of a nearby village who said he would show us the shortest way to the mountain top. He carried an elephant tusk, dark brown with age, into which a sort of mouthpiece had been carved at the narrow end. Through it he was able to produce a deep throaty sound which, he said, could be heard by his fellow villagers and tell them that he was on his way. We arrived at the village through a series of cotton fields. The capita gave us four men to show the way to the top of the mountain. This required a lot of machete work as the path—if there was one—was completely overgrown, especially the part through the forested areas. It looked like the rehearsal for a King Solomon's mines film. After another stretch through high grasses, the climb started in earnest. It was hard going, but I enjoyed myself immensely. We reached the summit at three in the afternoon. We had lunch and a well deserved rest. Like the previous ridge, the mountain top was a wide denuded area, a sort of carapace of consolidated laterite polished by time and weathering, so smooth that it reflected the sun like a dull mirror. In one of the many depressions that held rain water, I discovered mosquito larvae. It was a strange place for mosquitoes, so high and in such a stark environment. Our four "pathfinders" were constantly talking to the villagers at the foot of the mountain, so well did their voices carry in the still air.

We left at four, back to Abiengama, where we arrived at five. We had a well deserved beer at the local "duka" (small village store) and were about to leave when a truck came to a screeching halt in front of the store and out stepped Mr. Lacour, the managing engineer of the Abiengama cotton processing center. We were invited to his nearby house for another drink. After a while, two of his friends also stopped by. They carried fresh meat from Paulis and it was not long before it was proposed to prepare the meat "so that it would not spoil." Everyone helped to put a complete dinner together and it was a great success. The meal was delicious! One of Lacour's friends had promised to take us back to Pawa in his truck. But it was close to midnight when he finally decided to move on. On the way, the floorboard caught fire, started by the hand brakes that had been left on! With 600 gallons on board it was a rather frightening moment. We managed to put out the flames with sand and the journey continued, with only part of the floorboards and minus the hand brakes.

Everyone at Pawa was surprised to hear about our long walk. No one had ever been to the mountain or had walked 15 miles, just for fun. We were sunburned, especially our legs and knees, which had also suffered multiple cuts from the elephant grass.

Friday, September 14, 1945.

I am busy collecting chrysops flies. Sometimes they fly inside the living room and try to get a blood meal out of me. Usually I spot their approach—they are slow but silent fliers—and usually settle on the window pane when I chase them away from my arm or leg. There they can easily be caught with an upturned beer glass. I've got only one glass left to drink from. They, the Chrysops flies, are carriers of *Loa loa* filaria worms, which sometimes end up in the eye when a person is heavily infected.

I had another long conversation with Mutima, the houseboy, who is anxious for you to arrive because, he said, everything would be so much nicer in the house! We would have proper cushions in the armchairs, curtains on the windows and a real tablecloth. He would do everything for you; you would just sit in a chair and tell him what to do. He would wash and iron your dresses so that you would look beautiful—his own words—so that I would be happy when I come home, and I would find someone to talk to. It would be nice to serve at the table for four, the table beautifully laid with good china and real silverware. "Mzuri, mzuri, mzuri kabisa," he kept on repeating (good, very good). So hurry up.

Saturday, September 15, 1945.

A disappointing week as there were no letters from you. Waiting anxiously for Friday. Today I "did" the market. Doc came along. This time I also had to buy palm oil for the hospital and the leper camp. Smelled of palm oil for hours, but I am getting used to the mixture of palm oil, plantain bananas, perspiring crowds, laterite dust and the musty scent of bark cloth. I am surprised to see so many men with bow and arrow. They seem to be part of the walking outfit, like a walking stick or an umbrella in Europe, I suppose. The bow and half a dozen arrows are carried in the left hand. Bows, about 34 to 36 inches long, are made of a special kind of resilient wood of a sapling; the shaft of the arrow from the rib of a palm leaf. When used for small animals, such as birds, the first inch of the shaft is simply barbed with a sharp knife. For larger game, the shaft is fitted with a metal arrow head. Stabilizers are made from tensile leaves inserted through a slit in the shaft.

Doc, much intrigued, asked one of the capitas if he could try his bow. It became the main event of the day with the whole market watching to see the white muganga (doctor) send an arrow to unretrievable distances. But instead of roaring away, the arrow slipped from the string and fell at Doc's feet. The market exploded in laughter. With his usual tenacity, Doc was not put off, but asked the capita to make us each a bow and some arrows so that we could practice and wipe out that first bad impression.

Wednesday, October 10, 1945.

I caught my first tsetse fly (*Glossina*). It is a big one as most forest tsetses are. I found it as I was inspecting an area behind the hospital, where we intend to build a few huts for expecting mothers.

Monday, October 22, 1945.

A warm, sticky day with intermittent rain that keeps one perspiring the whole time. Moreover, I had to do a lot of physical work, unpacking and sorting out a big shipment of chemicals and pharmaceuticals from the United States. Was impressed by the neat and efficient way everything was labeled and packed.

Dr. Zanetti came back from Stan with a brand-new Ford pickup truck. The other health officer has arrived in the Congo, but will have to spend two months with a mining company to be trained in census work. In urgent need of a health officer at Pawa, Dr. Zanetti decided that my first two months here would be considered my training period. They couldn't have chosen a better place! Freddie Wouters, the new chap, was a member of the underground army during the war. He was caught by the Germans and sent to Heidelberg, where he was tried and sentenced to die by the firing squad. Why the sentence was later revised and how he escaped will make a good story for several nights once he joins us at Pawa.

Had a long conversation with Doc last night. Subject: the speed of light! Seems we are running out of conversation items.

Sunday, October 28, 1945.

Yesterday was a hectic posho (market). Around three in the afternoon as I was leaving to "do" the posho, I received a written message from the Brother informing me that his brick-making team had refused to carry newly made bricks from the oven to the drying shed under the pretext that they were brick-firing specialists, not ordinary "mpagazis" (workmen). The note said that I as station manager should do something about it. My presence being continuously needed at the market, his plea came at a most unfortunate time. To make matters even more confusing, Chief Ndabani arrived at this very moment with his complete entourage, meaning that it was an official visit that I, as chef-de-poste, could not ignore. As I greeted the chief, a heated argument broke out between two capitas and the presence of Mdabani became a godsend. I left the affair in the chief's hand, which, I am sure, he appreciated, and went to see our director, Dr. Zanetti, about the "mutiny." I must say, he handled the situation in a very diplomatic way, persuading them that carrying bricks was as honorable as their skill of firing them.

By the time I resumed the posho it was five. That day we had been allowed the use of the CRC car to go to Paulis, see a film, stay overnight and do some shopping the next day. Therefore, Doc had promised to help me with the posho, but it was all done when he came to the market. I finished the posho by the light of a lamp, hurried home, had a bath, dressed and arrived at Doc's house at a quarter after seven to find that *he* was not ready, having overslept during a nap! We were finally off at twenty to eight, I doing the driving, making the distance of 35 miles in 56 minutes. Awfully fast when you know the one-track bush road. After the pictures, we met Mr. & Mrs. Sacré, the previous chef-de-poste of Pawa, and Mr. Zotos, manager of the only European store in Paulis. We finally went to the CVC hotel at one in the morning! The next day we went shopping at Zotos, the general store carrying items from acid drops to zinc nails.

Monday, November 5, 1945.

Yesterday, Sunday, Doc and I had another of these unplanned, innocent adventures. I say innocent because it often starts with a casual walk that later evolves into a major expedition. Doc and I decided to walk to a mountain not far from Pawa that we were told by Kiberiti was "mbali kidoko" (far a little). We followed an easy path that led for a long while through textbook rain forest. We carried our newly acquired bow and arrow, traditionally kept in our left hand and felt very much "native." The tone changed somewhat when we came to a long stretch of swamps where we needed the real natives to help us keep our balance across slippery boughs. After fording a 30-yard-wide stream by means of a raft, one had to pull along a vine, and after still another swamp, we arrived at a slight rise at the foot of the mountain. It was two in the afternoon. But the top seemed so near that we decided to go on. It was four when we reached the summit. Kiberiti said that there was shorter way to return to Pawa. But as the sun set, at six as usual, we were still very much inside the forest and in pitch darkness. Then a severe thunderstorm broke. And although the almost constant lightning helped us occasionally to find the way, the accompanying heavy rain soon penetrated the canopy and drenched us thoroughly. Remaining dry-shod was no longer of primordial importance. We sheltered and rested for a moment at a village where Kiberiti bought a bunch of bananas of about 50 pounds, which his wife carried all the way to Pawa. We plodded on, now completely unconcerned where we stepped as long as it kept us going forward. On two occasions we waded through water that reached up to our hips, not bothering to remove clothes or shoes. On two other occasions we warmed ourselves at the fire of a hut. Each time we would resume our odyssey by the light of burning torches. But that did not last very long. After a 5-hour long march and the crossing of a last river, we arrived at Pawa at ten, exhausted and soaked to the bone.

Sunday, November 11, 1945.

Doc moved to Ibambi, where he is now in charge of the other CRC hospital and center. It means that I have started my own full-time medical work: (1) weekly visits to Abiengama dispensary; (2) daily clinic, together with Sister Fidelia, of the outpatients of the Pawa hospital. This is in addition to, not in lieu of my administrative work. In spite of these additional responsibilities, I am looking forward to start doing things for which I have been trained. With Doc gone, my conversations are now mostly in Swahili—the best way to learn a language, of course. Brother Nicolas had gone to Stan to pick up a surplus army lorry. Imagine my nostalgic shock when he drove in with a British Army vehicle still showing the corps badge of the Royal Engineers! Tomorrow, Dr. Zanetti is coming back with Dr. Gillet, the director-general of the Congo Red Cross. To prepare for the occasion, I ordered the Red Cross flag hoisted this morning at roll call. To my great stupefaction and embarrassment, the capitas of the various work teams turned it into a ceremonial show ordering their team to attention while the trumpeter tried the "hail to the flag." I didn't know whether to cry or to laugh. I must confess, it was all very solemn and I let it go at that. I do not know if this is going to be a daily performance and how Brother Nicolas is going to take it next time he attends to morning call.

The dry season has started. No more clouds, higher temperatures, but drier air. The early mornings and the evenings are actually cool and very refreshing. Sometimes a thin layer of morning fog spreads from the forest over our small community; like early autumn in Europe.

A new doctor, Dr. De Paepe, has arrived to stay for a few weeks in Pawa for his training period. His wife, a certified nurse, is also waiting for a "priority pass" to join him. They will later take up the administration of the CRC post at Medje, about 40 miles northwest from Pawa.

I got a long letter containing the sad news that George Judels died in a German concentration camp only last March, a few days before it was liberated!

Saturday, December 15, 1945.

The carpenter shop is turning out an occasional piece of furniture for the house. (Carpentry for the new wing of the hospital has higher priority.) A few days ago I received twin beds in replacement for the camp bed I have been sleeping on so far. Sister Fidelia is sewing the mosquito net to cover both beds—less material than for two single beds, I said, blushing. I have drawn plans for a bookcase to fit along the wall next to the open fire.

Yesterday a Pygmy brought me a small forest antelope he had killed on his way to Pawa. Fresh meat being a rare commodity, I bought it for 40 francs—too much I was told later. Anyway, the meat was delicious and, considering I had only two meals out of it, so it must have seemed to Kiberiti.

I've got one more job: soap maker! At Pawa we make our own medicinal soap from cottonseed oil. But the oil has become very expensive as it is in great demand in overseas markets. So, Dr. Zanetti, knowing about my chemistry background, has asked me to try local palm oil instead. To make a good job of it, I need to know the degree of saponification of the local palm oil, which means that I shall have to prepare a series of exact solutions for titration and testing. Our "soap technician" is Sukari, who also operates the tam-tam. He is a slippery character! Ha!

Thursday, December 27, 1945.

The whole Pawa community was in high expectations because they all knew that I had received a telegram, and everyone, including me, hoped that it included THE news that you were on your way to Pawa. It was a telegram from Hans and Odette wishing me a happy new year! How very kind of them, but how disappointing for me!

Monday, December 31, 1945.

The last day of the year . . . and what a year it was!! The flying bombs, the liberation of Europe, the end of the war with Germany, the first atom bomb, the end of the war with Japan, my contract with

CRC, my first flight, my arrival in Africa, a new career. How much more can you cram into a single year?

I have invited Freddie, the new health officer, to spend New Year's Eve at my house. But as he had just arrived from a grueling two days' journey almost without sleep, he promptly dozed off at ten.

From the village comes the beat of many drums and loud rhythmic chants and stamping feet. I went to watch as discreetly as possible, standing in the circle of onlookers. There were dozens of dancing clusters, each marked with a ring of palm leaves, a huge campfire and a team of ecstatic drummers. Thus ends 1945!!

Tuesday, January 8, 1946.

Dr. De Paepe, who has to stay for two months in Pawa to complete his training period, is sharing Freddie's house (previously Doc's) during that time. We three are now spending most of the evenings together. We get along very well. It is amazing to learn how many mutual acquaintances we have although we ourselves never met.

Paid for by his father, DP (De Paepe) received a new Ford today! This gives him—and Freddie and me—a greater degree of freedom and we can drive around on weekends. I said a degree of freedom because no member of the medical profession is supposed to leave his or her center of attachment without permission or informing his superior. This is to ascertain the whereabouts of all medical personnel in case of medical emergencies.

Yesterday evening DP, having an urgent letter to mail for Europe, asked Freddie and me to accompany him to Paulis in his new car. Being a beginner driver and never having had to negotiate Congo roads, he had difficulties keeping to the middle of the road. I should explain. All roads are single-track, cut out from the jungle vegetation the width of a car, with a narrow strip of grass supposedly kept short separating the roadbed from the draining ditch at either side. With no artificial surfacing of any kind, these types of roads are deservedly called "dirt roads." In the Nepoko, as in many other parts of the Congo, surface soils are of the red laterite type, usually good rolling surfaces, unfortunately quickly deteriorating under heavy rain, intense traffic, and quite treacherous when the laterite is of the gravel type. All traffic following a single driving lane in both directions, the roads are soon hollowed out, leaving a raised dome in the center. Covered with grasses, they may hide hard surfaces or solid rocks. Low-riding cars constantly scrape their bottoms on these raised ridges mostly without serious damage, but a rock may cause a hole in the crankcase, and the end of the drive for an unforeseeable time as traffic on the back roads is extremely light, help far away and available spare parts a matter of luck.

At sharp bends, the road is usually widened to double tracks, divided by a hedge of citronella grass—a good place to pass another vehicle, which in other places has to be negotiated by delicate maneuvers on the "shoulder" while avoiding slipping into the ditch. In places where maintenance has been neglected, tall grasses grow in the middle and on both sides of the road, giving the impression of driving through a tunnel. Grass seeds soon cover the inside and outside of the car with visibility approaching zero and engine temperature soaring with a clogged radiator. Maintenance of the road is left to the capita of adjacent villages who delegates a team of men, called "cantoniers," to keep the road free of overgrowth, trim the ditches, level the ridges in the center and fill potholes. According to the season and the mood of the cantoniers, one will find conditions along a stretch of road fair, poor or downright impassable.

Wednesday, January 23, 1946.

Yesterday was very hectic. The three of us did the outpatient clinic at the Pawa hospital. The largest numbers of cases were of syphilis and yaws, all requiring intravenous injections of "Arsenol." Of the 110, 86 were for syphilis. We worked from ten to half past one. But working with DP was a real pleasure and very instructive. We also had several witty moments during the interviews with patients, sometimes leading to the history of previous times.

After five we drove in DP's new car to a coffee planter eight miles this side of Paulis where Freddie wanted to have a look at a motorbike for sale. The house, Mediterrean style, was beautifully located in a beveled valley near a small lake formed by the damming of a stream. The coffee plants are of the variety "robusta," grown in all lowland locations of the Congo. A better variety, "arabica," can be grown only at higher altitudes such as the Haut Ituri. Fredi bought the motorbike, but as it was now well into the night, decided, wisely, to come back for it at some other time. So we set off back to Pawa. A few miles later, the motor started faltering and laboring. As neither DP nor Freddie had any previous experience with motorcars, it was up to me to make a diagnosis. "The carburetor," I said resolutely, hiding my uncertainty. We drove a few more miles hoping against belief that the trouble would go away. And then the motor quit altogether. Here we were halfway between Pawa and Paulis with odds for help before the next day close to nil. With the aid of a flashlight I located the carburetor—first success—which was of a simple design. I unscrewed the top, thereby giving the impression that I knew what I was doing, and found the filter-washer at the intake clogged with dirt. I cleaned it, reassembled the parts, DP switched on the ignition and—oh, miracle—the motor purred with sweet music. We had no more trouble—which shows what instinct and luck can do.

Freddie let me ride his motorbike. Some sport!!

Friday, February 2, 1945.

Stanley had trouble with porters. We had trouble with motorcars. It started last Wednesday. In the morning, went to Paulis with the army truck to load ten drums of gasoline and other materials, and mailed various parcels. I had to rush back because I had been asked to follow, in a CRC pickup, DP in his car, who was going to meet Professor Dubois at Wamba and drive him to Stan. The reason for this "security"—besides the fact that at the same time I would acquire a load of old tires to be made into footwear for lepers—was to see Dubois safely across the Nepoko river ferry which, in certain seasons, is sometimes difficult because of either high or low water. The ferry is simply half a dozen dugout canoes tied together broadside, across which a wooden platform has been attached. By means of two planks one drives from the bank onto the ferry, which is then pulled across by four boatsmen by means of a cable. Driving a vehicle onto the narrow planks is the critical phase: the planks are slippery, often steep, and require precise driving skills.

When I arrived back at Pawa, DP was just leaving. I snatched a hasty "lunch" of bananas and by driving fast managed to catch up to him well before we came to the ferry. The crossing of both vehicles went smoothly, and soon we were on our way to Wamba, about 30 miles away. Here I left DP and loaded my seventeen tires and seven bottles of wine for Doc.

I returned to Pawa via Boma so that I could pass Ibambi and deliver the wine. By this time I was very thirsty and hungry, having had only a few bananas for lunch and I was looking forward to a good drink, a good meal and good conversation at Doc's when suddenly the motor stopped. Just like that. Completely dead. Not the least forewarning. Not the faintest idea what might be wrong. I had reached a road junction at the end of a small village. I stepped out and started fumbling with the car's insides to make it look routine to the children and other inhabitants who were gathering around me. I took the carburetor apart because that seemed the easiest thing to do although, from the way the motor quit, I did not believe that was the trouble. I did find a fair amount of dirt, but when after cleaning and reassembling it, the motor still would not fire, my fears were confirmed: something more than a dirty carburetor was the culprit. It was getting dark. Petrol lamps were produced and an old African ex-driver joined the fun of taking things apart. Then I discovered the prime reason for the breakdown: the sparkplugs didn't spark, but that knowledge did not help me solve the problem. It indicated, however, that something was wrong with the electrical system. But, as far as I could ascertain, all wires seemed connected properly and in place. The trouble was obviously something that could not be found or repaired by the light of a storm lamp or with a screwdriver. I was indeed marooned. True, together with the old driver, we had found many things to tighten, wires that could be better connected or insulated, and a few missing screws and bolts, making us wonder why it had taken the car so long to break down. Yet none of the repairs seemed to impress the engine, which stodgily refused to fire. I clearly needed outside help. I asked for someone with a bicycle and soon a young boy came along to volunteer. I gave him a note for Doc—about 25 miles away—explaining my predicament and asking him to contact the Protestant Mission at Nebobongo, where, I knew, a good mechanic was living. Soon thereafter, an askari (a kind of policeman) appeared out of the dark, lit a fire, and sat down on a folding chair close to the car. I was in for a long wait, it seemed. The askari suggested that I spend the night in a nearby "resthouse," but I preferred to stay with the car. I doubled up on the front seat, my head resting on my upside-down pith helmet, and went to sleep. Though I woke up every few hours, I spent a restful night otherwise. I was glad to see the sun rise and was somewhat furious that Doc had not yet responded to my S.O.S. (I learned later that the messenger had left only early that morning.) At around eleven, Doc showed up in his panel pickup and towed me to Ibambi, after long deliberations about how to attach the towing rope. I needed all my driving skills to keep a safe distance behind the speeding car in front and to keep in the middle of the slippery and twisting road.

At first, Mr. Williams, the Nebobongo mechanic, was as baffled as I had been; then he declared that there was something wrong with the distributor. In a way I was glad that it was that serious and not something trifling which I could have fixed in five minutes. In the meanwhile Dr. Zanetti arrived with Freddie, looking for the remains of the car and me, in that order. Finding the former intact, he was so relieved that he actually forgot to fly into a rage, as he usually did when something went wrong. Williams found an old distributor that fitted and the engine started right away. Back to Pawa, but on the way, the motor once more started to behave badly and I was glad to reach home and have a shave, a hot bath, and something to eat. I had missed four meals. Then I went to bed, but did not sleep as well as the previous night!

The next day, Friday, I returned with the car to Ibambi, where Williams was to install a rebuilt distributor. One mile before reaching his place, the car broke down once more, so that I had to walk the rest of the way. But even the installation of the new distributor could not persuade the engine to fire. Williams worked on it for the rest of the afternoon without success. In the end he diagnosed the trouble as a faulty fuel pump. Once more, Dr. Zanetti arrived at the scene and, once more, I was towed at great speed, hanging on for dear life!

Saturday, March 2, 1946.

Today I put on my "delivery man" hat. First I took medical supplies to Ibambi on my way to Medje. I also collected the 12-gauge shotgun I bought from Doc. It was a real old-timer's hunting weapon: double barrel with an outside hammer, the type carried casually in movies or magazine ads in broken barrel fashion by a graying gentleman standing at the fireside with a glass of alleged whiskey-on-the-rocks, bearing the legend: ". . . whiskey for men of distinction." Mutima, who sat next to me on the front seat, held the gun casually like that "man of distinction" so that it was plainly visible to anyone along the road and in the villages.

At Medje, I loaded the trunks of Ms. Vandensteen into the truck. She is leaving next Sunday and has been in charge of the CRC center. Dr. and Mrs. De Paepe will replace her. I arrived at Paulis, my next stop, just after noon. While the pickup was being checked at the garage, I had lunch with Zotos, the Portuguese general-stores owner. Afterwards, I worked on the shopping list everyone had given me, leaving little time to do my own shopping. I had agreed to meet the De Paepes and take some of the heavier things they had purchased in my CRC van. Among the items was a second-hand kerosene-operated refrigerator.

Then, I rushed back to Pawa, stopping on the way at Abiengama to deliver items from Freddie's list. When Freddie saw my shotgun, he insisted on trying it out. He looked in vain for a bird to practice his skill on and when, disappointed, he wanted to remove the cartridge, the gun fired by mistake. Luckily, it was pointed downwards, but the recoil and shock threw him backwards to the ground. At the noise of the explosion, hundreds of birds took to the air.

That night we had a farewell party for the DP's, with Professor Dubois and Dr. and Mrs. Zanetti. It was a marvelous evening with Professor Dubois the soul of the party with his detailed, colorful stories about his colonial career and later research on leprosy—which had made him one of the leading leprologues. A narration of wit and wisdom.

Back home at ten-thirty. I finally had time to read my mail.

Sunday, March 3, 1946.

This morning the DP's left for Medje. I helped move their belongings from the house they had temporarily occupied onto the CRC army lorry. Then came their two houseboys with *their* belongings, which soon swamped all and included two goats and a large cotton basket full of chickens. Finally, the noisy expedition left, the DP's in their new car in lead. I was left wandering in the empty house like a desolate, forlorn ghost. But once I had locked up and sat down to tea in my own home, my spirits picked up and I was ready to resume the lonely life that had been interrupted for exactly two months.

This afternoon, I had the visit of Chief Karume, who is in treatment for gonorrhea at the clinic. He is heavyset, sixty years old. Chief for the last 22 years over 5,000 subjects, he has 50 wives and 40 children. His chefferie produced 750 tons of cotton last season, sold at 2.50 franks per kilo. Proudly, he showed me his bank account with a balance of 185,000 francs—not bad for a forest-bound native chief. Eyeing my collection of a few throwing knives, he said he would send me some real nice knives with ivory handles. In exchange, I proposed to take his picture, which seemed to please him. He speaks a slow clear, simple Swahili, of which I understood every word. He asked me about life in Europe, and with the help of bystanders, I tried to explain. Each description was met with long aaah's and raised eyebrows of disbelief. A skyscraper became 20 or 30 "nyumbas" (huts) on top of each other; the ocean was like the river Nepoko except that the expanse of water was wider than the eye could see; the ships that crossed the seas carried a hundred times the crew of the largest canoe; "ndeke kwa wazungu" (literally "bird of the white men") he sees sometimes flying high in the skies could carry his entire family with room to spare for dozens of goats; and so on. With our beautiful cities, radios, streetcars, automobiles, cinemas, airplanes, electric lights, paved streets and roads, piped water and fantastic houses, why, Karume wanted to know, do white people come to bury themselves in the jungle, face horrible diseases and sunstroke, look daylong through microscopes, load and unload large ships, build hospitals and churches, march long distances to put things on maps, import expensive drugs to dispense them free and many times live in huts like the natives? I had no answer.

After Karume left, I went with Mutima and the "moke" (small boy, helper) to the forest to try out my shotgun. At one point, Mutima stopped in his track and excitedly pointed into the trees above, whispering "makako, kule, kule" (monkey, there, there). Of course, I saw nothing and disappointed he announced "nakwenda" (it left). Then I spotted a big bird and let go. The explosion shook me in no small way, but the bird flew away, unharmed it seemed. Another big bird, a kind of hawk, landed near the same spot. Probably because I was less nervous than the first time, my second shot brought the heavy bird crashing through the lower canopy to the ground. My first hunting success. Mutima said it was a "ndeke mbya" (bad bird) because it steals our chickens, "lakini mzuri kukola" (but good to eat). I let him have it.

Thursday, March 7, 1946.

I woke up, as I often do, as the forest awakens. But it was still dark. I had hoped that there was something wrong with the birds' biological clocks. There was not. Soon Sukari's gudugudu (tom-tom) shattered my dreams of another half an hour in bed. I found out the reason for the discrepancy: it had rained! The rains have come! The vegetation has recovered its fresh colors! The air has that titillating smell of dusty soil wetted by new rain! Nature is turning a new chapter! Akunai hill has gained another dimension with a layer of dense clouds separating its lower slopes from the emerging top, so that it looks like a miniature Fujiyama.

It was still raining at the time I started my clinic at Abiengama and I only finished at five. The reason for the long days—disregarding for the moment the flattering assumption that I draw increased "clientele"—is that the director has asked me to install a postnatal service. I have on the average 15 children—aged one week to one year old. Each has an individual index card giving his or her age, weight and length marked every month, and anything worth mentioning, such as first teeth, diet, and so on. To make the procedure less boring and somewhat merrier, I gave each of the children a small piece of chocolate. This reward was a great success. Last week I forgot about the chocolate, and this provoked a riot by the angry mothers, who wanted to know why their babies had been excluded from the chocolate program. Live and learn. The mothers also receive a piece of soap and soon complaints were heard that it was too small.

Friday, April 5, 1946.

I received so much and such good news that I don't know where to begin answering. Moreover, there is only a small chance that you will receive this letter if indeed you sail on the 19th. But you never know and also your sailing date may be postponed. It has happened so many times!

In my previous letter I included a list of priority items that would be the most useful to bring with you—if you find the space! For advice about shots and other things, see Dr. Rodhain at the Tropical Institute (and ask him if he has received my parcel with blood smears and liver sections from red-tail monkeys). Mrs. Zanetti is in Europe and perhaps you could arrange to meet her at the Red Cross so that you could have news from Pawa at first hand and from the point of view of a housewife, not from an enthusiastic, romantic mosquito hunter.

Awaiting news about your arrival at Leopoldville and, later, Stanleyville, I keep up my daily diary. Of course, I shall need the exact day of your arrival at Stan so that I can arrange to meet you there and drive you the 320 odd miles through the rain forest to Pawa.

After a separation of ten months, my wife and our two daughters, then six and five years old, finally managed to get a sea passage to join me. They spent a most terrifying four weeks on board an ex-troop ship that had been chartered to transport in a single voyage some 600 wives and children of the first group of war relief colonial officials who had volunteered to leave without their families, some as much as two years before.

I tried to imagine the progress of the ship by estimating her speed and her position day by day. It was a kind of self-inflicted punishment to realize that many days still separated us, but it was better than to be left completely in the dark even if my calculation later proved to be too optimistic.

Family Reunion

It was early April when I got news that my family was part of a "shipment" of 600 women and children who would travel in the old S.S. *Elisabethville*. I do not use the word "shipment" loosely because that was what it was. The odyssey of the "600" will remain a blotch in the annals of the Belgian colonial service. The ship left Antwerp on 22 April. It would take her 26 days to reach Boma instead of the normal 15-day passage. One can imagine—or can one?—the conditions on the ship with a normal contingent of about 125 passengers when the greatest number of the "600," many packed in hammocks in the holds, became seasick at the first pitch-and-roll. Great must have been the courage and the love of the wives for having endured the conditions during that voyage of the "hell-ship" as it was later described by some passengers.

On 17 May, the radio announced the arrival of the "E'ville" at Matadi. A letter from Mr. Davreux, director of OTRACO in Leopoldville, to Dr. Zanetti informed us that my family had already been booked on the riverboat *Berwin*, leaving Leopoldville for Stanleyville the following day. One of the slower riverboats, the trip would take about 17 days. After a frantic exchange of telegrams I learned that the *Berwin* was expected at Stan on 5 June.

I received permission to meet my family on their arrival at Stan with the CRC pickup van. The trip was further justified by all sorts of official errands and a long shopping list for materials and equipment for the workshops, not to speak of the bits of paper Pawa inhabitants pushed into my hands, occasions like this being rare and in-between.

The distance between Pawa and Stan is about 320 miles, but that doesn't mean a thing unless one is familiar with Congo roads and the hazards of ferry crossings, wooden plank bridges, the long stretches of mud and mire, toppled trees and the number of deep potholes along the "good" parts. The road runs over its entire length through tropical rain forest, every bit of it going up or down with a small plank bridge at the bottom of each vale, and includes the crossing of four major rivers: Nepoko, Ituri, Lindi and Tshopo. Although most romantic, ferry crossings always presented some kind of risk when the rivers were in flood or when the level of the water was too low, and driving onto the platform on two slippery planks a bit chancy. "Modernization" of the ferry system was not always an improvement upon safety. A few months earlier, the ferry across the river Lindi, previously operated by a team pulling it along a cable, had been speeded up by the use of a motor launch, less entrancing but a lot faster. All was well until, one day, the motor quit in midstream and the ferry, loaded with two lorries and a number of passengers, drifted downstream in the strong current. A near catastrophe was avoided when the frantic boatswain managed to get the motor going again for a short while, long enough to beach the ferry onto the riverbank, less than a hundred yards from the rapids. As it was, some people lost their lives as one of the lorries overturned in the water when the ferry landed broadside. Such were the hazards of travel in the Congo.

I left Pawa one bright early morning, accompanied by Kiberiti, the cook, who had found some unrefutable arguments to come with me. I refused, however, to take also his two wives and his uncle, not so much for the room they themselves would take as for the household stuff they planned to take along, such as beds, mortars and pestles, a complete battery of pots and pans, a large sack of manioc in a questionable state of freshness and two goats. I managed to bring down the load to: Kiberiti, one wife and two suitcases. After a long palaver, Kiberiti seemed satisfied with that arrangement. I wondered whether it was what he had in mind from the start, the extra load being just a bargaining chip.

I hoped to make Stan in one day, which would leave me plenty of time to run all the errands before the arrival of the *Berwin*. Making good speed, I crossed the Ituri River at about ten in the morning. The road, although somewhat slippery in several places, was relatively smooth and on straight stretches I was doing up to 50 miles an hour. I was going full speed down a nice straight downhill stretch, a couple of miles past the ferry, when suddenly there was a sickening irresistible jerk that threw the vehicle uncontrollably to the right just as I was overtaking two men carrying a large box under a pole. I heard the thud as the back of the car struck the box between the two men. For the next seconds I fought hard to keep the car on the road and had some very close shaves with the edge of the deep ditch that bordered it. I used the brakes as much as I dared without spinning the car, a tendency I could feel all the time until I managed to bring the vehicle to a halt, still upright and still on the road. Then all was quiet. Kiberiti's color was more that of a sunburned Caucasian than that of a MaBudu and I was shaking all over and my knees felt like unvulcanized rubber. Then my thoughts went to the two men I was almost sure I had hit and possibly killed. As soon as I was able to make use of my legs, I jumped out and ran up the road. Imagine my relief when I saw the men standing, dazed it is true, but without the box. They were trembling and I could sympathize with their reaction. The big box lay upside down in the ditch, the pole by which it had been carried broken in the middle. The men were speechless but otherwise unhurt. After Kiberiti and the two men had regained use of speech, a lively description of the accident in Kibudu followed, translated by Kiberiti: the back of the car had hit the box right in the middle, the impact had made the car bounce back on the road, the pole had broken and the box was thrown into the ditch. Very possibly, the heavy box had saved their lives, I thought. The box contained medical supplies for a nearby hospital. Opening the box, I found two bottles with bismuth emulsion smashed, the glutinous contents dripping on cotton wool and bandages. Finding themselves alive and back to normal speech, the two men started complaining bitterly about what had happened and their fear that they would be punished by the muganga for the loss and the damage. I quickly wrote a note explaining the accident, signed it and turned my attention to the vehicle. I expected to find a burst tire but none were. The vehicle was sagging on the right rear and I expected a broken spring, which would have been bad enough. To my horror I found something far worse than that. The support that held the master spring leaf to the underside of the chassis had broken clean off so that the bottom now rested directly on top of the spring-leaves. Butterflies started fluttering in my stomach and I felt completely at a loss. I tried to persuade myself that time would eventually take care of our troubles. But time was precisely something I could not spare if I wanted to arrive in time to meet my family. Such a breakdown would have been dreadful in a city, in the midst of the rain forest it seemed hopeless.

Slowly I began to think more positively. The mission of Avakubi was on this side of the river and I figured about five miles away. I turned the car around and, driving at something like ten miles an hour, I made my way back, stopping now and then to check underneath. I arrived at the mission and explained my predicament to one of the missionaries. Unfortunately they had not the means to help me. They suggested that I cross the river again and try to reach Nia-Nia, an important depot of the CVC (Compagine des Vicinaux du Congo). Gingerly, I drove the car onto the ferry, crossed the river once more and reached Nia-Nia, about ten miles further on. The European mechanic was absent, having been called away to salvage an overturned lorry between Mambasa and Beni, some 150 miles from Nia-Nia. The African mechanic tried to soften the bad luck by saying that even the head mechanic would not have been able to do the repairs without first getting the parts from Stan. Some consolation! The butterflies started fluttering again. Then the African mechanic came up with an African idea that would never have crossed the mind of his European boss. What he suggested was that he would call a couple of mpagazis to cut a piece of soft wood and tie it between the chassis and the upper spring-leaf. A banana trunk would be best, he said, because it had "spring" and would be less subject to shifting. It sounded like madness, but as I could not come up with a better idea, we proceeded. By the time the mpagazis had returned with a suitable piece of banana trunk, and after we had secured it with wire and rope between the spring-leaves and the bottom of the chassis, it was dark. But the job was done, and the car was on an even keel. How long it would stay that way along the remaining 190 miles to Stan I did not dare to contemplate. In any case, I decided not to risk driving during the night, but to await the morrow to try the crazy contraption. Luckily, Nia-Nia had a good hotel so there was at least no problem where to spend the night. The next day we were off at five. I am not going to dwell at length on this singular journey. To portray it succinctly, "how to travel not on a shoestring but on a banana trunk," comes to mind. I did the 190 miles to Stan in 12 hours, driving at 20 miles an hour, trying to avoid every possible pothole, and I can vouch that there were more than a few, each causing heart flutter. Of course, I stopped often to check the repairs and to make adjustments with the wedges to take up the slack. Once we stopped in a village for major repairs when several wedges had worked loose and were lost. They were replaced by short pieces of branches cut by Kiberiti from a tree. Kiberiti kept quiet during the driving, but chattered away with the onlookers when we stopped—no doubt, giving a colorful account of our journey and discussing the odds of ever reaching Stan. I wouldn't be surprised if the story of how "mekono ngufu" drove a "mashua" (motorcar) to Kisangani on a "miti ya ndizi" (banana tree) joined so many other stories told along this famous trade route.

We arrived at Stan still in time to take the pickup to the garage.

"Very ingenious," said the Ford mechanic. "Where do you live in Stan?"

"This," I replied nonchalantly, "was the repair done at Nia-Nia, where I left this morning at five."

The man's exclamations of disbelief and admiration also held a strong undertone of "how crazy can you be?"

I left the garage well content. I had been assured that repairs would be completed by the next day. I had reached Stan still two days ahead of the estimated arrival of the *Berwin*. The mishap of a hopeless breakdown in the forest had been outbalanced by the enormous amount of luck of having reached Stan on a banana trunk.

What a moment of joy it was when, two days later and right on schedule, the *Berwin* docked, my wife and two daughters standing on the upper deck. I jumped on board before the ship touched the wharf, a feat that was loudly applauded by the African onlookers. The trip back to Pawa was, luckily, less adventurous. The whole family enjoyed the drive through the forest immensely in spite of the cramped space on the front seat. Kiberiti sat in the back with our luggage and his large basket of chickens.

The arrival at Pawa was a triumph. The house was in immaculate order. Freddie had set Mutima to work to red-wax the floor, polish the furniture, decorate the vases and pots with fresh flowers. The impression on Dora was overwhelming. No doubt, it contributed enormously to her love for Pawa at first sight.

Settling Down

For those employed in the colonies, too much work and too many responsibilities may have been a fair reason for complaint. Boredom might have been one for the wives who chose to accompany their husbands to live in the African bush. They came in increasing numbers during the period following World War II. Lassitude was especially to be feared in families the majority of whom lived in isolated outposts. Pawa was certainly a case in point. Luckily, Dora adapted readily to life of utter social isolation, helped, as she discovered, by a natural inclination for gardening and by self-imposed duties that ranged from sewing, which she hated, to the weekly control and tallying of the food store, a paramount necessity. She also took up hunting with a 22-automatic, providing an occasional pigeon for the pot, complaining at times that the gun did not shoot straight. She started a vegetable garden in a plot cleared at the edge of the forest across the road. Growing vegetables proved to be a constant uphill battle against weeds, for which the timid shoots were no match, as a variety of gnawing insects preferred by far the tender leaves of the vegetables to the ones they had to contend with before this golden opportunity came. The climate, too, seemed unsuitable to produce edible vegetables as we know them. Most of the plants shot up so quickly that they blossomed into flowers before their culinary age. In the dry season they just sulked and withered. Those that showed any promise were promptly eaten during the night by foraging animals or devoured by the many kinds of leaf-eating insects.

Dora also started raising chickens, but this too proved discouraging when, one night, a column of fire ants cleaned out the whole chicken coop, leaving only immaculately picked bones. Another time, ants and predators were not the enemy but Newcastle Virus disease took over and the chickens died one after the other. The chicken coop had to be burned. With great determination, Dora started all over again. In spite of these many setbacks, we were seldom without chickens, our prime source of animal protein during our three and a half years' stay in Pawa.

One by one, aspects of colonial life, so euphoric during the first halcyon months, received occasional rude awakenings. We found out that, without vigilance, the water carriers would not be seen for most of the day, thus bringing the normal household operations to a halt—and the same for firewood. Pawa, like thousands of other outposts in the colony, had no piped water. Water was carried from the nearby river by a team of two natives into two 50-gallon drums, one for consumption, the other for bathroom and other household use. After the first weeks of systematic testing, the carriers developed the habit of filling the drums early in the morning and then disappearing for the rest of the day, making perhaps one last delivery near sunset. Loads of firewood delivered by another mpagazi dwindled daily until the pishi had to be content with just a few sticks. Fierce arguments between the two usually restored a proper quota, at least for a while.

Pawa was not provided with electricity. Only a few large cities in the Congo boasted at that time of such luxury. Complexes of houses belonging to a commercial, manufacturing, mining or similar institution usually produced their electric current from their own generators. A few individuals possessed small gasoline generators, but in the 1940s the majority of the inhabitants of the Congo, black or white, depended upon oil or pressure lamps. The most popular pressure lamp was the "Coleman," of which we had two. They gave a very bright, white light, unfortunately generating a lot of heat, while the high-pitched hissing sound overpowered every other noise. We could actually hear the silence when the lamps were turned off, and it took a while before our ears adjusted to the whispering of the forest from across the road. Due to the heat generated by the lamps and the hot climate, all doors and windows were left open inviting every night insect of the surroundings to converge on our lamps, burning themselves in the flame, the stench mixing with the kerosene fumes. Large night moths, their wings beautifully decorated, would bash themselves to death against the chimney or, if inside, destroy the mantle in their last death throes. Equally annoying and destructive were the "flying sausages," the winged form of a two-inch-long species of ant which, during certain seasons, arrived in large "kamikaze" formations aimed at the destruction of the lamp mantles. During our first weeks in Pawa, Doc and I, with the enthusiasm, illusions and progressive ideas of newly arrived colonials, made a brief survey of the small stream that ran along the northeastern limits of the Pawa "plateau," a tiny branch of the Gadagada. We calculated its amount of flow in view of its possible use as a source of energy to spin a generator to produce electricity. Our hopes were dashed when, submitting our savant calculations to the director, he informed us that the depth of the stream was extremely variable and uncertain and almost nil during the dry season. Thus ended our plans for streetlights and a drive-in theater!

In spite of her discouraging results with vegetables, my wife tried her hand at flower growing. The garden at the time we occupied the house consisted of two patches of "lawn" one on each side of the fifteen-yard-long laterite driveway bordered by colorful but vicious "épine du Christ." The "lawn" was nothing more than the gallant survival of scraggy, sparse blades of cynodon grass. Two frangipani trees, one on the right and one on the left, relieved the bareness of the open space somewhat, their waxy, pinkish flowers sweetening the night air with delicate fragrance during most of the year. Dora set out to replace the puny "épine de Christ" with a border of zinnias. Agbobo, the garden boy, was instructed to dig up the spiny bushes and replace the laterite pebbles, which seemed the main constituent of Pawa's subsoil, by soil from the forest floor. Agbobo's prime task, thus far, had been the trimming of the 3,627 blades of grass of the lawn and removal of those that seemed to do well in the driveway. The rest of the time he spent weeding in the shade of the frangipani trees, a task that seemed somehow related to the position of the sun. After the replacement of the soil, he seemed eager to return to his grass-cutting activities although this exercise could easily be followed, even from inside the house, by the telltale noise of the flying laterite pebbles.

The flower border was only a partial success and Agbobo was soon able to resume his weeding in the shade of the frangipanis.

Besides the garden and livestock (we had added ducks and a goat) food supplies and storage also required my wife's constant attention. Not long after her arrival, Dora became alarmed at the speed by which supplies of butter, salt, sugar, coffee and tea had to be replenished. When information leaked out that Kiberiti conducted a small business of these commodities in the camp, we had more than a strong suspicion that the source of his business was our pantry. From then on, the door to the pantry remained closed, day and night, and Dora portioned out food ingredients for every meal. This measure reduced our food bill to a fairly reasonable level—but not quite. We discovered, one night, that Kiberiti's "moke" (small boy) had found a way into the pantry through the small window, which was usually left open for aeration. The replacement of the window with wire netting brought Kiberiti's business to a sudden halt.

The next crisis in the food department was our concern about the small number of eggs produced by our chickens, and even the disappearance of small chickens. All sorts of natural causes were suggested by Mutima, Agbobo and the "moke," each with plausible tales of a smart mongoose, civet cats, and rats with a particular predilection for our chicken coop. It is true that we had witnessed ourselves the temerity of a hawk as it swept down from behind the roof to snatch a young chick before our very eyes. Still, allowing Mutima half of the production of eggs and young chicks, as an incentive if he could solve the problem, greatly reduced the number of mysterious disappearances. Only Agbobo persisted in his mongoose tales.

The stress of suspicion can reach extraordinary proportions among colonial housewives. One lady, who had been in the colony for fifteen years, had developed her vigilance to a high degree of sophistication, suspecting her servants of the worst as soon as or if ever she dropped her guard. Most of the rooms in her house were kept locked except during the time the servants had to be there for their chores. Her dress always hung lopsided because of the weight of the keys in one of the pockets. The pantry in particular was under strict security, opened once during early morning when the houseboy received his cleaning kit, and the ingredients for the day's cooking were precisely measured in the presence of the cook with his instructions for preparation. The laundry boy would then be called, each piece of washing counted and a proportional lump cut from the long bar of soap. Later in the afternoon when the laundry boy returned, everything was counted once more, each piece of clothing was inspected for cleanliness and signs of wear. The buttons were also counted and, if missing, a strict interrogation would follow.

In most homes, the spirits cabinet was a major concern. The level of each bottle was marked on the label, holding the bottle upside down. There was a story of a bachelor who, annoyed by the constant decrease of brandy from the decanter, replaced the liquid with his own urine, it being of somewhat the same color. Still the level kept on lowering. Holding out no longer, he asked his houseboy point-blank for the reason. "I use the brandy occasionally to flavor your fruit salad, bwana," came the reply.

Traditionally, on Saturdays, posho day, the three Pawa housewives gathered at Mrs. Zanetti's house to buy chickens and eggs from the villagers. The exercise was a kind of game whereby the seller demanded outrageous prices he knew he would never get, countered by the buyer's offer she knew would never be accepted. The barter went on for a while mainly between the villagers and the houseboys to work out the fine points and until a price was agreed upon which, on the surface, seemed to satisfy nobody. The housewives, however, had an additional edge when they could "sweeten" the bargain with a bonus of an empty bottle or tin can, items that were in great demand in this part of Africa. At the start of the transactions, the respective pishi would evaluate the worth of a chicken by weighing it in the hand and from its nutritional condition, while eggs were placed in a basin with water to test their freshness, floating eggs being immediately discarded. The pishi was in a somewhat knotty position having to please his mistress while not offending the villager to whom, in one way or another, he might be related.

It was clear that with all the difficulties of purveyance, housewives had to call upon the greatest culinary imagination to compose the daily menu. Dora tried various local plants, such as taro (*Colocasia esculenta*,) on which the villagers seemed to thrive, to replace our traditional vegetables with variable degrees of success. Palm oil, however, abundantly available locally, played an important role in some of our dishes while chicken was our prime source of meat. The combination of chicken cooked in palm oil and manioc leaves, generously spiced with pili-pili (local pepper), was one of the most delicious dishes, called "moambe," a kind of national dish now available in some of the best restaurants in London or New York. Potatoes, always in short supply, were replaced by rice, beans or banana chips—thin slices of plantain banana fried in oil. Manioc leaves also were prepared and tasted as good as spinach. Kiberiti was a master in preparing many of these dishes; one of his inventions was cooked rice rolled into small balls and fried in oil. Our favorite vegetable dish was a delicious salad made from the heart of the palm tree. It could only be prepared, however, when a palm tree had been struck down during a storm or by other natural causes. Cutting a palm tree without valid reasons was illegal and rightly so. We had limes and oranges from wild-growing trees, and pineapple also from wild-growing plants. The top of the fruit was cut off and planted again. After a while we had a productive patch of pineapples. We dabbled into the science of wine-making from oranges after a recipe from the Catholic mission. But when our first batch exploded in the jar, we gave up the attempt.

Among the many other things that required Dora's attention was the never-ending fight against insects. Her campaign against cockroaches was mainly in defense of our wardrobe—to keep them out of the kitchen was hopeless. When walking into the kitchen at night, one could literally *hear* them scurrying away by the hundreds. The weekly *total* cleaning of the kitchen with water and disinfectant seemed not to affect them at all. Perhaps it prevented them from dying from bacterial infections. Tiny red ants infiltrated all foods, sugar being the main objective of their foraging. They were kept out of the food cabinet by the immersion of the legs in water-filled tin cans topped with oil or kerosene to prevent the breeding of mosquitoes. In spite of all these precautions, we had to shake the sugar bowl to dislodge the ants before taking a spoonful.

We were in constant fear that, somewhere, termites were insidiously chewing up one or another of our belongings, as indeed they were as we occasionally found out. Dora tried to reduce the damage to an acceptable level by regularly removing books and bookcases, chests, boxes, files, clothes and so on. I have related earlier our complete defeat when half-digested roof beams were about to collapse and we were forced to abandon the house. Shoes and other leatherwork seemed impervious to termite attack, but not to mold growth that covered all leather items with thick green grime if not taken out every week to "bake" in the sun.

With no motorcar, our outings during the weekends and holidays were restricted to long walks or a bit of hunting confined mostly to pigeons. But we were not completely deprived of transportation. In this land of old cars, few roads and widespread villages, the tipoy was the traditional way to travel, for chiefs and government officials. The tipoy, or carrier-chair, is essentially a chair attached onto two long poles—ours were made of raffia midriffs—suspended by ropes onto two shorter poles carried at each end by two "runners." At first, we felt a bit self-conscious being carried when, one day, all of us made a tipoy safari to the village of capita Akunani at the foot of the mountain about 10 miles north of Pawa. It was the same hill Doc and I had visited earlier in the year. Its dome-shaped peak, rising a thousand feet above the surrounding marshy lowland, seemed composed of solid high-grade iron ore. From Pawa we could often observe how, during electric storms, lightning seemed to strike the top again and again. The danger appeared not to have deterred the people from building their village at the foot, attracted probably by the fertile alluvial soil of the surrounding large depression.

The village boasted a government resthouse built from local materials in traditional MaBudu fashion. Here we stayed for a while and had our picnic. We admired the outside pillars supporting the overhanging roof, carved in the shape of a MaBudu man and a MaBudu woman. With Mutima's help we asked if the craftsman could make smaller replicas of the figures and, if so, we would be glad to buy them. Akunani was quite enthusiastic about the project and said he would put the craftsman to work immediately.

Weeks went by and we had almost forgotten Akunani's promise when one Sunday morning as we sat on the front barza, a column of a dozen or so mpagazis approached, weighed down by something long that they carried in a sling between them. They were two magnificently carved poles like the ones we had seen at the resthouse. We were embarrassed explaining that we would not be able to carry these beautiful pieces back to "bulaye" (home). They were very disappointed, but said that they now understood what we wanted. They promised that they would bring back smaller statues. Again several weeks went by but one day two Akunani people arrived with the marvelous figurines of a male and female Budu, the man complete with the traditional bark cloth between his legs and a tiny square raffia hat with a little chicken feather on his head; the woman in equally traditional skirt and "negbe" (small raffia plate worn on the buttocks). They were truly wonderful pieces of art. After forty years, the MaBudu couple still occupy a niche in our home and in our hearts. They were once cataloged and exhibited at the Lowie Museum of the University of California, Berkeley. I still regret, however, that whatever the difficulties and cost of transportation, we did not accept the large pieces.

As time wore on, Dora, estranged from any social activities and outside contact, grew very eremitical. She confessed that, one day, when a strange car stopped at our driveway, she instructed Mutima to tell the occupants that she was not home while she herself hid in the chicken coop.

The director, well aware of the social problems of the outposts, was immediately receptive to an idea I one day formulated that perhaps we should have a tennis court. "Sure," he said, "you build it with my blessings but without impinging on the CRC budget." The challenge was enormous. Here I was in the middle of the Congo forest set to build a tennis court without spending any money and without using CRC equipment or materials. It was really "the challenge of adversity" and only my fierce enthusiasm for tennis made me accept it. First: how to avoid expenditure. By "diverting" some of the men from the grass-cutter teams, I set them to gathering and transporting stones of the proper size to the open space near our house, the right size for a tennis court, I argued, because it was a nice flat area of about the right dimensions. I explained to the director that the removal of stones from the landscaped areas would be an improvement. After the base of the court was laid out and leveled, I had to tackle the playing surface. Hard courts are usually built from layers of crushed bricks or similar materials. I could hardly ask Brother Nicolas to sacrifice a month's production from his brick oven and, besides, we had no crusher. But I had a far better and highly original material: the smooth soil from the inside of the termite hills so assiduously removed by Makakaru during his demolition of termite mounds. So, Makakaru became chief surfacer—still without spending a penny, or so I explained to the director. Now came the problem of leveling and packing the surface to the proper hardness and compactness. This was solved by filling a 50-gallon oil drum with water and rolling it back and forth and across the surface, probably the most strenuous and difficult work thus far. It had to be while the surface was wet and the only way to do that was to wait for rainy days, which soon came. Then came the finishing touches, the most difficult to solve: making the net and fencing of the court. I was in luck. The manager of one of the COTONEPO posts "loaned" me an old but real tennis net he had discovered months ago while doing the inventory of his storeroom—"a silly dream of one of my predecessors," he assumed. After repairs, the net was as good as I could hope for. I saw no possibilities of "scrounging" a wire fence. A makeshift fence was therefore made from "matete" (elephant grass)—by no means high enough, but we had plenty of young spectators willing to retrieve balls! Mutima, our first African pupil, did so well that he must be considered the MaBudu champion, certainly at that time and perhaps for some time to come.

One of our major concerns was schooling for our daughters. From information gathered, it seemed that the Catholic mission at Fataki was the best, if not the only, choice for their education. The institution provided boarding and schooling up to the fourth grade and had the great advantage of being located in a region called Haut Ituri, a high plateau part of the western rim of the Rift Valley, at an altitude of 6,000 feet and therefore considered a healthy climate. So, to boarding school Winnie and Jessie went. The 370 miles from Pawa, converted in Congo miles, was quite a journey. Therefore, they came home only for Christmas and New Year's holidays, and for the long vacations at the end of the school year. A CVC bus did the journey in two days, stopping overnight at Watsa, about halfway. One of the mothers would travel up to Fataki and accompany the twenty to thirty children on their return home. This role once befell Dora. Going up, she traveled the odd 370 miles sitting in front next to the driver of one of the CVC "car-courriers," a very rough journey, it turned out, because of the extremely heavy rains.

It was many years later, long after we had left the Congo, that the girls started telling us about the dreadful time they had spent at the boarding school—as if they only then realized that the treatment and even the quality of the food had not been quite up to the standard one might have expected in an institution of that kind. They probably grumbled when they came home, especially when they were about to return after holidays. But then we expected some kind of protest even had the conditions at the boarding school been perfect. Perhaps we should have heeded their complaints more—not that there was much choice except for sending them to a boarding school in Europe. Luckily for Winnie and Jessie, their boarding school lasted only three semesters. During the first year after their arrival, Dora taught the girls and it was only after she felt that Jessie did not seem to make any progress that we decided boarding school was the only sensible solution.

It was just as well that during the first fifteen months in Africa the girls spent their adaptation time with us in Pawa. Of course, Pawa and the Congo were exciting experiences for five and six-year-olds. They were a big hit when, together with their mother, they visited a village or the labor camp, where they were followed by a horde of children and women particularly intrigued by their very long blond hair. Upon their return from their walk in dusty villages, they all had hot baths generously sprinkled with Detol disinfectant. The cleaning was especially thorough when, a few times, they visited or traversed the leper village.

As my wife loved to visit the camp and talk to the women, always busy with—to her—unfamiliar activities, she developed a kind of "entente cordiale" with several of them and she became an "accepted" regular visitor without causing the suspicion or animosity against whites one sometimes felt in the inhabitants of certain villages. Having shown a great inquisitiveness for all things locally grown or produced, she was invited, one night, by Mutima to go to a secret place, "somewhere in the forest." It all sounded a bit foolhardy to me especially when Mutima strongly suggested that it would be better for me not to come along because, if I interpreted his Swahili correctly, "it might compromise me." Dora's curiosity was far too much roused to consider any objections from me. So, dressed in my old raincoat and wearing my field shoes, she stepped from the back door. At my suggestion that she should also wear my old felt hat or pull a silk stocking over her head, the flash from her eyes nailed me into my armchair. Following Mutima to a secluded area behind the camp, so her story went later, she arrived at a low hut in which she could distinguish two dark figures crouched in front of a small wood fire above which a kind of iron kettle rested on rocks. The top of the pot was connected by means of a sort of gooseneck to the hollow stem of a banana leaf the far end of which rested on a narrow-mouthed calabash. The hollow sound of continuous dripping indicated that something was being distilled from the kettle into the calabash. What Dora witnessed was the illegal moonshining operation of "arak," a high-proof alcoholic drink obtained from the distillation of "malafu" (palm wine) or, even more potent, of that obtained from the fermentation of bananas. Dora was allowed a sip which, she said, would classify my gin as mouthwash. Mutima's delicate suggestion that I be excluded from the night expedition was, of course, because as chef-de-poste I would have had to report this activity had I seen the operation with my own eyes. I had not.

Missionaries, Religious and Others

Liberal thinking about colonialism has generated downright condemnation, and the introduction, role and spread of Christianity in Africa has not escaped the wrath of the critics.

Personally, I believe that the influence of the Christian religion upon pagan Africa has been both beneficial and detrimental. Beneficial because it has instilled, to some degree, a common orderly morality that is shared by all tribes in the "Christian areas." This has helped to generate unification and mutual understanding. On the other hand, it has disrupted, at the level of tribal life, the relationships that are essential to traditional African social organization. Each religion claims unquestionable verities of its belief. Hence, the credibility of each can be questioned. Fanatic believers and leaders have been responsible for century-long human conflicts, leading to holy wars, of which the Crusades were historically the most dramatic; the Middle East region, the latest and bloodiest of them.

If one is allowed to judge from the practical consequences rather than the spiritual presence of Christian missions in Africa, then we have to admit that a tremendous amount of good social work was accomplished by the hard-working "mo-pes"—that is, the Congolese pronunciation of the French "mon père" (Father).

As in many other Congolese medical institutions and outposts, Pawa too had its small Catholic enclave run by a head Father, two "working" Brothers, one head nun, and two "working" Sisters. Both Brothers were fully occupied in general construction work and making continuous improvements and additions to our small, secluded community. As chef-de-poste, I was administratively responsible for these activities, but the Brothers pretty well ran their own show, and rightly so. Some 320 miles away from Stanleyville, the closest big city, and 35 miles from Paulis, the end of the Aketi railway line, we relied almost entirely upon our own resources: we made and fired our own bricks, cut trees in the forest for processing into construction timber and furniture, blacksmithed our simple iron implements, planned and built our own houses and other structures.

As for the two Sisters, their devotion to the sick was of the first order. Sister Fidelia ran the hospital with the help of Benjamin, the African head male nurse, and three African dressers. She was also in charge of the surgery room, where Dr. Zanetti, the director, operated two times a week. She also ran the maternity ward. Sister Cypriana administrated the leprosaria attached to Pawa, one village located at the far end of the Pawa community, the other four miles away. These types of leprosaria had been developed during the war years and went by the name of "V.A.I.L." (Village Agricole d'Isolement de Lepreux - Agricultural Villages for Isolation of Lepers). She organized the division of work in the vegetable gardens, distribution of supplementary food, such as rice, dried fish and palm oil, was in charge of the routine treatment of leper patients, and saw to it that the Hydnocarpus fruit was harvested and processed into Chaulmoogra oil used in the treatment of leprosy.

Without all this benevolent help from the Catholic mission, the medical center of Pawa could simply not have functioned.

Mass was held every Sunday morning in the small church, attended by the Red Cross personnel and people from nearby villages. Outlying villages were routinely visited by the traveling priest, Père Laar. Père Laar was a liberal-minded preacher. He loved to travel and visit villages tucked away from from the beaten path, and to spend the night in the nearby rest houses. He willingly attended village festivities, even participating in dances. He was loved by all. Without doubt, his openmindedness contributed to his success as a preacher of the gospel. He knew and understood more than anyone else the way of life of the African villager, its social intricacies and intrigues, the illegal arak stills, the mesmerism of the witch doctor. From his casual remarks, we felt that he had some knowledge about the organization and perhaps some of the members of the secret society of the "anyota," the leopardmen who killed people during the night for ritual purposes and left leopard claw marks on their bodies. For his own sake, we never questioned him about the subject. We felt that he was in a far better position to judge if and how to make use of his knowledge.

Another religious group also collaborated with the Congo Red Cross medical program: the Protestant Mission of Nebobongo, near the CRC Ibambi center. As they too were engaged in leprosy work, they received financial and material support from the CRC. This was mainly in the form of medical and pharmaceutical supplies obtained from Pawa through me as keeper of the stores. As such, I was in touch with the Nebobongo people more than anyone else in Pawa, and Dora and I befriended the members of the Protestant Mission, a bit to the annoyance perhaps of those of the Catholic Mission. With parsimonious financial support from their sponsors, the members of the Protestant Mission lived very frugally. Their buildings were made of local materials in the wattle-and-thatch style. Somehow, however, they managed to bestow their quarters with an unmistakable atmosphere of English charm, especially in evidence during the four o'clock tea we shared at times.

I had met Freddie Wouters only once at the Tropical Institute a short while before he was arrested by the Gestapo and taken to Germany to stand trial for betraying and sabotaging the German war machine. He was condemned to death. As mentioned earlier, he escaped by miracle both from death and imprisonment. This experience left him slightly acerbic and with a great desire to leave Europe, physically certainly, spiritually perhaps. With his diploma in tropical medicine, Africa was the obvious choice and he joined the CRC in the capacity of health officer. He was assigned the unenviable job, but one which he loved, of the medical census of the whole of the Red Cross territory, specifically the census and detection of new cases of leprosy. Freddie was a sworn bachelor—it took him no time at all to integrate with the regional group of die-hard Nepoko bachelors. He spent an average of three weeks every month, traveling "in the bush," visiting every village in the vast territory. The one week "at home" was spent in his pleasantly arranged wattle-and-daub house in Ibambi. No doubt inherited from his mother, a well-known sculptress, Freddie found beauty in shapes of the most common objects. He took immense pleasure admiring hand-shaped things, such as the roughly finished plastered walls, a pillar polished by passage and time, the glossy patina of a tar-covered beam above a wood fire, or the simple design in implements.

Freddie's somewhat cynical outlook towards life did not soften with time. On the contrary, his work, requiring strong determination to meet the vicissitudes of rough and constant travel under primitive circumstances, enhanced certain traits of his character. When roused, he would suddenly flare up - as when he threw a small wooden stool at the head of a capita or when he emptied the contents of the coffee pot on his servant's head because the temperature of the brew was not to Freddie's liking. His strong reactions may well have created awkward situations, traveling all alone, as he did, in isolated areas. On the other hand, the reputation of his firmness and quick flare up, undoubtedly relayed by tom-tom messages in the areas of his travel, may have been an asset to his task.

Arriving in a "chefferie" (chief's district), Freddie would, first of all, pay a formal visit to the chief who had been informed in advance through an official notice, delivered by "runner." After greetings, and perhaps a gift, Freddie would explain the reason for his visit and ask the chief's co-operation by instructing his capitas to see that all inhabitants of his village be present at the time and day requested by "muganga kidoko" (the small doctor - Freddie was very short). Official business finished, Freddie would unpack and settle in the "gite d'étape" (rest house). It was customary for the chief to instruct his village capita to see to it that the official visitor be looked after: gift of a "kuku" (chicken), a full water drum, adequate firewood. Depending upon the importance or specific request from the visitor, previous acquaintance or reputation, and the phase of the moon, the chief might call for a supply of "malafu" and organize a dance.

But the next day, Freddie would be all business, setting up his table with his boxes of index cards, having the inhabitants lined up, his "askari" in attendance to keep the line straight and moving, his assistant translating his questions into Lingala. (During his training period at the mines, Freddie had learned Lingala, a sort of Lingua franca used all over the Congo basin and by the army, rather than Swahili, a language spoken in eastern Africa countries and eastern Congo.)

From the information on the index cards, noted in the course of previous censuses, Freddie reviewed every single inhabitant, making changes for deaths, births or migration. The primary purpose of the census, however, was to assess cases of leprosy, to note eventual changes in the evolution of the disease in old sufferers and to detect new cases that would be registered for treatment at a nearby field dispensary or for long-term treatment at the leprosaria of Pawa, Zatwa, Ibambi or Babonde. All this did not always work out smoothly. Many times, lepers, especially new cases, would hide to prevent being recorded and being continuously pursued for weekly treatment. Other health officers might have accepted absenteeism as an unavoidable inadequacy of the census process. Not Freddie. He would search personally, accompanied by his "askaris," all dwellings and follow up all clues that would lead to the discovery and arrest the dissenter. House searches were extremely unpopular with most villagers, some because inspection might disclose things they preferred to hide, such as arak stills.

Besides leprosy, Freddie complemented his surveys with extremely useful recordings on the prevalence of other communicable diseases, such as syphilis, yaws, clinical signs of intestinal worms, enlarged spleen or liver, and other symptoms indicative of pathological conditions.

Freddie, no doubt, had the most colorful life of us all, and his notes and diaries, if indeed he kept them, would be a marvelous record of the life style of many health workers who toiled, unrecognized and unsung, in the steaming forests of the Congo basin.

To the Mountains of the Moon

We wouldn't have seen much of the Congo during our first four years if it hadn't been for Doc and his car. After his misfortune with the CRC panel pickup, Doc had accepted the director's "offer" to buy the wreck. Doc had not made such a bad deal after all when it proved that only minor repairs, mostly performed by one of his mechanic friends, had put the vehicle back in good running order. Signs of previous mishaps were still, however, very noticeable. Doc was delighted with his new freedom of movement, no longer depending upon the "ayes" or "nays" of the director for the use of the CRC car. He traveled far and wide and upon return from one of his long safaris told us about the marvels of the eastern highlands, the volcanoes of the Kivu, the wildlife of the Albert National Park, the snows of the Ruwenzori, the expanses of the Rift Valley lakes and the wonderful shops at Costermansville (now Bukavu). He pressed us to take our accumulated vacation time and make a similar trip, offering us the use of his vehicle. I showed due gratitude, but hesitated to accept his kind offer. I was reluctant to undertake such a long and difficult journey with Dora and the children and, I was somewhat doubtful whether Doc's car, having weathered more than a normal quota of abuse would perform still another miracle and survive one more arduous journey. But our ambition to strike out after many years of virtual isolation and our strong desire to see more of the Congo was too great to ignore. Therefore, when Winnie and Jessie returned for their long summer vacation, we decided to take off. Having been promised the delivery of his car by his driver one early Sunday morning, we all rose at five. Mutima was packed to go, his face showing both eager expectation, but also sadness for leaving his family behind. His immediate family and more distant cousins, numbering more than a dozen, occupied the front lawn, making it look like a busy market place. At eight o'clock, no car. At nine, nothing, nor at ten or eleven. Knowing Doc, I had feared something of that sort. Around noon, I managed a lift to Ibambi. Finding the pickup virtually dismantled, I called: "Hey, ho, something wrong?" Doc greated me in a dreamy way as if he wasn't quite sure of my existence and asked if I had time to see some of his new syphilis cases. If I hadn't known Doc well enough, I would have turned around and forgotten all about the vacation. Instead, I reminded him of our agreement of the previous day; to use his car. "Oh, yes, the car," he said, suddenly remembering, "Just some minor repairs. You don't want to take off in an unsafe car, do you?" he added innocently. I eyed him and almost burst out laughing. "No, that would be silly," I replied. It was no use arguing and asking why the "minor repairs" had not been done the previous day. I had already made up my mind that the day was shot and that, with luck, we might start the following day. So I took it philosophically and went to see his new syphilis cases. Fascinating.

Later that afternoon the car was ready. At least, Alphonso, Doc's driver, said so as he disappeared quickly inside his quarters. I didn't wait much longer either, in case Doc wanted to show me some more cases. I jumped into the car, and was agreeably surprised that it started right away. I drove off, the noise of the rattling body an excuse to ignore what Doc was shouting accompanied by vigorous arm waving as I shot out of hearing. Pretending it to be a gesture of good-bye, I cheerfully waved back. After all!

The next day we set off early as planned, but one day late. Except for the creaks and groans as we navigated in and out of potholes, the car seemed to work fine. Dora sat in the passenger seat while in the back, Winnie, Jessie and Mutima "made themselves comfortable" on top of trunks filled with our clothing. For someone not familiar with the Congo roads it may be difficult to imagine the torture of driving long distances on dirt roads with recurrent pits and hollows, deep ruts, slippery shoulders, sunken driving lanes, sharp rocks, loose laterite pebbles, deep mud or treacherous sand—fallen trees and washed-out bridges being among the most annoying hazards. Later, much later, we would accept such vexations as an integral part of African travel.

We were in the middle of a dry spell and the dirt roads were just tracts of packed dust. The crooked back door acted as a very effective vacuum aspirator and we were soon covered with samples of Congo soil. Having passed alternately stretches of black-cotton soil and of fine kaolin dust, our perspiring faces had collected some of each so that when we arrived at Watsa, our first overnight stop, Mutima, covered with whitish powder, looked like an albino while we, faces covered with dark soil, came close to the local skin shade.

The next day we passed Adranga, where Stanley had camped some 50 years earlier. There is also a monument commemorating Baron Dhanis's expedition to the Nile and his war against the Madhist bands who were continuously invading the northeastern part of the colony in those times. Up to this road junction, we had been driving across flat lands covered with woodlands and denser patches of forest. Now the road wound up the foothills of the Congo-Nile divide and the mountain range that formed the "wall" of the western Rift Valley, to a mean altitude between 5,900 and 6,600 feet, the highest part at about 8,000 feet.

We stayed overnight at Nioka. One of our concerns at each overnight stop was to find lodgings for Mutima. Most hotels provided quarters for servants of travelers. In other places, we had to inquire at the local police station or some other government agency or one of the merchants. It was cold and misty when we woke the following morning. The road wound along the high ridges and was pleasantly smooth, composed of yellowish quartziferous gravel, and bordered by mountain forest dominated by treeferns and bamboo. Grassy glades opened to marvelous vistas, to the west onto the tropical rain forest stretching all the way to the central Congo basin, to the east onto the plains of the White Nile (Bahr-el-Jebel), the outlet from Lake Albert—below us, but out of sight—and with occasional glimpses of the Ruwenzori range. We picnicked near a grove of cool arboreal ferns mixed with tall bamboo so outstandingly beautiful that King Albert, in 1932, had his car stopped at this very spot to admire the luxurious vegetation, a fact we learned from a historical marker. We passed Bunia—looking very much like an "Old West" cowboy town. Passing Komanda we drove once more through lowland rain forest. At Beni we turned east on a narrow road that climbed towards Mutwanga at the foot of the Runwenzori, Africa's second highest peak at 16,795 feet. On the way we met and chatted with a dozen or so Hindu boys seated on top of a well-laden lorry. Of particular interest to us was that they were field hockey players, once our own favorite sport, on their way back from a tournament at Mbarara.

The Ruwenzori, named by Stanley in 1871, means the "rainmaker" in local Kikonjo, but is known from ancient times as "the Mountains of the Moon." Unlike Mt. Kilimanjaro and Mt. Kenya, it is not of volcanic origin, but is formed in the course of the massive geological upheavals also responsible for the formation of the great rift valleys. The Ruwenzori is actually composed of a number of ranges, of which the Stanley group has six peaks above 16,000 feet, with Margherita the highest at 16,795 feet. Of great geological antiquity, Ruwenzori's fauna and flora are of immense scientific interest including that of the adaptation of life forms over a wide range of conditions from the level of the tropical lowlands to the arctic.

The hotel at Mutwanga had just been built and operated by a Swiss couple. Whereas the growth of a single *Zinnia* in Pawa seemed to need the combined effort of Dora and Agbobo, here flowers of all sorts and colors grew in profusion in every nook, niche, and receptacle. They cascaded from every wall and trellis. The place did not look like Africa at all, nor feel like it for the temperature, was on the chilly side—a pleasant change for people living in the sultry lowlands. Our first evening was gratifying too. With two couples from East Africa, we were invited to partake with the Ingles, the hotel owners, in a "fondue," a Swiss national dish, served in a huge steaming casserole kept simmering over a flame. The "fondue" is made from a blend of various cheeses melted in brandy and other "secret" ingredients. It is eaten by dipping lumps of (French) bread at the end of a fork into the bubbling mass, each mouthful to be washed away with wine. Our wine glasses were kept full and soon lively conversation and merry laughter set the tone of the evening. I dare say that we all immensely enjoyed the cheerful casual meal that seemed to release unrestrained happiness in everyone as happens during a reunion of long-lost friends.

While our new East African acquaintances slept off the late night, we started immediately after breakfast, the next morning, for Albert National Park along the west bank of the Semliki River, which traces the border with Uganda. We somehow missed the entrance of the park and noticed our mistake only when we came to Kasindi customs border post. It was now too late to go back and start the loop inside the park from the main entrance. So we persuaded the guard at the Kasindi exit to let us through so that at least we could visit the end section of the park. A guide grudgingly agreed to accompany us. About one hour into the park, in the middle of a vast plain where we had stopped to watch a herd of elephants, the engine refused to restart. I cleaned the carburetor, blew out fuel lines, racking my brain for causes of breakdowns that seemed to beset motorcars in the colonies—to no avail. At times, the engine started to die again as soon as I put the car in gear and released the clutch. Afraid that spending more time in the, so far, unsuccessful attempts at finding the cause of the breakdown would make it impossible for us to walk the ten miles to Kasindi before dark, we abandoned the car. It was past noon when we set off. Mutima and I alternately carried Jessie, and sometimes Winnie when she, too, got tired. Wearing only thin sandals that soon blistered their feet, we took them off and wrapped a piece of towel around their feet which made walking less painful, they said, and greatly improved their progress.

We followed a faint footpath which the guide seemed able to read—the motor road would be much longer, he said. It took us across a wide, treeless expanse. A recent bushfire had turned the grasses and bushes into puffy black ash, adding to the heat. We were soon covered with the stuff making us all seem to belong to the same race.

The guide complained repeatedly to Mutima in Swahili (he knew we understood) about the folly of the white people and whimsical behavior of cars (kitu ya matata = things of trouble) in particular. Dora's main concern were the elephants which moved in the same direction as we did keeping the same distance. Luckily, the distance widened as they veered towards a dense forest gallery. We saw no other animals.

We trotted on under the merciless sun. The water in the canteen was nearing the bottom but we did not dare to empty it completely, sparing the last drops for Winnie and Jessie. They showed the greatest courage, amazingly never complaining besides asking whether we would soon arrive. We did not know.

The day wore on, the shadows lengthened. But then the guide stepped up our wearisome pace as he said he recognized that we were nearing the end of the park, repeating excitingly: "Sasa, iko karibu" "Sasa, iko karibu" ("Now it is close by.")

The sun was low when we at last reached the customs' bungalow, a sight we had so desperately longed for during our five-hour walk. We spent the next half hour trying to re-hydrate our system, just drinking plain water in small amounts. After our water-balance was restored, none of us seemed to be the worse for our adventure. It is amazing how much a human body can take, but it could have ended otherwise! A passing lorry gave us a lift back to Mutwanga. What a relief it was to be back at the hotel and wallow in a cool bath! What a wonderful feeling having rinsed away the grimy dust, to be in clean clothes and to sit down to supper! We never thought we would some hours earlier! Let the worries for tomorrow come. . . . They did.

The next day I made contact, through Mr. Ingles, with a local planter who was going up the Semliki valley and who was willing to take me back to the car. The afternoon was well advanced when we pulled up behind the stranded car. I noted with a bit of shock that the car had been moved a few yards—by elephants, I presumed. But such a detail was irrelevant when our combined efforts—the planter was a bit of a mechanic—failed to get the car going. Night came on and we decided to tow it all the way to Mutwanga by means of a steel cable attached to the rear of the planter's truck. I remained in the car to do the steering. When we reached Kasindi and the main road, it was dark. Then the real hazards started. In broad daylight it would have been very difficult to keep the car at a proper distance and correctly lined up with the truck driving at a good pace over the treacherous 40-mile-long twisting and roller-coaster road. At night it felt like suicide. Things did not improve when suddenly the headlights failed as did everything else electrical, including the horn. I had no way of warning the planter of the changed situation that now approached the level of inevitable destruction of both me and Doc's car. The planter, unaware of my real peril, kept the (to me) reckless speed. Perhaps he was late for supper. I expected the car to bump into the truck at any moment or swing off the road or miss the numerous narrow bridges. Whichever angel steered the car that night knew his or her business. I cannot believe that I myself was doing the driving. Never in my life have I felt so completely helpless in the face of such great danger—except once, when during the liberation of Antwerp I opened the door of a room in a supposedly empty house and looked into the muzzle of an automatic rifle held by a neatly dressed German SS officer. As I said, how I managed to steer that car to Mutwanga during that infernal ride is something that will puzzle me forever. When I arrived, I was completely numb in mind and physically weak. When Dora pointed out that I was late for supper, I just stared at her.

The following day the planter came back to "have another go at it." We went over everything once more, mechanical and electrical, finally changing the firing order of the plugs and got so mixed up that the engine would'nt even turn over any more. We found an old Chevy owner's manual and put the firing order back as it was supposed to be. At least, the engine started up again, but the car still refused to move more than ten yards when the gears were engaged. The planter had another bright idea.

"Let's see what actually happens when the car moves," he said. "If you lie along the fender while I drive you might see something unusual."

To me it looked like another attempt on my life, but I couldn't come up quickly enough with another plan. He started the motor and while I lay alongside the open hood, he engaged the gears and drove the car a couple of yards before it stopped, as in previous attempts. I hadn't seen a thing. Perhaps I was too busy trying not to fall beneath the front wheel or getting mauled by the fan-ventilator. We did this exercise a couple more times. And then I yelled. I had seen a spark jump from one of the electric cables connecting the spark plugs to the distributor and at that moment the motor stopped. The cause for all the trouble now became quite clear and stupidly simple: each time the motor picked up speed and began to vibrate, a bald spot in the wire touched a metal part on the engine block, causing a short circuit that cut the ignition. We laughed like children at the end of a story when the imposter-prince is beheaded and the princess is finally free to marry the real one. Two inches of electric tape took care of repairs!

Of all the Congo provinces, the Kivu Province has the greatest variety of scenery, from grass- and woodland savannas to rain and mountain forests, lakes, rivers, wildlife reserves and the Virunga volcanoes, some still active. Its eastern borders include the crest of the western Rift Valley wall, of which the Ruwenzori range is part. The region of Lake Kivu itself is a center of attraction well known to most colonials, especially those living in the sweltering lowlands, for the cool climate at 5,000 feet is a welcome relief.

Lake Kivu's geological history is somewhat different from the other lakes that formed at the low points in the rift valleys. During the volcanic upheavals near the end of the Pliocene that created the Virunga range, lava flows blocked the upper part of the drainage basin of the Rutshuru River. With no outlet, the waters rose ever higher inside the basin until they forced their way across a ledge and into a valley on the southern end of the lake and drained the overflow (today called the Ruzizi River) into Lake Tanganyika, 170 miles away and 2,660 feet lower. At present, Lake Kivu occupies an area close to 1,000 square miles, has a maximum depth of around 1,500 feet and, at 4,600 feet above sea level, is the highest lake in central Africa.

We were duly impressed by the splendor of the magnificent mountain scenery, awestruck by the towering masses of the Virunga volcanoes, and moved by the placid grandeur of Lake Kivu. Our admiration of all these wonders came several days after we had left Mutwanga, however.

We left Mutwanga in the morning, early enough to see the sparkling snows of Ruwenzori before the daily cloud cover blocked out the peaks. Doc's car was running smoothly and we had no trouble on the way to Lubero and Luofu, where we spent the night at the Trois Canards, a small inn at the rim of the Kabasha escarpment. When the following morning we drove down the winding but beautifully engineered escarpment road, we had magnificent panoramic views over the Ruindi plains, Lake Edward and the hills of the Ruanda. At the bottom of the escarpment, the road continues southwards into the wide, flat valley of the river Ruindi. This entire area is included in the Albert National Park, 185 miles long, 12 to 30 miles wide, an area of some 2,000,000 acres embracing the entire range of the Virunga Mountains, the lava plains, Lake Edward, the Semliki Valley and the Ruwenzori Mountains. It is the only park containing gorillas and okapi. The plains are well stocked with wildlife associated with eastern Africa savannas: topi, waterbuck, buffaloes, elephants, warthogs, lions, leopards and hundreds of hippopotamuses in the river Ruindi and other water courses. We had no chance to see gorillas, secure in their bamboo forests on the slope of the volcanoes, nor the furtive okapi hidden in the deep forest.

The limit of the park is reached a few miles before Goma, a small, pretty town, together with Kisenyi in Ruanda, a well-known resort area on the shores of Lake Kivu. Here the uninformed traveler has two choices to reach Costermansville (now Bukavu), usually abbreviated to "Cost": the "normal" road along the western shores of the lake or the "spectacular" one in Ruanda skirting the eastern lake shore. The informed traveler does not hesitate to take the western side. We, at that time, belonged to the former category and opted for the "spectacular" road, winding for 180 precarious miles cut from perpendicular mountains dropping into the lake.

Starting from Goma in brilliant sunshine, we ran into solid rain and thunderstorms as soon as we started the ascent from Kisenyi to the Kibuye escarpment. The heavy rain soon turned the micaceous-laterite soil into slippery slime, making descents like riding a toboggan, ascents like going up a grease pole. The precipitous edge of the escarpment was never more than a few yards away, the surface of the lake perhaps a thousand feet below. There was not a single straight section of road of more than 300 yards. Numerous narrow bridges of uncertain age and solidity barely allowed passage for the torrents rushing from the mountain side. The intense rain reduced visibility to 50 yards or less—our only consolation being that it was very unlikely that anyone else was mad enough to use the road under the circumstances. Had we encountered another vehicle, (and seen it in time), chances are that neither driver would have risked making room for the other until the weather improved.

But there had been another car on that road the same day, under similar circumstances. When after the miracle of our arrival at Hotel du Lac we booked in and later sat down to a late supper, we found our East African friends sitting at the bar. We looked at each other and Charles started the conversation with:

"Did you by any chance come by . . . ?"

"Yes, we did," I said before he could finish his sentence, "you are looking at the result of a miracle."

Charles shook his head:

"We are too. Halfway Bobby vowed to burn 12 candles in church if we came through alive. She just came back from fulfilling that obligation."

Costermansville, those days, was for the colonials of the eastern lowlands as London or Paris must seem to sheepherders in the Pyrenees. One could find the latest imports not only of clothes and materials but also of food we lowlanders had craved for years; smoked beef, Swiss cheeses, French wines, chocolates, fresh vegetables, apples, pears and grapes. We, "from the inland," in sunbleached shorts, faded short-sleeved shirts, and uncertain headdresses, looked definitely "provincial" compared with the locals in long trousers, proper dress shirts and ties, and jaunty panama hats; the women in flower dresses, stockings and smart light bonnets, looking as if on their way to a garden party. Sleek shiny new cars whizzed along *paved*, yes paved, wide streets. At night, the streets were lighted with electricity, and gay neon signs colored the main avenues. How different from Coleman-lamped Pawa!

The great pleasure we derived from spending those wonderful days in the "pearl of Kivu" were not the only significant part of our vacation. Another highlight was my encounter and conversation with Dr. Louis vanden Berghe, my ex-professor of protozoology at the Tropical Institute. Meeting him made our Kivu holiday remarkable and greatly influenced our future. More about that in due course.

The day we were to leave "Cost," the car developed new trouble: a boiling radiator. It was easily diagnosed and fixed with a new fan belt which, however, we had difficulty finding because of the uncertain age of the Chevy. Thankful that the problem had been spotted in town, we started the return journey with renewed confidence, this time choosing the western shore road around the lake. It was not only easier to drive because it followed the contour of the lake at the water level but was also 35 miles shorter than the Kibuye road on the Ruanda side.

The weather was clear and we made good progress. Once we reached Goma, we could follow the same road as the one we had come by. Indeed, there is no other direct road to the Ituri. Now that we had reached our destination in the estimated number of days, we felt that we could linger a bit longer at scenic places such as the volcanic plains north of Lake Kivu and the seven volcanoes of Virunga Range with peaks between 10,000 and 14,000 feet.

Five months earlier, on 1 March 1948, Gituro, a side crater and offspring of the Nyragongo volcano, had erupted, sending two separate lava flows across the more ancient lava beds, cutting the Goma-Rutshuru road in two places. When one of the flows reached the lake, it made the water boil—"shamuka kabisa" (really boil) as a native witness told us—sending a huge plume of steam high into the air. A "temporary" road had been traced across the solidified lava streams. Traffic has soon reduced this one to washboard design that shook Doc's car to its very last bolt.

We stopped frequently and walked the hardened lava that was still warm to the touch. We were surprised to see that vegetational growth was already actively colonizing the new soil. It was also interesting to compare the different types, height and density of the vegetation communities and stages of development according to the age of the various lava flows over the last decades.

It was on the day before reaching Pawa, a few miles before Watsa, our overnight stop, that we discovered how thankful we ought to have been for our safe return. Earlier that day, we had come down the twisting and precipitous road from the mountains of the Haut-Ituri. Some time after passing Adranga, the road had turned really muddy and at one point I stopped the car to examine a stretch that looked particularly malicious. As I stepped out, a distinctive "plop" sounded from below the car. It could have been mud detaching and falling from the fenders, but I was curious. I peeked underneath and immediately noticed that the rod linking the steering to the front wheels by means of a ball joint was lying loose on the road, attached only at one end. Judging from a piece of wire still dangling from the chassis, I presumed that "repairs" had been attempted before. Imagine the outcome had the wire parted as we came down the mountain road! I managed to reassemble the ball joint using new strands of wire. Thus we reached Watsa. A garage mechanic improved somewhat upon my repairs, assuring me that it was the best he could do, but that the repairs would hold until the whole steering system was replaced.

I had taken dozens of black-and-white pictures with my old camera, but when, several weeks later, I found time to develop the film in an improvised "darkroom"—dark because I processed the film during a moonless night—several films were spoiled when the emulsion separated from its base as a result of the high temperature of the developing solution and the wash water. Imagine the Johnsons coming home from one of their African safaris and Osa telling Martin: "Sorry, darling, our films did not come out as well as expected—in fact none were exposed!"

Pulling up Stakes

Life at Pawa was never dull for me. On the contrary, I was under constant pressure, particularly during the first two years when my duties included that of station manager. After I was replaced in that capacity, I was given more responsibilities for medical work, including that of running the laboratory. My routine schedule then became: weekly visits to the dispensaries of Abiengama and Budubudu; bi-weekly visits to the government dispensary at Vube, 50 miles from Pawa. The rest of the time was divided between mornings at the pharmacy to prepare requisitions for the other CRC centers. The afternoons were spent in the laboratory examining blood smears, stools and urines, and performing serological tests for syphilis. With Dr. Zanetti, I was studying the incidence of malaria parasites in newborn babies and their mothers at the Pawa hospital. I had the doubtful privilege of attending many births, during which I made blood smears from the mother, from the newborn baby and from the placenta. Without really trying, watching babies being born taught me how to assist in birth and how to handle the baby and afterbirth. This would come in good stead at a later date.

I sat for many hours at the microscope placed in front of the window that faced Akunani's mountain. When I felt like dreaming or resting, I turned the mirror underneath the condenser so that it projected the scenery in front through the eyepiece. The inversed image had a wondrous, dreamlike quality, soothing to the mind. I was fascinated by the frolics of a lizard I had christened "Billy," recognizable by its mutilated tail. In the quietness of the drowsy afternoon, "Billy" would come out from under the table and climb up in the corner of the window frame, in ambush for flies, smacking its lips after a successful catch.

Pawa was a major center for leprosy research in the Congo, insignificant as it may look on the map, and it was often visited by authorities "on tour." Professor Dubois, the well-known leprologist from the Tropical Institute in Antwerp, was a regular visitor who stayed with us for weeks at a time. Journalists came wanting to "cover" Pawa as part of a series of social studies in the Congo. Some, in their enthusiasm for details and close-up photos of lepromatous cases, had to be warned of the danger of contamination by contact. Higher political authorities, ministers and governors, loved to be photographed next to advanced cases to show their concern for the unfortunate and their impetuosity for danger.

As 1948 advanced, we started thinking about our home leave due in August. The usual colonial contracts were for three years service and three months home leave, with an additional three months leave if one renewed the contract. That year, however, our placid life and immediate plans were rudely shaken. On Friday, 13 May 1948, a DC-4 SABENA flight from Stanleyville to Brussels crashed during a heavy thunderstorm in the rain forest before reaching Libenge, its first stop. Among the 69 victims was our director, Dr. Zanetti. Their home leave long overdue, Zanetti's wife and two children had left some weeks earlier while he had stayed to insure the smooth transition to his temporary replacement, Dr. Micholovitch, a government medical officer. Friends had teased Dr. Zanetti about flying on Friday the 13th. The greater was the shock when they heard about the crash. It was a stunning blow not only for us at the Red Cross but for most residents of the Nepoko region, where Dr. Zanetti was a well-known and popular figure. For the next several days we at Pawa and other CRC stations, traveled to several small outposts where religious and commemorative services were held in his memory. It was all very sad. We were dazed and perplexed by the events that remained for a long time inconceivable. Dr. Micholovitch was asked to extend the interim period until another candidate for the position could be found.

Before Dr. Zanetti left, he had proposed that we occupy his house so that ours, irreparably damaged by termites, might be rebuilt. In view of this, he had packed and stored his belongings in one of the small rooms. The district officer, Mr. Suain, inventoried and sealed the boxes and trunks so that we could move in. It was a large house, dark, and we didn't like it, although it was cool because of a constant breeze from the large verandah that faced Akunani mountain.

We were due for home leave three months later, but in view of the new circumstances I was asked to extend my stay for another year. I could not accept this proposal because of my commitment to join the IRSAC Institute in early 1949, but agreed to stay on until the new director arrived or for a maximum of six months. This would bring us to February 1949.

After what seemed long delays, especially to Dr. Micholovitch anxious to resume his government post in Stanleyville, the new director, Dr. Swerts, arrived in October. He was just out of medical school and the school of bacteriology,—young, enthusiastic, extremely likable and goodlooking. We took to him immediately and during the brief five months of our acquaintance became very good friends. We knew that in him, the CRC had found a staff member of exceptional qualities, as proven later throughout his 16 years of service, the longest stretch of service anyone had ever given in Pawa. Dr. Swerts was a symbol of devoted medical care, unequivocably pledged to the welfare of his patients and that of the whole region. His unselfish affection for the people gained him their wholehearted confidence, particularly among the leper patients to whom he had dedicated his life.

[Dr. Swerts was gunned down by Congolese rebels in November 1964, 19 miles from his beloved Pawa and his leper patients. "In killing him, the Congolese killed the very man who stood as a symbol of dedication to their own people. Only a miracle can give them another Dr. Swerts," I wrote after I heard the news.]

While we lived in the Nepoko region, we did not realize that this was Africa still in its "primitive" form. I do not use the word in a derogative way. Perhaps I should say "pure form," but that would leave anthropologists aghast. Unconsciously, we held Kibali-Ituri as a standard against which we would later judge subsequent African residences: whether we preferred the sweet, heated grasses of the eastern savannas to the musty dampness of the forest; the cool winds of the Aberdares to the balmy breeze through the oil palms; the expanse of the Okavango Swamps to the shady forest seepage pools; the herds of wildlife on the plains to the bands of monkeys in the canopy; the westernized African in second-hand clothes to the MaBudu in bark cloth.

It was with great expectations for new horizons, literally and figuratively, that we said goodbye to Pawa on 19 February 1949. We retraced the slippery 320 miles to Stanleyville, uneventful this time, and embarked on the Congo river boat *Reine Astrid*, a paddle-wheeler which had plied the Mississippi River many years earlier, before being purchased by OTRACO (Office de Transport Riverain au Congo).

I contend that those who have not made the trip on the Congo River have not seen the Congo. Besides, it is the only way to see 1,000 miles of rain forest from an armchair. For two weeks, the river boat glides on the mud-colored waters, at times so close to the trees that one can see monkeys eye to eye, or so far distant from the banks that the river seems a shoreless lake. The forest unfolds before the passengers at a speed of seven miles an hour, hour after hour, day after day, for 15 days going upstream, 12 days going down. Many think it is boring. We found it fascinating. At this snail's speed one can leisurely observe the intricate structure of the tropical forest of vines, aerial roots and saplings contesting the space between the floor and the canopy. Occasional glimpses of small groups of huts along one of the banks caught people unawares going about their daily chores, as in a candid snapshot. It is like going back half a century, and with a little imagination, one feels like a member of a pioneer team exploring darkest Africa. Isolated on a raft floating on an uncertain stream and, even responsible for its safety, we steer the craft, hoping the captain is with us. Every incident is shared by all. The rumor of a crocodile or a hippo sighting ripples from bow to stern. The cackle of a disturbed monkey is heard by all. The buzz and bite of an occasional tsetse fly completes the African scene.

Meandering between seasonally shifting sandbanks and channels—marked by white signs nailed against a tree—and occasionally guided by calls from the man in the bow with the sounding lead, the boat feels its way cautiously and unhurriedly. Nevertheless, river boats get stuck at times on an unexpected bank. The placidity of the journey is temporarily shattered as we approach a large village where dozens of canoes meet the river boat like metal slivers attracted to a magnet. Brisk and brief transactions are conducted, cut short when the paddle-wheel picks up speed once more. At scheduled stops, local craftsmen have built up a tourist business, their merchandise displayed at regular stalls. Bolobo, one of the oldest stations in the Congo (1882), was famous for its fine ivory craftsmen. "In the old days," prices were ridiculously low, but with the influx of dollar-tossing tourists, prices in later years reached international market values. The most exhilarating stop, however, was at the end of the day at the "station de bois," (coaling station if you will) where the stoke holes of the wood burning boilers were replenished with firewood, cut and prepared in advance by OTRACO laborers. As soon as the boat was made fast at the wharf, more often the beach, an incredible shambles would follow, during which crew and passengers tried to get ashore while villagers pushed to sell their goods to those still aboard. Trade was lively and noisy. Fights were not uncommon, especially later at night when most of the locally brewed "pombe" (spirits) had been consumed. In the meanwhile, a thunderous clatter was added to the general pandemonium when bundles of wood carried on the heads of the "mpagazis" were dumped one by one into the hold. This went on during most of the night. When, at first light, the boat slipped its moors, few of the crew or the passengers had closed their eyes for more than a few hours. During the first hours of the morning cries of crocodiles or hippos went unheeded. Later in the day, the heat under the deck canvas was almost unbearable and it was only in late afternoon that life stirred among the passengers.

As we neared Leopoldville (now Kinshasa), the forest dwindled and more open grassland prevailed. At the same time it became possible to judge the real width of the river, which, in certain parts, seemed a vast expanse of water that stretched to the horizon. Such a place is the "Stanley Pool" at the northern limits of the capital city.

After spending one night in Leopoldville, during which Dora had a frightening nightmare, we boarded the train to Matadi, where we were booked on *M.S. Armand Grisar* with destination Antwerp. And this would have been the end of our nearly four years of African adventures. Not quite. Near Moerbeke, about halfway on its ten-hour journey, the train was stopped. We were ordered to disembark with all our luggage and to carry it a mile to another train waiting across from a large gap in the railbed where a sudden recent flood had washed away the soil. In Matadi we were told of a 48-hour delay in the date of sailing. With no available lodging to be found, we had to endure two days on board the overheated ship, where none of the generators providing power for the ventilation systems was functioning. Matadi lies in a deep trough through which the Congo River, near the end of its course, moves its massive volume of water laden with tropical moisture. Thus Matadi has probably the most constant unpleasant climate in the Congo. During the two days in our small cabin below deck these unpleasant conditions were concentrated within a four by five-square-yard space. During the day we tried to escape the stuffy cabin by walking the broiling Matadi streets, but did not dare to leave the cabin unattended too long having heard rumors that thefts in ships docked in Matadi harbor were very common. The nights were the worse when, dripping wet, we tried to sleep.

It was, therefore, a relief for everyone when we cast off and moved out of the cauldron. A breeze, hot as it was, replaced the stagnant air. After a two-hour stop in Boma, once capital of Congo Free State, private domain of King Leopold II, we soon reached the mouth of the Congo River and the open sea. In spite of a short but nasty storm in the Gulf of Benin, we reached Antwerp within the scheduled fortnight.

It was, of course, wonderful to see family and friends, although, at first, conversation was restricted to answering the repeated questions of "How are you?" Then the excitement settled down and we could look around and absorb with satisfaction the feeling of places long remembered, pleased to find that our love for them had not waned. To submerge myself in *the* atmosphere, I went alone to the nucleus of old Antwerp, the cathedral, and stood in awe, once more, before P. P. Rubens's triptych "Descent from the Cross." I walked along the streets and stood on a streetcar among the "ordinary people," feeling like some kind of unsung hero back from the steaming jungles of central Africa. We had picked up a tan that made many people stare at us (it was still wintry in Europe) probably associating it with some expensive spree to the Côte d'Azur or ski resort in the Alps—although our out-of-fashion and mothball-smelling clothes denied such a thought. We often felt the urge to let them know that ours was a genuine tan, the result of four years' exposure to the African sun. We derived some secret satisfaction by conversing in Kiswahili in the presence of strangers. It was all very childish, I am sure, but in the 1940s, Africa was still very much the stomping grounds of the adventurers and not the fashionable hunting and tourist attraction it became later on. Having left Antwerp in 1945 only a few months after Hitler's last V-1's and V-2's had hit the city, it seemed strange to walk in the streets where everything had returned to normal as if nothing at all had happened. We were alarmed to hear for the first time the screech of low-flying jet planes that brought a brief instinctive reaction of looking for a nearby door—or hallway, waiting for the explosion of a V-bomb.

We seemed to have lost the ability of easy conversation that characterizes ties between old friends—this causing us some distress. Perhaps *we* had changed as a result of four years' estrangement from the "civilized" world. Or had a sort of aftershock with the return to normal life after World War II affected our friends? We thought that perhaps, when we spoke about Africa, our friends not being able to visualize the circumstances, missed the essence of the story. Perhaps we were inexperienced storytellers. Their rare questions seemed trivial to us, indicating a complete lack of comprehension about conditions in the Congo. We wondered if they were interested at all in what we had to say about the colony. To use a cliché, but one so true, "we lived in separate worlds." After the first weeks of our home leave we stopped referring to Africa altogether and, instead, discussed the local news and the performance of the old hockey team and the tennis club. This seemed to bring us back to the level of mutual communication.

After some red-tape delays, I was appointed "technical assistant" with the newly formed IRSAC Institute, with a first posting as station manger to Uvira, the new research station that was being built on the northern shores of Lake Tanganyika. Undeniably, Kivu with its diversity of landscapes, its climate and, yes, the easy access—compared with Pawa—to a choice of daily commodities, had made a favorable impression upon us. But it was by far the attraction of new ground, the excitement of creating, the prospect of research work, the opportunity for travel, the anticipation of team work that incited me to accept Dr. vanden Berghe's proposal to join IRSAC (Institut pour la Recherche Scientifique en Afrique Centrale = Institute for Scientific Research in Central Africa). As I was due to take up my new position sometime in May 1949, our home leave was reduced to three months. After a crash course in medical entomology, and a two-weeks' vacation in Switzerland and Italy, our leave was up. I had found time, however, to participate in a field hockey tournament in Folkestone, England, as center halfback of my old hockey team. It was the last hockey match I would ever play.

Part II
The Winds of the Savanna

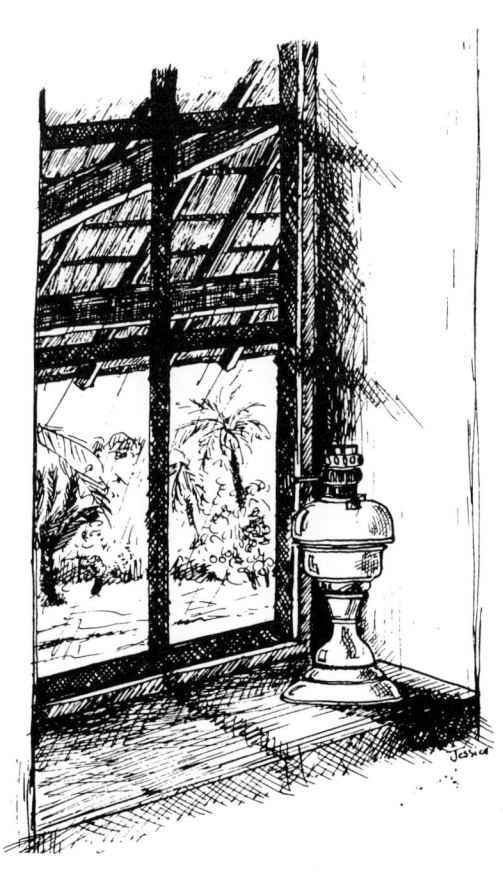

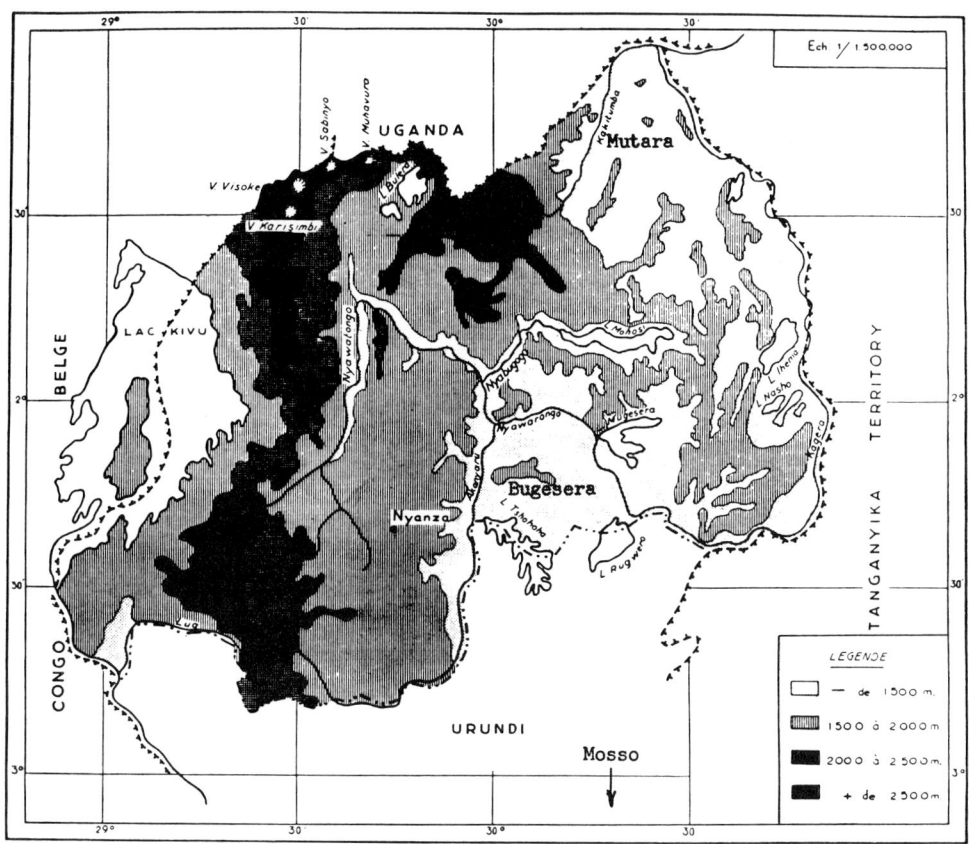

The Kingdom of Ruanda (1950)

Home on the Lake

On 10 May 1949, Dora, our two daughters, now nine and eight years old, and I were on our way back to Africa on board a SABENA DC-4 flight to Leopoldville via Tripoli. At the time of boarding there was a moment of commotion. We learned later that it was caused by the official leave-taking of King Charles Rudahigwa II of Ruanda, who had been in Belgium on a state visit.

The plane refueled at Tripoli around midnight. Bullet holes in one of the hangars were vivid reminders of the African campaign during World War II when the town was lost and retaken several times and finally liberated by Montgomery's Eighth Army in its final push to victory in Africa.

Daybreak saw us floating, ever so slowly it seemed, above the limitless forest, recalling, once more, the now familiar broccoli pattern. Then, suddenly, we saw the Congo River and landed at N'dolo, Leopoldville's airport. We spent the evening with our old friends, Hans and Odette, with whom we had been crocodile hunting only three months earlier. As usual, we had a great time together—a great part of the conversation having to do with reminiscing about our "clandestine" parties during the German occupation, now safely a part of personal memories. They were the last hours we would have together. A year later they migrated to Australia.

Our connecting flight—a DC-3—left at seven for Usumbura, capital city at that time of the Ruanda-Urundi Protectorate. The King of Ruanda and his Belgian adviser, Mr. Dreyfus, were once more among the passengers. Through Mr. Dreyfus, the Mwami (King) learned that I was a new member of the IRSAC Institute. The Mwami was much interested in our institute first because one of IRSAC's research centers was located in Astrida (now Butare), not far from his official residence at Nyanza, and, second, our director, Professor vanden Berghe, was a personal friend. We got into a conversation about the potentials of research in Africa. Until then, most research in biological and other sciences concerning Africa had been carried out in European universities and other institutes. Professor vanden Berghe's plan was to build research centers in Central Africa itself by providing modern facilities equipped to perform research *in situ* by a team of scientists of different disciplines, who would strive towards a coordinated goal in both pure or applied sciences.

We refueled at Luluabourg, a small, hot, dusty airfield where gasoline was pumped by hand into the DC-3's wing tanks. We hoped that the drum held only genuine aviation gasoline and not palm oil sold in similar drums in the local market. After a couple of snapshots of Winnie and Jessie with the Mwami, we were back in the air on our last lap to Usumbura. Lake Tanganyika and the majestic mountains of Ruanda-Urundi came into view as we descended for landing, near the tip of the lake.

Relaxing after refreshing baths, we sat at the hotel's barza enjoying the splendid scenery, glad to be back in Africa.

The next day we were whisked away by car to Costermansville, now officially called Bukavu. We stayed a full week for instructions and briefings and to receive my official post designation: Uvira, on the western shores, the Congo side, of Lake Tanganyika, opposite Usumbura. Apparently, the week in Bukavu was meant to "soften" my posting to Uvira. Indeed, Uvira had developed a bad reputation among the IRSAC people as being terribly hot, humid, dusty and uninspiring. A little settlement of disillusioned government officials and thieving merchants, they said. The native Bavira and Bafulero were rumored to be among the most unmanageable peoples of the whole Kivu Province.

It was a great change from Pawa, indeed. When leaving Pawa, we also left our beloved forest, an area that probably was still to be considered part of "le vieux Congo." But in spite of our love for the forest, we looked eagerly forward to meeting the savanna. So it was with great expectations that we climbed aboard the IRSAC van which, together with the driver Ernest, would be at my disposal to exercise my duties as station manager. After driving through a desolate high plateau, locally known as "moon scape," we arrived at the Kamaniola escarpment. Possibly excluding Kibuye, the Kamaniola road may be one of the most dangerous. It winds and twists precariously along the face of a perpendicular escarpment over a distance of 20 miles. The occasional spectacular views have entranced many a driver who, hypnotized by all that splendor, did not live to tell about it. The road is either cursed for its inches deep chalky

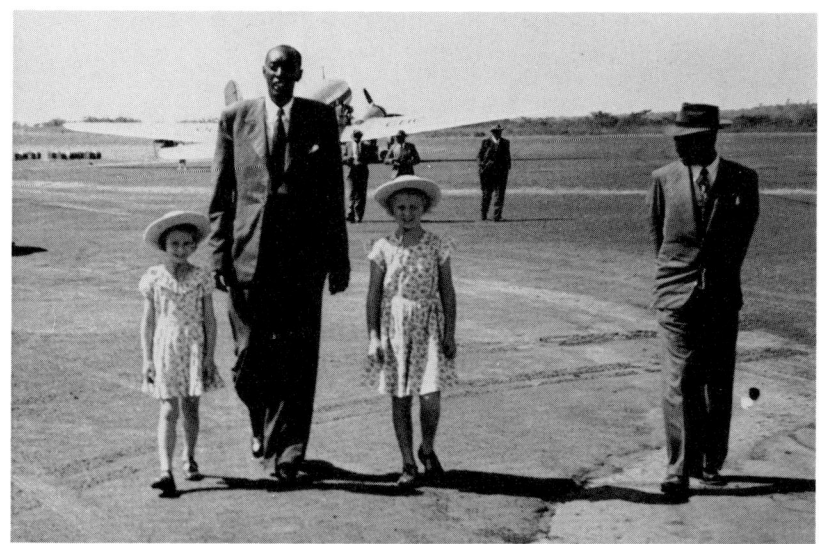
Rudahigwa II, King of Ruanda, with Jessie (left) and Winnie (right) during a stopover in Luluabourg.

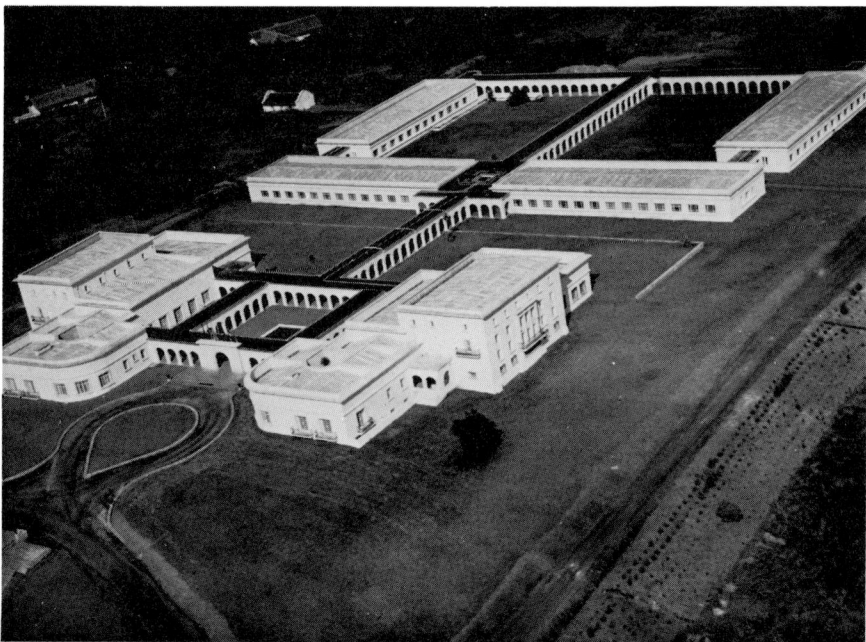
Main Center of I.R.S.A.C. (Institut pour la Recherche Scientifique en Afrique Centrale) at Lwiro, Lake Kivu.

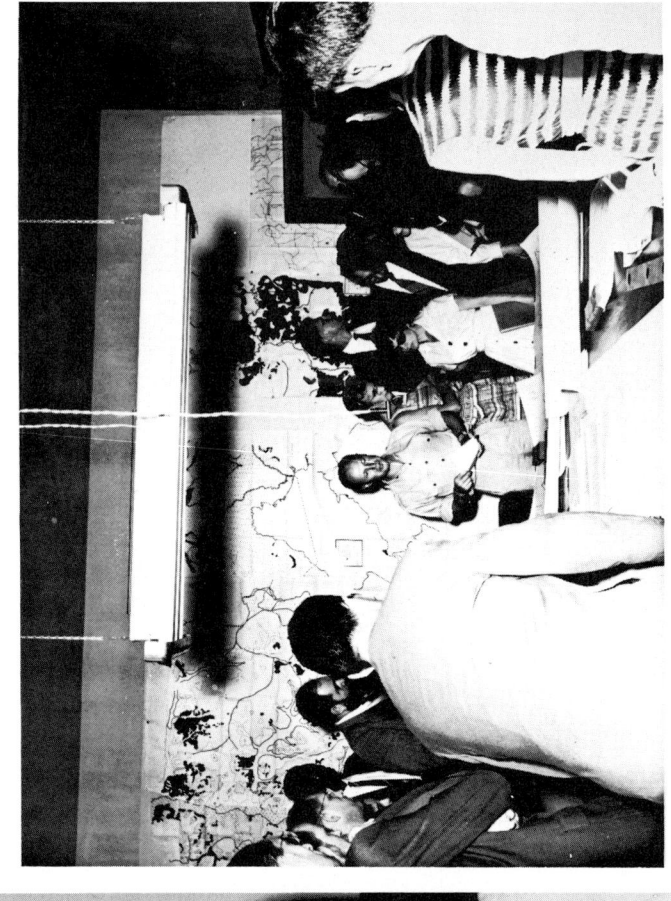

The author explaining his correlation maps project to other participants of the first meeting of specialists in vector-borne diseases (Lwiro, 1957).

Ignace Vincke showing "the ropes" of malaria research to two French W.H.O. trainees.

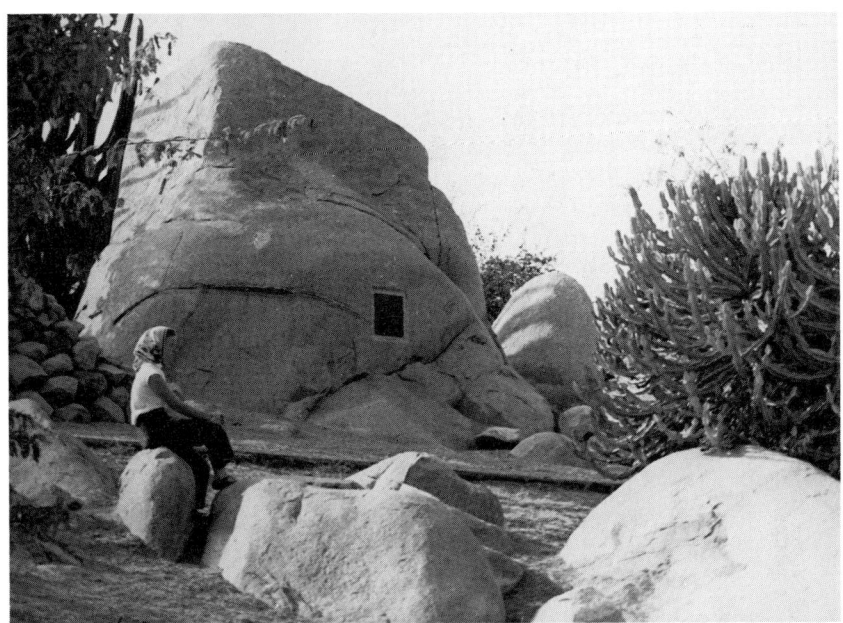

Jessie at the memorial for C.F.M. Swynnerton, pioneer glossinologist of the early 1920s who died in the crash of a survey plane near Shinyanga (Tanganyika) research station.

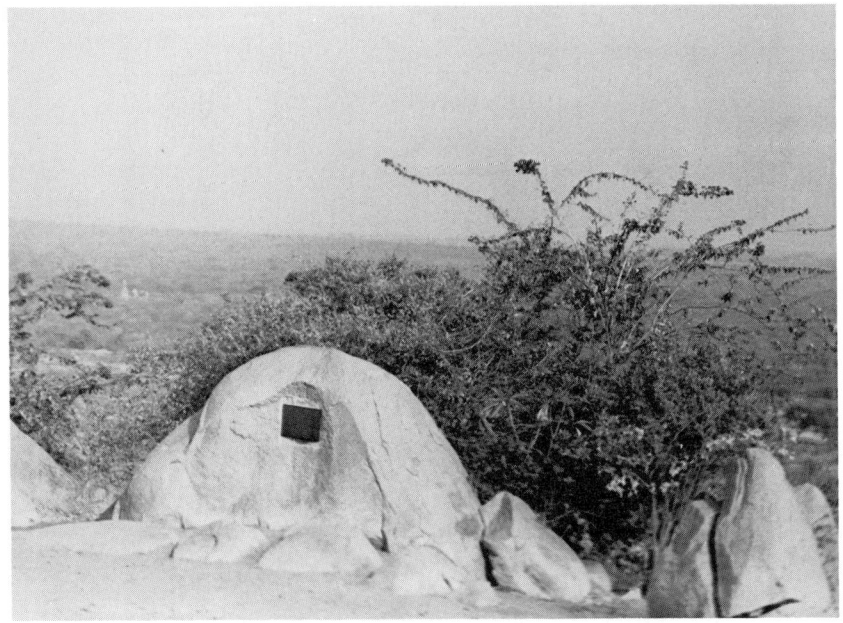

Memorial of C.H.N. Jackson, "father of tsetse research" in Shinyanga hills.

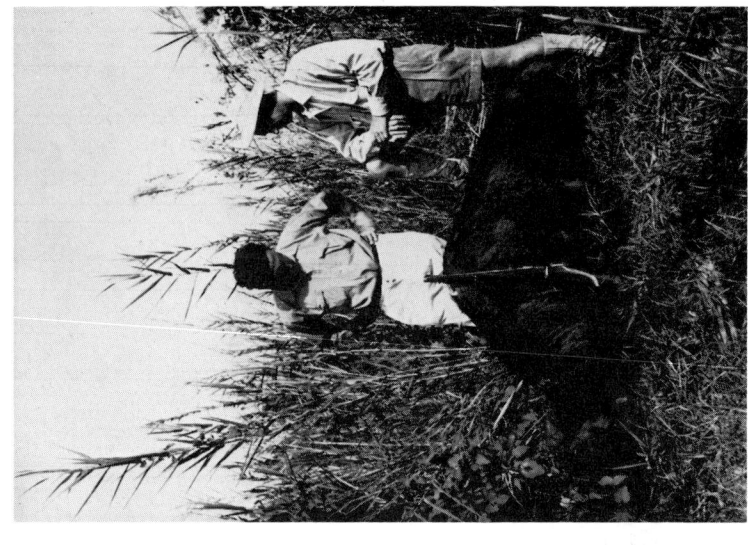

Author's (right) first buffalo hunt in Ruzizi Valley. Monsieur Cloosen still seems to ponder who shot the animal.

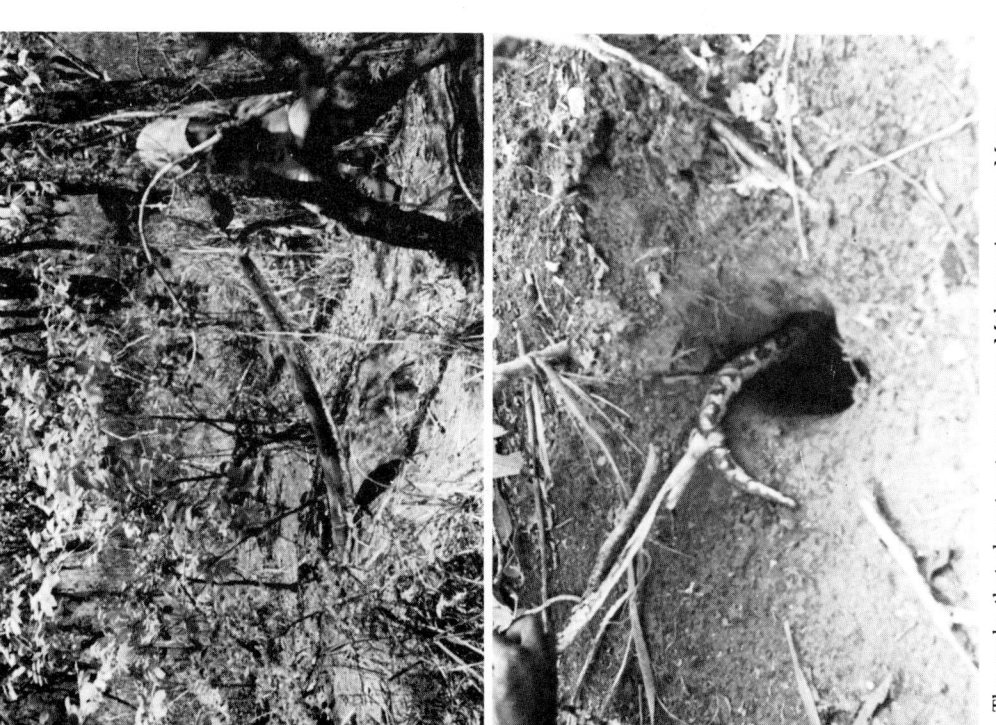

The snake that almost got away near Malagarasi camp, Mosso.

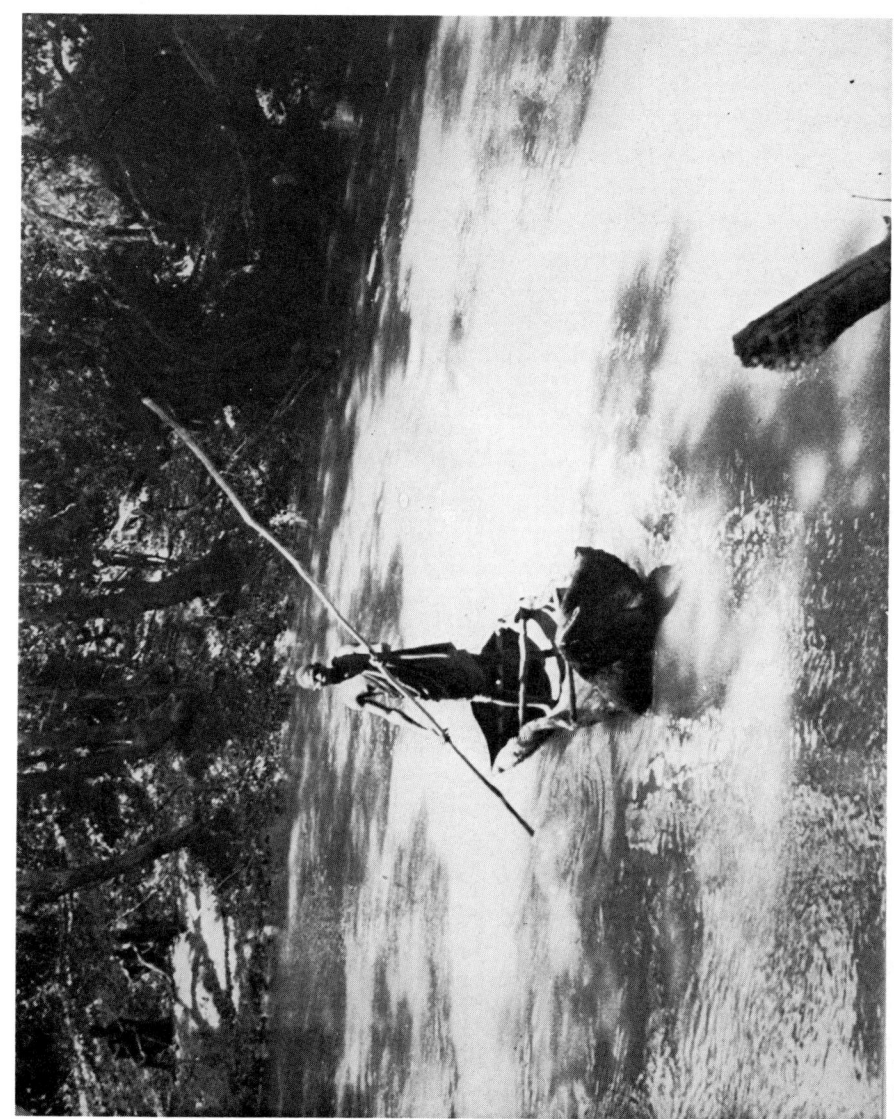

Bark canoe trip on the Malagarasi River.

dust or damned for its treacherous soapy mud. Under either condition, one hopes that when the car skids, it will be towards the mountain side. The Kamaniola road is one track over its entire length, except for a number of "turnouts" where vehicles have to wait until traffic from the opposite direction has passed. The flow of traffic is then reversed until a signal from the next control station indicates the approach of another convoy. At these strategic points, signals are given by beating an empty drum or, in clear weather, by hoisting the drum on a high pole that can be seen from the other control stations. Generally, the system works fine. The road leads from its highest point at 5,300 feet to the valley of the river Ruzizi at 2,300 feet and from a cold, damp, green agricultural land of tea and coffee to a hot, dry and bleak, stunted savanna. By the time the weary and thoroughly carsick traveler reaches the valley, he is only mildly interested in noticing the Ruzizi waters rushing down its gorge. From then on the only hazards are deep ruts and potholes, mad drivers of huge transport vehicles, and an occasional washed-out bridge—and, at times, a herd of elephants leisurely walking across the road near Luberizi. Cultivated land alternates with meager savanna and secondary growth, dotted here and there with small groups of huts until we reach the more fertile Ruzizi delta at its outflow into Lake Tanganyika.

Encased between the Ruanda-Urundi high plateau to the east and the Mitumba range to the west lies the 490-mile-long Lake Tanganyika, the longest lake in the world and, 4,800 feet deep, the second deepest after Lake Baikal in Central Asia. The altitude of Lake Tanganyika's surface is 2,500 feet, so that its bottom is 2,300 feet below sea level. The lake originated from the drainage waters of the surrounding high ridges formed after the creation of the Rift Valley. For a long time, the level of the lake was regulated by an outflow of a river system draining the waters to the *north*, into the valley now occupied by Lake Kivu. About 20,000 years ago, lava flows from the newly formed Virunga volcanoes blocked the valley at both ends—creating Lake Kivu—while the same tectonic movements further lowered the Lake Tanganyika basin. After a while, the rising waters in the newly formed Lake Kivu found an outlet in its southern end, giving birth to the river Ruzizi that now flowed *south* into Lake Tanganyika. With its previous outlet flow now reversed, the level of the lake rose steadily until, during man's memory, the waters forced an outlet by bursting into the Lukuga valley, a low point along its western shores, and joined the Lualaba, as the Congo River is called south of Stanleyville. From a tributary of the Nile, the waters of Lake Tanganyika thus became a tributary of the Congo basin. When, in 1858, Burton and Speke discovered Lake Tanganyika, the basin was still without an outlet. The rising of the lake's level was still observed at Udjiji at the time Stanley met Livingstone in 1871. But a naval officer, Edward Coode Hore, who had established a limnograph in 1879 began to register a sudden halt in the level and then a decline. From March 1879 to August 1880, the level fell more than ten feet. When he toured the lake to investigate, he found that the natural, narrow dike that separated the lake from the Lukuga valley had eroded, creating an outlet, the present Lukuga River.

The Ruzizi—Tanganyika complex was the physical environment in which we would spend the next two years. We had little contact with the local Bavira or Bafulero inhabitants or the so-called Baruanda, refugees who had fled Ruanda during one of the uprisings earlier in the century, and lived in the mountains above Uvira, all different from "our" Ma(Budu). The easy-going relationship we had enjoyed so much with the Pawa population was totally absent here, as it would be everywhere else we resided afterwards. And we missed Mutima.

When we had sadly said goodbye to Mutima when we left Pawa, he had eagerly begged us to call him after we settled in a new place. We had made a vague promise to do so, not certain ourselves where we would land during the next years. Once in Uvira we were afraid that transplanting Mutima and his family into an alien, even possibly hostile environment among other tribes, might not work out so well. But the experience with Felix, a local Bavira houseboy we took on during our first months in Uvira, made us realize how much we missed Mutima.

Felix understood and spoke Swahili but was terribly slow in doing certain things, forgetful in everything else. A typical scene was laying the breakfast table. He would stare for some time at the bare table as if planning his strategy. Then, piece by piece he would put on the table cloth, the plates and, after much more planning, the saucers and cups. As we sat down we reminded him to bring the bread, the butter, the cheese or jam, the spoons and knives.

"Iko wapi chai," we would ask. ("Where is the tea?")

Felix boiled water and made tea. Then came his greatest performance: Felix would come sailing in with the tea pot and put it on the table. As we reached to pour he changed his mind and turned the spout about SSW, eyeing the position for a moment. Then he would swing the spout slightly south by west. Not satisfied, he rotated the pot firmly northwest. With a sigh of satisfaction he would leave, after we had watched the performance with fascination.

A lengthy correspondence in Swahili to Bafwagada, Mutima's village—how the letters got there, I have not the faintest idea—resulted in Mutima's arrival in Uvira a few months later. We had managed to pay for the fare through the local CVC transport company. Suddenly, Africa felt more familiar.

Uvira was a bit of a letdown: a single dusty road lined with typical slovenly ndukas (native shops) and dilapidated houses. The only colorful notes were the blue, choppy waters of the lake and, in season, the brilliant scarlet flowers of the flame tree or flamboyant tree (*Delonix regia*) that bordered the road. According to colonial tradition, the town was divided into the "white section" that included most of the shops, the hotel, the government offices, the houses of the D.O., of Dr. Jungelson, Mr. Kemp, a planter, Mr. Meeus, the bar and delicatessen shop and Mrs. Duvivier. The second part included the native quarters that lodged all those employed by the local business or trade and, since the start of the construction of the IRSAC center, those employed by this institution. Dispersed along the lake shore were a few huts of fishermen.

We put up at Hotel du Lac managed by a Maltese couple. It was the only imposing and reasonably well-kept structure in Uvira. Past the dukas, just beyond the government offices, a neat little public square faced an unencumbered view of the lake and led to a clean, narrow beach reached by stepping across the railway track which linked the harbor at Kalundu, a few miles further south, to the Kamaniola escarpment road.

IRSAC had bought the massive skeleton of a hotel under construction but abandoned when the company went bankrupt. Judging from the gigantic hulk, it would have been a grandiose undertaking. The square, two-story building enclosed a large central patio. A balcony ran all along the inner side, overlooking the patio. The front balcony, part of a huge room no doubt intended for the dining hall, provided an unobstructed view of lake and mountains. At the time of our arrival, the rehabilitation and modifications to transform the structure into a series of research laboratories, dependencies and living quarters had already been started by a team of a constructor, a cabinetmaker and a mechanic. The property also included three houses, occupied by the three technicians, and a large storeroom used as a machine- and woodwork shop. Two small annexes had been built, one to house experimental animals, the other for an electric generator. With no piped water anywhere in town, water for the three, and now four, households had to be hauled from the Kalimabenge River, two miles down the road, in 50-gallon drums on an old pickup truck. In all, we employed from 80 to 100 Africans. I was in charge of all but the scientific activities. I was payment officer, supplies overseer, administrator and complaints department all rolled into one. It was Pawa all over again, but on a far larger scale and in a far less pleasant environment.

On the opposite side of the lake was Usumbura (now Bujumbura), the administrative center of the Ruanda-Urundi Protectorate. The kingdoms of Ruanda and Urundi were once part of German East Africa. After World War I, the League of Nations handed the administration of the two kingdoms over to the Belgian Government under the supervision of the colonial administration. The rest of German East Africa became a protectorate under British colonial rule. The traditional authority of King Rudahigwa II of Ruanda and Mwambutsa of Urundi was recognized by the Belgian government. The balance between the traditional monarchical system and the colonial administration, however delicate at first sight, seemed to work well until, the civil war, in 1961, following independence, completely wrecked the old kingdoms, and the Watutsi overlords were brutally murdered or evicted.

As the administrative manager of the IRSAC center, I had the doubtful pleasure of visiting Usumbura on official business once a month, my pocket full of shopping lists that had me jump from shop to shop in an effort to find all the items—an impossible task it seemed to me in this forsaken corner of the African continent. Construction materials were either available in oversupply or scarcely to be had at all. If there was a glut of cement, one could be certain that rod iron was unavailable. Plywood seemed abundant when the lake boat with a nail shipment ran aground at Kigoma. When desperately in need for white paint, all that the shops carried was blue in various shades. By the time the shops closed for lunch "hour"—at least a two-hour affair in these parts—I was in a state of utter exhaustion and a nervous wreck. Closing my mind to the vexations that would meet me as I checked off the missing items upon my return to Uvira, I was glad to jump in the van and escape Usumbura's bustle and heat. On the way back it was always soothing to admire the majestic 10,000-foot-high Mitumba Mountains full of color and shadow, the ravines cut with geological precision, the white clouds capping the peaks with delightful perfection, and the deep-blue waves of the lake whipped in a fury by the afternoon breeze. Metal-plated bridges spanned the two arms of the Ruzizi River near their outlet in Lake Tanganyika. Their loud clamor as one drove across had long since chased the large crocodile population further upstream. Towards Uvira, the small fisherman's village of Kilomoni occupied one of the sandy beaches, a group of square huts made from reeds growing in profusion in the seasonal swamps farther inland. The village would play an important part in my later research on malaria.

My duties as station manager were in constant conflict with my desire to spend more time on research. The duties were rendered the more difficult because of the scarcity of supplies when cement was rare, bricks a bargain commodity, wood unseasoned, transport infrequent, and meeting the demand for water a constant headache. To alleviate this water shortage at the construction site, I diverted the water of the Kalimabenge River from a place upstream into a ditch running through the IRSAC grounds, watering a small garden on the way, and through a culvert under the road and the railway into the lake. As the water gushed happily across the IRSAC compound, I sat back awaiting enthusiastic congratulations from my colleagues. The constructor seemed happy enough, but one researcher stormed into the director's office in Bukavu complaining that his research project on the lake shore was utterly ruined by the influx of fresh water. So the water supply was closed and we went back to the old water-hauling days. Yet, although the water supply system had been shut off, arguments for or against it were not. Consequently, the sluice was opened or closed several times according to whether one side or the other came up with convincing arguments. The story, now lost perhaps in Uvira's historical records, at that time provided welcome material for the gossiping inhabitants—until the Greek shop owner once more threw out his daughter and this more important subject had to be discussed. As time went on, the limnologist became interested in other organisms and the water was allowed to run again through the ditch. On several occasions, however, I had to protect my system from owners of gardens who diverted the supply into their "shambas" (fields).

Other problems had to do with human conflicts and frictions between members of our own group, which, besides the three technicians, all now included three scientists: a limnologist, an entomologist and a herpetologist. Common complaints concerned their lodgings or inadequacies thereof, personal and professional use of IRSAC vehicles, nondelivery of water or firewood, and so on. Conflicts between the African supervisor and the white technicians were often caused by a lack of understanding and communication, especially because most technicians were new to the colony and did not speak Swahili. In addition, there were the usual difficulties with African labor: absenteeism, drunkenness, mutual debts, family problems, unreliable performance and sometimes theft.

Our own accommodations during the first year were hardly compensating for the hardships on the job. We were lodged in two rooms above an African shop, with no bathroom or kitchen. Dora cooked on a kerosene stove; we washed ourselves in a basin as if we were camping. The toilet was in an outdoor hut in the backyard, reached by walking down an outdoor stair—quite unpleasant during the night or a rainstorm. Mutima, who had joined us after the first few months, was living in a chicken coop minus the chickens, but not the remnant fleas and other ectoparasites. Our furniture consisted of four camp beds, a camp table and camp chairs, and some packing cases. We, too, had to deal with fleas, no doubt because of the two dogs that had been kept in the room for many months prior to our occupation. How Dora and Mutima stuck it out for all that time proves their respective devotion to me, for which I should be eternally grateful. As for me, my daily worries on the job probably kept me from realizing their hardships.

But not all members of the family had a bad time, if one believes a diary Jessie kept and was recently rediscovered about her and Winnie's Uvira days. It tells how wonderful it was to be back in Africa and to have a large backyard in which to play without upsetting anyone! How they could watch Nyama-na-poli, Mutima's wife as she prepared food and cared for her babies, but how sad it was when one of them died of malaria. Riding their bicycles up and down the street, they came to know most of the Uvira inhabitants. From our balcony, they watched the customers of the shop below, among whom were the Baruanda women in their traditional dark blue cloth knotted over one shoulder, and their simple but very effective adornments of necklaces, arm and ankle bands made from pink and deep blue beads. They talked incessantly and laughed a lot, so Jessie's diary goes. Among the regular onlookers in front of the shop was a young boy in ragged clothes, his hair made up with beads and match sticks, who sang and played the likembe (thumb-piano). At times, a very old woman would come out of the Greek nduka across the street, shaking her long white hair that covered her shoulders and upper part of her body, and walk on high-heeled silver shoes up and down the street, to disappear once more inside the shop. From Jessie's diary, one gains the impression that half of Uvira's population was slightly unbalanced. Half of Uvira's population admitted that the other half was. The climate, they said.

In September of that year, we enrolled Winnie and Jessie, now ten and nine years old, at an excellent boarding school in Astrida (now Butare) in the Ruanda highlands. Although this meant another separation, we were happy to know that they were well taken care of and that they were in a healthy climate. Another reassurance was that over the weekends, they could visit with friends at the IRSAC center in the same town. Furthermore, Astrida was only 150 miles from Uvira. Nevertheless, it took five hours driving, taking reasonable risks, or four and a half hours, taking unreasonable risks. The reason was that the narrow mountain road had few straight stretches and most bends were close to 90 degrees. At a place, called "kitchwa saba" (seven heads), seven curves could be seen in the road higher up. In the dry season, the surface was a tender pink dust; in the rainy season, a dark pink mud, its high mica contents making it particularly soft and slippery. Landslides were common during heavy rains, at times cutting the road in more than one place. The road hazards also affected our own operations as the IRSAC center at Astrida was dependent for certain supplies on our Uvira stores.

From Usumbura, the road winds straight into the Ruanda-Urundi highlands with elevations between 5,000 and 6,000 feet, dipping a few times to cross deep valleys where swift running streams drain the high rainfall. The first ascent takes the traveler to the Nyongwe forest at about 6,000 feet. For some ten miles, the road follows a fairly uniform contour, traversing the magnificent mountain forest reserve where often black-and-white Colobus monkeys (*Colobus polykoimos*) can be seen. In the dry season we often drank from a seepage spring at the side of the road and ate the refreshing acidulous "monkey apple," a sort of Anona fruit that grew wild in the forest. After a plunge into the valley of the river Akanyaru, the road climbs once more, twisting its way from hill to hill and into reforestations of eucalyptus and "black wattle" (Mimoseae) trees, until Astrida is reached at an elevation of 6,000 feet.

Our lodging conditions improved markedly after the first year when the rehabilitation of the upper floor of the IRSAC building neared completion and we could occupy the front rooms of the right wing. The floor plan was somewhat awkward in that all the rooms ran into each other as in a railway carriage. But the rooms were all very sunny, airy and a tremendous improvement on our quarters above the native shop. We had a marvelous view of the lake and the mountains on the far shore. At night, after the generator was switched off at ten o'clock, we could hear the soft sound of the short waves as they broke ashore. The wind would shift and the murmur of my Kalimabenge diversion that ran underneath our windows became louder. In the background, the cicadas sang their never-ending chirruping medley. The curtains moved gently in the breeze, noises became distant and thus we fell asleep.

While in Pawa my problems as station manager were confined to the immediate "family" of the Red Cross personnel and the headmen of the nearby villages. As station manager in Uvira, my duties seemed to require some kind of public relations with the town's inhabitants, colorful to say the least. The IRSAC presence was not readily accepted by the white settlers and officials. We were intruders in the sedate, everyday, slumbering life of a small, drowsy, dusty and dull post, whose population hadn't changed for the last decade except for forgotten deceased and ignored births. Suddenly, a half dozen newcomers moved in, new to the colony—already a first offense—with ideas very different from the "old colonials," and with them more than a hundred Africans from various tribes. The balance of relationships—already delicate because of the abolition of corporal punishment—was disrupted, secrets were in danger of exposure, isolation from the outside world was shattered. Whereas the town had struggled on a meager budget, IRSAC came in with new vehicles, glittering equipment, a labor force not seen since the building of the railroad, and well-dressed white personnel with no apparent restrictions upon their shopping sprees. Between them I stood, a step above the "damned new colonials," but far from belonging to the staunch old guard. It was like walking on a fence on the one side being loyal to IRSAC and personnel, while on the other side understanding the resentments of the inhabitants. Conflicts occurred frequently; complaints were almost daily routine. It was the first time I came under fire from a government official, the administrateur territorial (district officer or D.O.), who called me into his office and accused me of paying my African personnel more than the official wages. It was also an excuse for him to find out what kind of a person I was and how to deal with me. I must confess that I had made the deadly mistake of not going to see him and introducing myself during the first hectic days of my arrival. He was not going to brush me off that easily. I tried to make good by going into some length over the ideals of our institute and how our local activities might benefit the community. I suppose that all this didn't make the slightest dent in his tough colonial hide, but I felt that, as I left his office after a grilling one-hour interview, I had not made things any worse.

At eighty, Mme. Duvivier was easily the oldest inhabitant of Uvira. She was the widow of a major who had fought in the victorious colonial army. He had died a few years before from some mysterious tropical disease, leaving her a small pension and an equally small house in Uvira. With no relatives, she was "stuck there." She said she wouldn't move in any case because it was here that her husband was buried, and so would she be. As was the case with other Uvirans, I became acquainted with Mme. Duvivier as a result of her complaints. Her garden wall bordered on the rear of the IRSAC compound near the place where our laborers used to have their lunch. Her wall made a convenient conduit for getting rid of wrappings, fruit offal and other litter. (I had warned) that littering the IRSAC compound would be punished by "kata franca: (cut wages). Mme. Duvivier sent me a short note that within few words managed to describe all the shortcomings of the new generation of colonials and the time worn maliciousness of the Africans. I went to see Mme. Duvivier for the first time. I was met by a small, gaunt, wrinkled old lady and by a flood of abuses that belied her meek appearance. After she had exhausted herself, I noticed with satisfaction that it would probably take a while before she could muster another outburst. I introduced myself, offered my well-meant apologies for the unforgivable behavior of my personnel and promising that I would see to it that it would never occur again. It never did. Somewhat appeased and back to normal breathing rhythm, Mme. Duvivier related her life "dans ce vieux Congo" with her husband and how, as the wife of an army officer, she had participated in the occupation and creation of the Belgian Congo Colony after King Leopold II, under international pressure, had to relinquish his personal domain. Dora and I had tea with Mme. Duvivier several times after my first conversation with her and through her, IRSAC gained a staunch promoter of its ideals.

Payday, held every fortnight, was another big headache. More than 100 laborers would line up in the central courtyard while I counted out their wages in the presence of their supervisor, Selemani. Arguments were frequent when their pay was less than expected because of absenteeism or penalties for various misdemeanors, usually reported by the constructor or by Selemani himself. The noise after payment was even louder when the men started arguing about return of debts owed by their fellow workers. Borrowing from each other on payday was a common practice—to get the money back was another matter altogether. At the end of payday I had the painful task of trying to balance the accounts. For reasons that remained obscure, many times the count did not tally and the only way to do so was to add money from my own pocket—as I had done before at Pawa. It was said that the bankrolls from the bank teller were not always accurate—on the minus side to be sure—which may account for the occasional deficits.

A Touch of Malaria

My official title with the institute was that of scientific assistant, but I was expected to fulfill the role of station manager until IRSAC personnel could be brought up to its full staff complement. I had an unwritten understanding with the director, however, that if I could find the time and opportunity, I would start a part-time research project. At first, this was a bit of a joke because we could have used two station managers during the first years. However, by working literally day and night I managed to squeeze in a few weekends away from Uvira and into the Ruzizi Valley, where I proposed to study blood parasites of the local fauna. Dora and I camped out in a small mountain tent, which was horribly hot during the day and unbearably cold at night. We slept in sleeping bags on the ground, and somehow survived. Limited in time, I concentrated on hunting birds with a small bore shotgun. For one thing, birds were far more common than mammals in the valley, and relatively little is known of bird parasites. I made blood smears of each bird killed and collected any ectoparasites present. The blood smears were later stained in the laboratory and examined under the microscope. It was low-key research, but it gave me the opportunity to practice field techniques and to explore various parts of the valley, which would be helpful later on. The blood samples showed a variety of parasites that may have belonged to still undescribed species, but I found no time to pursue their study any further. For that reason, the project was "integrated" into that of the regular parasitologist, rightly so perhaps. In any case, this preliminary work and the interest I showed in carrying it out was good enough to show the director that I was eagerly waiting at the starting line for a full-time research career.

The big chance for more sophisticated research came sooner than I expected when Dr. Ignace Vincke started a malaria research project in the Ruzizi valley. Dr. Vincke, a government researcher from Elisabethville (now Lumbumbashi), was a well-known malariologist. His fame spread worldwide with his discovery of *Plasmodium berghei*, a rodent malaria parasite now maintained in every medical laboratory engaged in parasitological research. The history of Vincke's discovery reads like a detective story, as in reality it was. Tracing the finding of an unknown plasmodium infection in a rare rodent to its vector—an undescribed "wild" mosquito that lives in secluded valleys of an isolated high plateau of the Kundulungu area in Katanga—led to the full description and life cycle of *P. berghei*, named after Professor vanden Berghe, our IRSAC director. The importance of the discovery was that it gave scientists the opportunity to study a malaria parasite in all of its phases in small laboratory animals, mice for instance, and that experiments can be made to find more effective antimalaria drugs or vaccines.

A greenhorn in malaria research and only a one-tour colonial, I was apprehensive working for Dr. Vincke. He was rather short-tempered when things were not going to his liking, and always impatient for results. We did not hit it off well during the first months. I found it difficult to please him when occasionally he came over from Elisabethville to check on the progress. Our research project concerned the evaluation of the use of DDT in field trials to control malaria by applications of the insecticide inside the huts in experimental areas to reduce or eliminate the *Anopheles* mosquito population responsible for transmission of the disease. The Ruzizi valley, a highly endemic malaria area with a number of separate, small villages, was ideal for such trials. This was the heyday of DDT, well before *Silent Spring* silenced its use in many parts of the world. It was in the late 1940s that DDT became commercially available in large quantities on the world markets. Preliminary trials had shown its great potential as a mosquito control agent and, therefore, of the diseases they transmit. Controversial reports, however, indicated that although DDT would kill mosquitoes at contact with surfaces sprayed with the insecticide, something, smell perhaps, had a repulsive effect upon certain mosquitoes which avoided landing or resting on sprayed walls and thereby escaped lethal contact. Our experiments in the Ruzizi valley were aimed to confirm or invalidate DDT's usefulness in the field as a mosquito and malaria control agent against the local malaria vectors: *Anopheles gambiae, Anopheles funestus, Anopheles pharoensis* and a fourth species, *Anopheles pretoriensis*, of which the vectorial capacity was unknown. Preliminary data on the malaria situation were obtained during several months of survey that included the examination of blood smears from the inhabitants of the various villages within the experimental zone of about 25 square miles; the spleen index, a measurement of the enlargement of the spleen of children under 15 years; the presence and relative abundance of the four *Anopheles* species in the dwellings; and the characteristics of the breeding places of these mosquitoes in nearby water courses. The relative density of the mosquito population was estimated by what became known as the "window trap." This consisted of a square-shaped box frame covered with mosquito netting, that allowed the entrance of the insects through a funnel-shaped cone that ended in an inch-wide opening inside the box. The trap was placed in a fitted opening cut in the east-pointing wall of a hut, the entrance facing the inside of the room. Female mosquitoes that take blood during the night from people sleeping inside will normally leave the hut at sunrise to rest outside or, in some species, will digest the blood while resting inside the hut and leave only a few days later to deposit their eggs in an outside water course. In huts fitted with window traps, the light from the rising sun passing through the trap was the most conspicuous escape route from the dark inside of the hut, so most mosquitoes landed inside the trap. This was placed on the outside with a sleeve to permit the removal of the insects caught inside. Collection was made every day just after daybreak, and the mosquitoes were tallied per species and in categories of four stages of repletion with blood and one for the carriers of eggs. Almost all mosquitoes caught were females since they are the ones to fly inside to take blood. The insects were then dissected and the salivary glands and stomachs examined for the presence of malaria parasites. We also made direct mosquito counts by fumigating a hut with commercial aerosol insecticide, after the floor and the furniture were covered with white sheets, and doors and windows had been closed. After ten minutes, we entered the hut and started collecting and counting the dead mosquitoes, later to be identified by species and hunger stages and dissected. Our record number in one of the villages was 1,792 anopheles in a single hut, and 1,812 in another!

Anxious to follow results, Dr. Vincke had asked me to report by official telegram the weekly findings. A typical telegram would read something like the following: "TWENTY SEVEN FEMALES TRAPPED IN KILOMONI STOP TWELVE WITH BLOOD FIFTEEN DEAD STOP DISSECTED SEVEN STOP ONE INFECTED SALIVARY GLANDS."

After a while, the postmaster became suspicious and informed the D.O. about this alarming exchange of telegrams. Once again, I had to appear before the D.O., but this time the interview ended with a chuckle. And still another good story joined the Uvira repertoire.

After we established the basic malaria pattern in our experimental square, DDT was applied to the inside walls of the huts and the subsequent incidence of malaria in the population and of mosquito densities was compared with previous figures. There was clearly a decrease of both, but many oddities had still to be investigated, and the whole question of eradication of malaria, which looked so promising with the discovery of DDT, had to be considerably revised in later years.

While I had been waiting during my home leave for the final IRSAC appointment, I had followed Dr. vanden Berghe's advice and taken a "crash" course in medical entomology under Professor Schoutenden, director of the Museum of Colonial Sciences. But it was my work with Dr. Vincke that set me on my way to making medical entomology the basis of my later career, which, to use a single denominator, could be described as a vector-borne diseases ecologist. As the majority of tropical diseases are transmitted by insects and other invertebrates, their study is an essential part towards the control of these diseases. As for me, it gave me the opportunity to spend many subsequent years in field research and to become intimately involved in the study of the many varied African biotopes and to appreciate their intricate biological communities. Further specialization made me part of that select group called glossinologists, expert in the study of tsetse flies (*Glossina*) and African sleeping sickness (trypanosomiasis).

Because of its location on the shore of Lake Tanganyika, the IRSAC center at Uvira was primarily dedicated to hydrobiological research. Other IRSAC centers specialized in their own but by no means only research objectives: at Elisabethville (Katanga), biochemistry; at Mabale (Equatoria), botany; at Astrida (Ruanda-Urundi), anthropology. The main IRSAC center at Lwiro (Kivu) covered several major subjects such as: biology, medical sciences, geophysics.

An advantage of working at the Uvira center was the Lake Tanganyika-oriented research. This labor translated for me into spending many hours in cruising or just anchoring off-shore, gently rocked by the early morning swell, while the hydrologist made observations, dragged fishing nets or collected plankton. We avoided late afternoon when strong winds would whip the lake into choppy waves. The warm waters were lovely to swim in, but we had always needed someone to stand by with a gun to keep the crocodiles away for they were very numerous along the shores.

Crocodiles, however, nearly cut short my colonial career. One late Saturday afternoon, Jean Michel, the mechanic-technician, came back from a hunting trip all excited because he had shot and killed a large crocodile near the mouth of the Ruzizi. Being too far from a place that could be reached with the pickup and too late in the day to get help from our center, he and a few natives had hauled the animal ashore with the intention of returning the next day to transport it by canoe to a point where it could be loaded onto the pickup. It was a huge animal, he said, with an old wound made by a spear with the metal point still sticking out of its side. The next day being Sunday, four of us went with the pickup truck to help retrieve the animal. As we approached Jean's kill, we realized that he had not spun "a-big-one-that-got-away" story. The crocodile was at least 15 feet long, so we chartered a large canoe. Several times we came close to capsizing as we stowed the animal, which took up almost the whole length of the craft. We clammered aboard, first the two owners of the craft, who would steer it from the stern, followed by Jean. Next was Henry, another IRSAC technician on vacation from the Ruanda center, and his wife, Milou. She and I were the only ones with standing room, all the others had no choice but to sit on top of the alleged dead animal. I stood in the prow ready with a .303 rifle in case we should have trouble with crocodiles that crowded the river. As we reached midstream, the "impossible" occurred. The "dead" animal, warmed up perhaps by the people sitting on top and annoyed by their weight, started moving and with its mouth wide-open advanced toward Milou. First in line of attack, she backed away towards the prow and I, perfect gentleman that I was and in her way for further retreat, saw no other solution but to fall into the river. The brain, it is said, works like a computer, not as efficient perhaps, but equally fast and with more imagination. During that split second, as I reconstructed my impressions later, I had decided not to try to use the rifle, first, because a bullet ricocheting on the hard hide might hit people; second, the shot might not be enough to stop the animal, judging from its present performance; third, I might miss the animal altogether during the commotion and blow a hole in the bottom of the canoe. I recall depositing the rifle, almost gently (I have always been careful with loaded weapons)—before I fell backwards into the river. In the next moments I was dimly aware of brown-colored water as I went under. And then, without effort on my part so it seemed, I popped up again and saw the lovely sight of blurred sunshine and a dark shadow, which, I presumed, was the boat. I grabbed it with both hands and held to the side of the canoe as it drifted by. I was hauled aboard before a bona fide live crocodile could get me. It flitted through my mind that to be back aboard was perhaps not the safest place either, but I was reassured when I saw that the "dead" crocodile was lying still. Not wanting to take any more chances, we instructed our paddlers to row back to the bank as fast as possible. They didn't need any encouragement. The crocodile was hauled on land without further trouble and to make sure, Jean shot it a couple more times. It was hard to explain how the animal was "killed" 15 hours earlier and had remained immobile during all that time only to revive suddenly and scare us out of our socks. Dr. G. Marlier, our zoologist, was overjoyed with the catch because he was interested in its stomach contents. Dutifully, I made blood smears. The story of the "dead" crocodile went around like bushfire and is now part of Uvira's oral history.

My own first success in Uvira as a hunter, beyond the birds I had collected during my parasitological survey, was to bring down a bushbuck (*Tragelaphus scriptus*) I shot in the Ruzizi valley while hunting with two other IRSAC members one late afternoon. Bushbuck are extremely shy animals, spending most of the daytime in dense thicket vegetation. They come out late in the day, often to eat young shoots in vegetable gardens if they live close to human habitations. I saw the animal in a split second—a vague shadow in the failing daylight—and aimed almost at random with my shotgun. Out of politeness, the two others helped me look for the animal in the high grass. More than anyone else I was surprised that we found the dead antelope, especially as it was now quite dark. The bushbuck was received with great enthusiasm by the IRSAC residents, who were short of meat. Even Mme. Duvivier received a share.

The next hunting party I participated in, (as an observer) was for buffalo. It was organized by Mr. Closen, a settler who lived quite a way up the mountains bordering the Ruzizi plain near Sange. I was invited one day to join him and two of his friends to chase buffaloes that plagued his sugar-cane plantation by trampling and eating young shoots, and possibly get "one for the pot." His friends failed to bring an extra gun as they had promised. So I tagged along "for the fun." The sugar cane was 10 to 12 feet high and it looked to me a rather unhealthy place for encountering, let alone shooting, a buffalo. But Closen was an experienced hunter and had shot buffalo before in defense of his plantation. We plodded along in a desultory way, stopping from time to time to listen. Seeing beyond six feet was out of the question. As we were about to resume our scouting after one of our halts, an unmistakable snorting, crashing of canes and pounding hooves quite close by, informed us that our search was over. The previous eager expression on the hunters' faces changed a shade towards "What the hell do we do now?" Who was to volunteer to take the first step towards the goal we had so ardently sought a moment ago? The question was answered precipitously when the buffaloes crashed out of cover. Being thrown into confusion by the "wall" of hunters—guns cocked—and one meek bystander, there followed a melee of panicking buffaloes, uncertain hunters, a scared onlooker, blazing guns and a lot of dust. When the dust settled, we were all accounted for, some still with smoking guns. And, of all miracles, one dead buffalo! Mr. Closen estimated that he lost more sugar cane during the brief six-second encounter than what the buffaloes would destroy in six days. But the heart of the hunter was satisfied. "We" had downed one. Who had shot the fatal bullet? Arguments are still ringing in the mountains.

On 26 May 1950, two years after construction had started, the IRSAC-Uvira center was officially inaugurated. Except for details that would probably take years to complete, the skeleton-hotel had been transformed into several research laboratories. The whole extent of the enormous downstairs front hall—planned as a reception hall by the hotel people, I presume—was now occupied by huge aquaria holding a variety of rare and not so rare fishes from the lake, part of the collection studied by the hydrobiologist. The renovated courtyard was a mass of tropical plants, collected and arranged by the botanist, their look of coolness enhanced by the gentle dribble of a fountain inside an unsymmetrical pond. The upstairs had been converted into four resident apartments, a guest apartment, a library and a meeting room that opened directly onto the wide balcony with its splendid view of the lake.

The inauguration was a big affair, attended by Mr. Petillon, vice-governor, and other high-ranking officials and, of course, the hierarchy of the IRSAC Institute, including members of the board of directors from Brussels, and several representatives of other institutions and universities.

Our two years in Uvira now drew to a close. A young chap had arrived some months previously to take over the station manager position and I was to be relocated to Astrida, where I would replace the station manager, due for home leave. We looked forward to the change because we would be in the same community as our daughters' boarding school.

Pleasant incidents marked our last days in Uvira. The first occurred on the day we left. We did the rounds to say goodbye and, when we came to the front hall of the building, were surprised to find all the African personnel assembled in that place. The head clerk stepped forward and read the letter he and others had composed to wish us good luck. We were very moved. The original text of the letter is given below. I refrain from translating it for fear of losing its color and meaning. I want to preserve it in its original form with its beautiful and so typical African expressions of devotion.

The other pleasant thing was that the coconuts I had planted personally to embellish the beach in front of the IRSAC property had started to grow into healthy saplings. Several years later, I was proud to learn that the trees had matured beautifully and that the beach looked like the shores of a South Sea Island.

The letter:

Monsieur et Madame Lambrecht,
    A l'occasion de votre départ pour Astrida je tiens au nom des membres du Personnel Africain, en même temps que vous rendre notre hommage le plus sincère, à vous souhaiter bon voyage, bon séjour à Astrida et bonne santé, bonne chance et courage aux nouvelles responsabilités du chef de poste que vous allez assumer demain au Ruanda, ce pays de merveille!
    Si je pouvais vous traduire tout ce que se laissent chicotter les oreilles, par les murmures de ces membres depuis qu'ils avaient appris votre désignation, je riquerais fort de finir par donner une somme à une brochure relatant ainsi l'événement de l'heure!
    Mais hélas, le temps n'est pas aux longs discours pour réciter toute une litanie due à l'émotion se transportent ceux qui hier vous

administrez. Aussi nous nous voyons dans la necessité de nous borner sur un seul point, qui est au-dessus de tout éloge: vous exprimer notre gratitude de reconnaissance.

D'ici peu, nous vous voyons, d'ici peu, nous ne vous reverrons plus, car vous nous serez dérobé, peut-être pour toujours et Dieu sait comment, par les rideaux des arbres plantés le long du chemin, et finalement, par les pentes des montagnes du pays que vous sentez maintenant notre émoi de partance!

Au cours de vos longs mois d'administration du poste d'Uvira vous n'avez pas manqué de constater l'inconscience professionnelle, l'ignorance notoirement marquée du noir, etc . . . Et nous espérons qu'en traitant ceux d'Astrida de la même facon que ceux d'Uvira, vous gagnerez, soyez assuré, l'estime indiscutable de tous les jours; que le jour de votre départ comme aujourd'hui ils diront: nous avons perdu un chef!

L'abre si petit qu'a planté l'auguste fondateur, le roi Leopold II, dont le fils de Belgique a pour mission l'entretien, a poussé ses racines jusqu'à une profondeur indeterminé et le Congolais ne fait que consommer les beaux fruits de la production à toute heure du jour. En aidant le noir se relever de son ignorance de choses juridiques, de sa faiblesse morale intellectuelle, lui faisant sortir de son abime de l'erreur et de respecter la loi, le droit de l'homme dans la vie sociale, économique et politique pour qu'il puisse se rendre apte a penser lui-même, vous verrez que, malgré certains points à considerer, le noir serait à même de seconder le Belge colonisation dans d'autres cas particulier qui, hier, pas plus qu'aujourd'hui, ne pouvait faire face.

Si au cours de cet entretien vous avez constaté un mot deplacé, veuillez bien m'en excuser, le cheval à quatre pieds, trèbuche parfois. Néanmoins, ceux qui s'adressent à l'âme at à l'intelligence doivent être guidés et rationnellement conduits dans toute la mesure du possible.

En continuant à donner des conseils précis au noir, en lui montrant comme par le passé le bon chemin intéressant son domain qui lui faciliterait un jour la réalisation de ses progrès vers l'idéal, afin de se rendre utile lui-même et toute sa famille et, ensuite, serviteur de sa patrie, nous verrons naître des nouveaux cieux et une nouvelle terre! C'est avec la douceur qu'il faut ramener les esprits égarés.

Adieux, Monsieur et Madame Lambrecht, si pas ici bas, du moins dans l'autre monde, selon la volonté du Maître de l'Univers.

Jean-Robert Bofuky

Steno-dactylo.

Uvira, le 15 février 1951.

"A Thousand Hills and Seven Volcanoes" (*)

The kingdom of Ruanda is located between 1°20′ and 2°50′ south of the equator; 28°50′ and 30°55′ east longitude. The entire country is part of the high plateau of the eastern wall of the western Rift Valley. Numerous streams drain the 60-inch rainfall, forming marshy valleys and a number of small lakes between the hilltops. A high ridge of 8,500 to 10,000 feet runs parallel over a length of 40 miles along Ruanda's western border, separating the watersheds of the Congo and Nile river systems. To the east, the plateau slopes gradually towards the lower savannas at about 4,000 feet. Here, the Kagera River forms the border between Ruanda and Tanganyika Territory (now Tanzania). Southwards, the plateau continues at a somewhat lower elevation but with the same physiognomy into the kingdom of Urundi, separated from Ruanda by the rivers Lua and Akanyaru.

The northern frontier of Ruanda is marked by the spectacular Virunga Volcanoes with seven peaks above 10,000 feet, Karisimbi, the highest, at 11,280 feet.

Of the dense forests that once covered most of the country, only three percent are left; the remnant of Nyongwe forest on the highest ridge of the Congo-Nile divide was declared a forest reserve under colonial administration. The gradual destruction of the former forests was the result of the progressive infiltration of nilotic cattle herders from the north. Avoiding the lowlands infested with tsetse flies, carriers of fatal nagana cattle disease, the herders led their animals onto the highland pastures, thus displacing the indigenous Bahutu agriculturists. These, in turn, were obliged to encroach upon the forest all the more because during the dry season the cattle occupied the fertile valleys. The peaceful but progressive and enduring invasion has been going on for the last four centuries, resulting in the present overpopulation of all arable parts of the country, with a population density of 233 per square mile (1952). The agricultural society of the Bahutu was replaced by the social structure of the pastoral Watutsi and resulted in the overlordship of the Tutsi (only 10 percent of the population) over the Hutu who represented 85 percent. The rest of the population, about 5 percent

(*) Title of a book by Marie Gevers: *Des Milles Collines et Sept Volcans*

is made up by Batwa, a group of people of pygmoid hunter-gatherers descent.

The Tutsi are usually elegantly dressed. Even before the arrival of the Europeans, high-ranking Tutsi had started replacing the former cowhide or bark cloth garments by large pieces of bright-colored or white cotton cloth imported by East African tradesmen, bought from east coast Arab merchants. Both men and women wore two separate pieces of cloth, one wrapped to form a narrow skirt, the other floating, knotted at the shoulder.

Both Hutu men and women wore bark cloth skirts, now replaced by dark cotton. The men sometimes covered the upper part of the body with a goat's skin, the women preferring a cow's skin, which also served to carry the baby. Both Tutsi and Hutu women like to wear bracelets and necklaces made from bright-colored beads.

Twa men and women covered the lower part of their bodies with goat skins. In all tribes, the traditional apparel is slowly being replaced by the increased imports of western clothing, noticeable in those living near commercial centers.

The first white explorers to set foot in the territories were John H. Speke and Sir Richard Burton, who crossed into Urundi in 1858. Thirteen years later, Livingstone and Stanley camped just south of present Bujumbura. Following the Belgian victory of the 1914-18 African campaign against the German troops, the territories of Ruanda-Urundi were entrusted by international mandate to Belgium in 1920. During its mandate, which would last only four decades, Belgian technicians, administrators and scientists managed to make good strides in improving the previous precarious economic conditions through introducing better agricultural techniques, new cash crops such as tea and coffee, the organization of public health care, the establishment of centers of education—formal as well as technical—the expansion of veterinary services, and research. The preservation of the remnant forests and wildlife was assured, the first by declaring government reserves and creating large areas of reforestation around locations of dense population, the latter by creating natural parks for the complete protection of fauna and flora.

We found the "mood" between Uvira and Astrida markedly different, commensurate perhaps with differences in their physical as well as their social environment. For instance, the stately, proud, six-foot-tall Watutsi and their superb long-horn cattle could hardly be put in the same class as the coarse, toiling Bantu goatkeepers around Uvira. The sound of the royal drums that penetrated the bodies of the audience like a sledge hammer was several notches superior to the casual, haphazard drumming that was lost in the Ruzizi night before it spoke. No chief of the Bavira or Bafulero could compare favorably with Bami Mutara, the seven-foot-tall King of Ruanda, dressed in immaculate long white robes, his head adorned with a wide band of multicolored beads, held high as he gazed over his domain of mountains grazed by majestic herds of long-horn cattle.

Because of the rather temperate climate, most settlers as well as government officials dressed in long trousers, many sporting dress shirt and tie. The D.O.'s name was d'Arianoff (lower case "d", apostrophe, capital "A".) In his impeccable uniform he certainly looked more imposing than his Congo counterpart in Uvira, who wore shorts and open shirt. Mr. d'Arianoff always traveled in great style when on official tour. While most D.O.'s contented themselves with a one-ton pickup or a Land Rover, d'Arianoff needed a three-ton vehicle. I had the opportunity of visiting his camp once when he was tenting in the Mutara region. It was early evening as I passed in my Land Rover on my way back to camp from a tsetse fly survey. I thought it would be proper to stop and say hello. As I approached his brightly illuminated tent, I couldn't believe my eyes. The scene was not unlike one from the "Arabian Nights." The interior of the tent was decorated with wall hangings; the floor covered with carpets and furnished with regular armchairs and other pieces of house furniture. I expected to see him in a tuxedo—I am sure he kept one in his wardrobe trunk. As it was, even in his bush outfit—immaculately pressed—he somehow matched the fashionable interior.

We never really liked Astrida—certainly not when on the day of our arrival, we were informed that the promised chef-de-poste house—a lovely cottage-style house with a beautiful garden—had been allocated to the mycologist—the result of active string-pulling at Brussels headquarters, we found out. *We* would move into the house *he* was supposed to occupy but, as a result of the multiple changes he had demanded, would not be ready for occupancy for some time. We had to stay at the Hotel Ibis, temporarily.

We got the impression that many Astridians were snobbish, at least towards us, coming from provincial Uvira—nor was the impression always imagination. Astrida's choice location and climate seemed to have acted selectively for a certain class of Europeans. Even the IRSAC center did not escape the general trend. It was a complex of angular, modern low buildings, quite different from the classical colonial type. The cottage-style houses made from natural stone were dispersed judiciously on the gentle slope of a hill at the town's west side. Plenty of lawn and flowers enhanced the parklike setting of the center which looked more like a country club than a place of scientific research. But then, the major theme of research of the center was anthropology, a "non-polluting" science if there was one. As such, the IRSAC center of Ruanda imposed a tranquil atmosphere, more "refined," let's say, than a center for zoological research where one would expect mud-covered researchers to tumble in from far-flung safaris, trailing behind smelly traps and cages with screaming animals. In Astrida, the mood in the laboratories, (rather offices) was sedate and one felt more like whispering rather than speaking in a normal voice. The mycologist even when whispering, could be heard all along the halls. Not only his voice, but spin-offs of his research were evident everywhere—spores from his fungi cultures, some new species perhaps, which dispersed insidiously and now occupied parts of walls and nooks in an explosion of grays, pinks and greens.

The mycologist was rather self-indulgent, giving little consideration to others. He had one laboratory, as did all the other researchers, but he persuaded authorities in Brussels that he was entitled to more rooms. He soon burgeoned into three. At one time, he decided that he needed an experimental mouse colony and that I, first as station manager and second as having some experience in mouse colony care picked up during my stay at the yellow fever laboratory in Stan, should organize a facility for experimental animals. Like so many who have never been involved in raising animals, our mycologist assumed that housing some mice in a couple of cages, putting them on racks would produce the desired effect. Far from it: cages have to be cleaned and sterilized, food prepared, pedigrees recorded, litters separated, dead animals disposed of, and so on. When he proposed that we organize all this activity in the two small toilets in the main hallway, I said that it simply could not be done. Moreover, the toilets, the only ones we had, were needed at times, if he knew what I meant. For an experimental animal colony, we needed separate facilities with all the trimmings. Soon letters arrived at my desk from high up asking me to explain my refusal. I let them have it. The storm abated when the mycologist lost interest in mice.

I was on better terms with the anthropologists. They were an interesting bunch of active people, each specializing in various aspects of the study of man: ethnology, musicology, physical anthropology, nutrition, genetics, linguistics, sociology and prehistory. Many of them were to become well-known authorities in their own fields.

When we arrived, most of the construction work of the center had been completed except for that of a permanent workshop. The administrative offices, together with the mechanic shop, were located at the bottom of the hill, reached by a self-made road that wound down its flank in proper hairpin fashion. Close to a fertile, marshy valley, the previous station manager and his wife had started a vegetable garden with some success. But as fresh vegetables could be bought locally from African small farmers, the project had been abandoned. More important was the nursery of small eucalyptus and pine trees intended for the reforestation of the IRSAC hillside.

Our director had insisted that in building the center, as much as possible local materials should be used, including granitic stones that could be quarried from a hill about 20 miles from Astrida. As an aside, the hill was the site for one of the scenes in the film "King Solomon's Mines," the first version, that is. During the filming, Stewart Granger and others "camped" in air-conditioned trailers in Astrida, with some large trucks filled with food supplies that included certified sterile water for daily household consumption. I accompanied the Greek constructor on one of his quarrying trips. One does not simply drive over to the hill and start loading stones. One has to use dynamite and hope that the explosion will reduce the huge boulders to nicely shaped blocks of the right size. Mr. Christodoulos handled sticks of dynamite, detonators, fuses and Bedford cord like a pro, but the first charge set did not explode. As we walked from behind the boulder where we had sheltered, I was a bit apprehensive that the explosion might occur as we drew near. Luckily nothing happened. The following tries were successful and we usually got home with a well-laden lorry.

I had previously alluded to Astrida's reliance on supplies that had to be fetched from Usumbura or Uvira. For this reason the center had a "fleet" of two 5-ton lorries. Every time we sent the driver down for provisions, we didn't have a moment of peace, afraid something might happen along the tricky mountain road. We were also more than suspicious that the driver would be tempted to arrange some transport business of his own along the way, if only by loading some passengers for a fee. This practice not only was a source of delay but also could become an insurance liability. Providing transportation for paying passengers, their goats, chickens, and other paraphernalia was a widespread common practice among African truck drivers. Many times when a road accident with a truck occurred, it involved dozens of illegal passengers. Mr. Hensens, our shop and transportation manager, tried to mitigate the abuse by installing a recording device on the transmission box that registered distance versus time, thereby also marking speed and stops. Hensens was a bit of a jack-of-all-trades, not always in the top ten of the trade-hat he wore. He was the one who had installed the electric circuits in the houses and it was not unusual when switching on the living room lights to find the toaster coming on. I can personally vouch for such mix-ups. The first time I stepped into the bathtub filled with hot water from the electric waterheater (what a change from Pawa, but how much more dangerous!) I received an electric shock that would have shot me right out of my socks had I not been undressed. Hensens came the next morning to check the circuits and everything seemed fine. A few weeks later, however, when a friend who was spending the night with us took a bath he too was almost electrocuted. Being an electrical technician himself, he found that the short-circuit occurred only when the porch light was left on!

Sloppy construction in these days, so often the work of amateur "constructors," was not infrequent. Moreover, building materials were usually in short supply and deliveries were hampered by transport difficulties and delays. During the time we lived at Hotel Ibis, one of the nearby rooms was remodeled. When they came to change the plumbing, it was found that the drainage "pipe" was made from the inner tubes of bicycle tires!

One had to admire the ingenuity of the ad hoc replacements of often rare orthodox materials. I have already mentioned the innumerable and widespread uses of 50-gallon drums as an almost indispensable item in the practical running of the colony.

The African drivers were the real wizards of the transportation system. Without their dexterity for on–the–spot auto repairs, transport would have been in a sorry state. The space under the hood of an African-owned car looked like an old, abandoned attic full of cobwebs. Crossed wires, adhesive tape and metal straps all seemed essential in holding the parts together and making them work. Batteries and generators were the major black sheep; cars and trucks were commonly started by being pushed in first gear, a task in which the "chauffeur-moke" played a major role. The "chauffeur-moke" was a young boy—12 to 16 years old—who washed the vehicle, filled the radiator, pumped the tires, blew out fuel lines, syphoned gasoline from the reserve drum into the gas tank, directed maneuvers in tight corners, tied the tarpaulin, jumped out of the cabin with a wheel block to prevent the lorry from rolling after stops, and retrieved it, quickly jumping back onto the running board when the vehicle moved off.

Sand and water were a common ingredient in gasoline, collecting while the drum stood in the open air and rain. Gasoline was delivered from a loosely fitted hand pump. Real service stations existed only in the big cities. Carburetor trouble was, therefore, an almost routine problem and was usually suspected at the first sign of engine trouble. One learned to fix it by cleaning the various parts, blowing out the fuel lines, and draining the gas tank.

Because of its favorable location, Astrida was the seat of several other institutions: the Agricultural Research Center and the Native Welfare Foundation. One section of the former institution managed an arboretum dedicated to research in experimental reforestation. The young chap attached to this center was a mountaineering fan. One day, boasting and eager to demonstrate his skills, he managed to climb the sheer wall of a tall chimney made of natural stone up to the high ceiling in one of our friends' houses. The couple of cocktails he had earlier may have prompted this feat. It looked somewhat odd, however, to the chief of the center, Dr. Maquet, who walked in at the moment our mountaineering friend had reached the high point and was hanging by his fingernails on the top stones, looking like an oversize gecko. Being a calm and collected person, Dr. Maquet's only comments were: "Are we insured for that sort of thing?"

We were very pleased, one day, to meet unexpectedly our good friend Dr. Swerts from Pawa. He was as surprised to see us as we were to see him. He knew vaguely that we were somewhere in Ruanda, but had no idea he would meet us in Astrida. He told us that not much had changed in Pawa except that Father Sabbe, head of the Catholic Mission, had died. Dr. Swerts was accompanied by a health officer, my replacement in Pawa, in fact. His wife had died from blackwater fever three months earlier. We suspected that this trip had been arranged by Dr. Swerts in an effort to try to soften the loss. We never saw Dr. Swerts again. He was shot by Congolese rebels ten years later.

It was amazing how many traumatic things happened during the short while we were in Astrida. At one time, I was awakened in the middle of the night by loud banging on the bedroom door that opened onto the terrace. Outside stood Mutima telling me in a shaking voice that his wife, Nyama-na-poli, was about to give birth to his fourth child—splendid news, I thought, but hardly a reason to tell me in the middle of the night. He could have told me the result the following morning, what? The plot thickened quickly when I learned that Nyama-na-poli had managed to make it halfway up the hill, declaring that she could not drag herself any further to the hospital or any other "proper" place and that birth was imminent. By now trembling myself, I hastily dressed, gathered some bandages and . . . yes, I remembered the Pawa maternity days . . . a pair of scissors. We found Nyama-na-poli sitting on the path obviously in the last stages of labor. It is amazing how, in a moment of crisis, one seems to be doing the right things. It would be impossible for me to describe all the details of that birth in the middle of the night, in the gloom of a flashlight, on a path halfway up the hill and under a dome of stars. Suddenly I found myself holding a baby, garroting the umbilical cord and cutting it off, dutifully turning the baby upside down and slapping its buttocks—noting "en passant" that it was a boy. A woeful cry indicated that all was well in that quarter. Mutima took his son and I turned my attention to the mother. The placenta came out all by itself and she didn't seem the worse for this impromptu birth. African women are tough. I took the family to the hospital, leaving instructions to improve upon my mid-wifery. Putting a few drops of silver nitrate in the baby's eyes, was a necessary precaution—a precaution against infection by spirochaetes while I also refined my crude sectioning and binding of the umbilical cord.

In the course of another night I developed such abdominal cramps that the pain made me crawl over the floor on all fours—not at all to look for a pajama button as Dora at first assumed. The pains lasted for two hours, during which I felt as if someone was dissecting my intestines inch by inch. Slowly, the pains subsided and disappeared altogether. The doctor, the next day, could find nothing wrong with me, but guessed that it might have been something to do with the kidneys, the passing of stones perhaps.

And finally, we suffered two burglaries. One, when a small boy, helper of our pishi, was seen by Dora to take a silver spoon and run off with it through the streets of Astrida, Dora in hot pursuit, but in vain. A second theft was more serious, but it could have been worse. It happened one late afternoon when we had friends over for a drink and the conversation turned on various styles of jewelry. During the discussion, Dora had taken out brooches and rings from the small strong-box we kept in the bedroom. When, after our friends left, she wanted to replace the jewelry, the box was gone. Someone outside the bedroom terrace must have watched her when she took out the jewelry, figuring that more valuables were inside. There were none, but unfortunately, the box contained all our official papers. With our imminent home leave, which we had planned to spend in the United States, this was a very serious matter. We knew that there was little hope that we would ever recover the box or the papers which the thief had probably destroyed after finding that the box contained nothing but, to him, useless papers. Hectic weeks followed—writing to officials and waiting for duplicates. Happily, these arrived well in time for our departure. Some of the stolen papers, however, were of great sentimental value: letters, original birth certificates and so on, which could not be replaced. Our material loss could have been much greater.

Within the same period for the first time we witnessed an earthquake. It was in the middle of the night when we heard an express train arriving from far away, thundering closer and closer until it seemed to steam into a station and the aftershocks rocked our house. It left a few cracks in some of the walls, but otherwise no damage.

I had been waiting impatiently for the arrival of a new station manager so that I could start full-time research. His arrival, scheduled for early 1951, was constantly postponed and I remained stuck with my managerial position. Afraid that it would become habit-forming both to me and to my directors, I started a mosquito survey project in the swamps of the valleys surrounding Astrida, at the same time building up the equipment for eventual later research. With that in view, I took on a laboratory assistant, Samson, a Usukuma from Tanganyika, who would later become one of my camp supervisors. My research position gained in strength with a request from the governor for a medico-entomological investigation of the lowland areas bordering Ruanda-Urundi in the east. These grass- and woodlands seemed ideal for cattle raising and suitable for large-scale agriculture and hence desirable for settlement of populations from the overcrowded highlands. It would be foolish, however, to start a resettlement scheme without preliminary knowledge of whether, indeed, the new areas were salubrious and economically habitable. We knew already that many of the lowlands were tsetse fly country that would exclude a population from keeping cattle and even present the risks of human sleeping sickness. Other health risks were most probably also present, certainly malaria, but not much was known about their distribution or incidence.

With the governor's request and my appointment by the IRSAC director to carry it out, I now became a recognized researcher in medical entomology. Only the delays in my replacement as station manager prevented the beginning of my full-time scientific career. Afraid that the opportunity would slip away, I made immediate preparations to assemble equipment, documents and maps of the Mosso region in southeastern Urundi, which had priority for my investigation. Continuing administrative involvement kept delaying the start of the project until I finally decided upon a date to which I stuck. THE day was the seventh of April 1951. It was the last month of rains.

Camp on the Malagarasi

It was beastly cold. The rain came down in solid streaks, blurring the view of the pines in front of the Rutana rest house. Water streamed from the sagging gutter along the brick pillar that supported the tin roof and formed a widening puddle in the lower part of the barza, threatening to run underneath the door. It would not make much difference because an enlarging dark patch in one of the corners of the ceiling was about to win the race. In the process of dissolving the bat guano that cakes every roof in Burundi, the percolating water would soon start smelling something terrible. Mutima pulled my camp bed away from the path of the flood. "Mvula napika mbya leo," he announced (The rains are bad today). I sighed—it was not a promising beginning for my work in the Mosso Valley.

The Mosso region is a long narrow valley that seems to have dropped away in a single tectonic break from the Urundi highlands, leaving a perpendicular wall 2,000 feet high. From this abrupt flank, the 3,500-foot-high valley stretches into Tanganyika (now Tanzania), the Malagarasi River forming the natural border between the two countries. The region of the Mosso extends from the shores of Lake Tanganyika for about 100 miles in the general northeastern direction. Nowhere is the valley wider than 20 miles. The vegetation is basically woodland savanna, but was strongly modified in several areas by past human occupation and agricultural activities. Many of the fields and pastures were abandoned as a result of human and cattle trypanosomiasis. The fallow land reverted to acacia woodland that further promoted the advance of the tsetse fly. The projected Ruanda-Urundi Ten-Year Plan was to help develop and resettle the valley and, with an improved road system, link its economy to the Lake Tanganyika water transport. Considering the well-watered alluvial soils, it was estimated that the area would be able to support some 125,000 settlers and their cattle, providing it could be made tsetse-free. This is where I came in.

Those who have hunted the savannas of Africa know the fly from bitter experience. Landing like a flash on an uncovered part of the body, it quickly inserts its almost invisible hypopharynx under the skin and starts pumping blood. If left undisturbed, the fly's abdomen fills with blood—human blood—until repleted as it attains the size of a small balloon almost one centimeter in diameter. The tsetse fly is the scourge of Africa.

The tsetse fly carries and transmits various species of *Trypanosoma,* microscopic haemoflagellates, two of which cause the fatal sleeping sickness disease in man while several other trypanosome species produce a similar disease in cattle and other livestock, called nagana. The fly can be found on 4.5 million square miles of tropical Africa, an area larger than continental United States. The concern and unrelenting efforts to control or eradicate it have been a major burden in colonial and later African administrations.

The story of the study of tsetse flies (genus: *Glossina*) and the parasite (genus: *Trypanosoma*) they transmit occupies a distinctive chapter in the history of Africa's development. Publications on the subject would fill a good-sized library. Research probes ever deeper into the fly's behavior, physiology, ecology and reproductive cycle. Tsetse ecologists give free reign to their imaginations to devise methods for analyzing these functions either in the laboratory or in the field. In this way, they hope to find a weak link in the chain of the fly's life cycle that could be used to halt its reproduction and interrupt the transmission of the disease.

At present, *Glossina* are found only in the African continent. Fossil impressions of four *Glossina* species have been found among the shales from the Florissant, Colorado, U.S.A., fossil beds, leading one to suppose that the fly was far more widespread during periods of the Miocene. Its absence from all other continents but Africa has been ascribed to continental drift, glaciation, changing climates and shifting fauna and flora.

Tsetse behavioral activity is essentially guided by its "hunger cycle." Both male and female flies feed on mammalian blood—the male only to satisfy its metabolic needs; the female, in addition, to feed its larva that develops and matures inside the female's "uterus" on an average every eight to nine days. The mature larva is dropped and burrows in the soil, pupates and develops into an adult fly in about 30 to 40 days.

Each time the fly feeds, on an average of every fourth day, it may pick up the trypanosome parasite from an infected animal or man. Development and multiplication of the trypanosomes take place in various parts of the fly's body, after which the insect becomes infective for man or animal—depending upon the trypansome species—at subsequent meals.

A large number of different African game animals carry trypanosomes in their blood without being affected by the infection themselves. One of these trypanosome species, *Trypanosoma rhodesiense,* is infective to man, causing acute Rhodesian sleeping sickness that may kill a person in a matter of weeks or months. Other trypanosome species are harmless to man, but transmit debilitating nagana to livestock. Tsetses seem to be more attracted to certain animals than to others; and certain animals are more effective carriers of trypanosomes than others. Tsetse feeding behavior is, therefore, of the greatest importance to the epidemiology of the diseases they carry. Because of the importance of game in tsetse ecology, the glossinologist is usually an ardent and keen observer of wildlife.

Roving, often crawling, through dense vegetation in search of tsetse resting or breeding places, the tsetse ecologist is many times confronted with awkward situations: stepping on snakes, facing lions or leopards, being caught in animal traps, being mistaken for game and shot at by nearsighted hunters. Falling in crocodile-infested streams from overturning canoes or makeshift river crossings is commonplace. At glossinologists' meetings, hair-raising stories are swapped about close encounters with rhino "chasing everything that moves including prams," as one of them put it, or being "treed" by a buffalo in a thorny acacia. Many adventures are the result of travel during the rainy season along stretches of quagmire—referred to as roads in the dry season—waiting at river crossings, drifts, for the water to subside or the thrill of "risking it anyway." To the outsider, a meeting of glossinologists may seem rather priggish, talk about "The Fly" being the centerpiece of conversation, but as the evening wears on, the talk drifts towards "the good old times," with anecdotes about departed colleagues and tales that become more colorful with each narration. Yet when the next day they gather at a scientific meeting, the tsetse experts are dead serious and many of last evening's stories appear to have occurred during well-planned surveys or experiments. Results are heatedly discussed and statistically torn apart if need be.

Rutana was a typical government post located on the flat part of a mountain ridge at about 6,200 feet. Common with other Ruanda-Urundi small towns, it boasted five to six bungalow type houses for government staff, extending from one side of the government offices, the post office, a rest house and a health clinic. A eucalyptus–lined road led to the central "centre commercial": a number of wattle-and-thatch structures that formed a quadrangle around the marketplace. Most of these were occupied by the traditional "nduka" (native shop), selling items from anchovy tins to zinc roofs. A wide, double door opens to the roomy interior, the walls lined with wooden shelves sagging with stacked merchandise. The floor is equally crowded with bags, boxes and barrels. The shop smells of Life-Buoy soap, paraffin, spoiled manioc flour, damp whitewash, jute sacking, rubber boots—but mostly of the offensive odor of dried fish heaped in square baskets near the entrance. A couple of Africans are in attendance while the owner, Arab or Hindu, reclines in a rickety chair under a barza gazing into the blue sky, or gloomily wrapped in a cheap, gray blanket at other times. He also keeps an eye on petrol (gasoline) sales from the 50-gallon drum in front of the shop. Fuel is dispensed by means of a hand pump that, alternately, delivers five liters from each of the two glass reservoirs in which the fuel is pumped from the pipe screwed into the drum hole. The glass of the five-liter reservoir is clouded with gummy stuff obscuring whatever is being pumped until it pours out of the hose. I have already mentioned the unpleasantness of water in fuel (sometimes added intentionally to increase volume) but often the result of pure negligence when the lead pipe into the drum is not properly tightened and rainwater finds its way inside. Rust is another common ingredient found inside a clogged carburetor. African drivers have found a way to avoid some of these problems. They line a funnel with an old felt hat that filters out rust and other solid ingredients as well as water. And, of course, felt hats are among the items sold in the nkukas. They are worn *and* used as filters when required.

The European quarters, on the other end of the eucalyptus drive, are less noisy, less smelly and less lively, rather morose, in fact. The small square, in front of the D.O.'s office is rigidly marked by white-washed rocks. The Belgian flag waves bravely on top of the tall pole in the center. White-washed stones also mark the driveways and garden hedges of the bungalows. Struggling coarse grass lawns are kept short by a gang of prisoners equipped with the "coupe-coupe." A zealous administrator's wife has started a geranium border, now sadly flooded by the long rains.

The morning after our wet arrival at Rutana dawned clear and bright—too bright perhaps because it could mean rain later on. But it was good to feel the sun. We, the driver, my two assistants, Zaghi and Samson, Mutima and I, started down the slippery road in the pickup van towards the valley, 1,950 feet below. About halfway, I got off and with Mutima started exploring the dense vegetation of a large gulley. I left instructions with Zaghi to follow the road downwards with the van and look for tsetse at suitable places, and to return around noon. Besides flushing two bushbuck, too swift for me to even raise my rifle, Mutima and I didn't find anything of interest: no tsetse flies.

We waited for the return of our vehicle, but when the sun reached the halfway mark in the western sky, we had to accept that something had happened to our men or our pickup and that we were marooned. Deciding against walking down at the risk of having to walk all the way back, we started reluctantly up the hot road. After a while we met the D.O. on his way to check on his limekilns. He promised to look out for our men.

It was close to five o'clock when, drenched in perspiration, we reached the rest house. By the time I had washed and changed clothes I heard the pickup coming up the drive. They had spent all that time digging out from a deep mudhole near the Musasa River. They had found no tsetse but a good number of Haematopota—a biting fly of the tabanid family.

And so ended our first day of Mosso research.

We tried again the following day, but when we reached the Musasa River, we found that the bridge was flooded. A half-hearted and unsuccessful attempt by Mutima to find the bridge underneath the flow persuaded us to turn back. The D.O. advised us to try the other road into the valley to the north of Rutana. "That is," he said "if the bridge across the Muyovosi is holding."

We loaded up and off we went. If the other bridge was out, we would be marooned in Rutana for the duration. As we reached the river, my heart sank to see only a few logs sticking above the water, the rest of the bridge barely discernible underneath the rushing flood. Gingerly, Mutima tested the structure by walking across. Taking Mutima's survival as an endorsement of the bridge's strength, our driver rushed the van across before it could find time to collapse.

We were the last vehicle to leave Rutana (we were told later) until the waters subsided one week later and repairs could be carried out.

The road we now followed skirted the edge of the abrupt cliffs below which the Mosso Valley stretched 2,000 ft. lower. Besides allowing occasional magnificent views of the valley, the road wound between short grass convoluted pastures dotted with huge scenic boulder outcrops. At Kayera, the cluster of buildings of the Protestant mission is snugly lodged on a wide ledge formed by a fold in a still higher mountain range. Lovely clear water from a spring runs through pastures covered with yellow flowers. The houses with their whitewashed walls and thatched roofs look very much like a small English village square. I made the acquaintance of Mr. and Mrs. Belknap, American missionaries who, with their four children, had lived in Kenya for five years. Mr. Belknap showed me the small plane he uses "to go shopping," but which was now out of commission with a broken landing gear. He had many interesting things to say about the Mosso and its wildlife, mentioning that I might have trouble with lions, numerous at times and not afraid to attack man.

The sun had come out, so we left in a hurry on our way to Kiharo where, Belknap told me, I would find a rest house. From the high ridge where the road made its plunge into the valley the view was breathtaking. Through the gaps in the clouds one could see every detail of rivers, fields, forest, and faraway hills. The greens were so bright as to be almost luminous. Rivers could be traced by their dense, dark vegetation, the Malagarasi standing out by the size of the forest gallery. We sped on and soon reached the Catholic mission at Mpinga and the village of Chief Kigoma. Anxious to take advantage of the dry spell, we did not stop, but resumed our downward plunge. The road builders seemed to have been in a hurry to reach the bottom of the valley in the shortest possible way, considering that the road ran along the flank of a deep gorge in a straight line from top to bottom.

We crossed several small streams on bridges surfaced with reeds. Like so many bridges in Africa, they were made of two or three tree trunks laid across the stream onto which smaller poles or rough boards were nailed crosswise. This makes a fine bridge as long as floods don't weaken the structure or the banks, or wood doesn't decay or termites do not sap its strength. Repairs or replacement is carried out when news reaches the D.O. that a vehicle has sunk through the bridge. Many of the Mosso bridges were topped with a thick layer of reeds—structurally as "strong" perhaps as a plank- or earthen-covered bridge, but psychologically inferior. One crosses the first reed bridge with many misgivings and with unsubstantiated faith that something of a sturdier nature lies beneath. Confidence is not improved when one feels the wheels sink into what seems like a kapok mattress. Nor do the creaking sounds and groans instill trust. After the first dozen reed bridges brash credibility returns. None of those bridges are very wide nor the streams very deep.

We reached Kiharo rest house around five, just in time to organize settling in, and start supper. The first night in the valley was uneventful.

Two African laboratory assistants shared my field work. They both stayed with me for the duration of my research with IRSAC, a term of ten years.

Antoine Zaghi was a tall, heavyset Baluba from around Elisabethville, about 23 years old when he joined my work. He had been trained in medical entomology, more precisely mosquito ecology and taxonomy, by Dr. Vincke. This and the fact that Dr. Vincke had not fired him after five years spoke for his integrity. I "inherited" Zaghi during my mosquito and malaria work in the Ruzizi Valley. When given a sensible research plan and schedule, he was a steady worker, a skillful mosquito and later tsetse fly dissector and microscopist. He was nonchalantly witty and devoted when he could be persuaded to be so. A sort of solid chap most of the time, he commanded respect from the team of fly-boys whom he supervised while I was away. Besides his native Kiluba and Swahili, he spoke good but sometimes stumbling French. I could tell when his answers to questions were somewhat ambiguous when he started with a dry cough or stuttered more than usual.

The origin of Samson, the other assistant, was somewhat vague, except that he said he was a Usukuma. He appeared one day in my office in Astrida with a long story of perhaps doubtful authenticity narrated in a strong East African—British accent about the miseries that had pursued him since the day he saw light in his Tanganyika village; his later experiences with the colonial army and how he had arrived in Ruanda with his wife to visit her parents, Bahutus; how, when his in-laws told him he could stay no longer, he found himself without a job, without a house and only a part-time wife. I suspect that he had been informed about my scientific interests because he immediately mentioned that he had served with the medical corps and had done some mosquito surveys. Had I been a surgeon, he would have emphasized his previous experience in amputation, I suppose. His military bearing that hopefully indicated a sense of discipline and perhaps of duty prompted me to take him on. Although a bit volatile and whimsical, he did not bely my first impression and I never regretted my decision. Finally, his continuous troubles with his wife and her family—which started to reflect on his work—made him decide to ask for his dismissal when he learned that I was leaving the Congo myself.

The entries and abstracts from my diary about the first days in Mosso are fairly representative, I believe, of what field work in Africa was, really is and will be for many years to come.

Saturday, April 21, 1951.

Leave Kiharo rest house at 7:30. After three miles reach Butetsi, an abandoned government camp of two huts, a kitchen and a sort of hanger. See the subchief and ask him to carry out some repairs to the structures so that we can use as a temporary camp. The river Mazimero, which, with its well-developed forest gallery I suspect to be a tsetse habitat, is about three miles away. A first early morning survey doesn't show tsetse, but a lot of tabanid flies. Fresh lion spoor makes us hesitate to enter the gallery at that point. Making a detour through well-wooded savanna, arrive in the forest gallery farther upstream where we capture our first tsetses. Back in the same spot later that afternoon find many more, including one large one. We are being bitten ferociously by large, beautiful anopheles mosquitoes, of which we collect several. From the examination of our collection today make the following identifications: the small tsetses: *Glossina morsitans*, the larger one, provisionally: *Glossina fuscipleuris*; the mosquito: *Anopheles implexus*. The latter, however, shows some important variations in wing design from the typical *A. implexus* and will require further taxonomic study. Ask subchief to designate ten of his men for tsetse collecting work.

Sunday, April 22, 1951.

This morning organized five teams of two fly-boys to start a long-term tsetse collecting schedule. While Zaghi throws his weight about showing how to use the fly catching net to men whose only occupation so far had been to till the chief's field, I explore the Mazimero all the way to its spring source, a low cave about three miles from the road. Find anopheles larvae, possibly of *A. implexus*, which should help in better identification. Attacked by many tsetse. Starts raining till two. Return to Mazimero at four accompanied by the ten fly-boys. Encounter large band of baboons. Shoot one, but when we reached the place where it fell, find only a large pool of blood. Assume the other baboons have carried him away. Hope to collect more large tsetse. Are attracted by loud baboon arguments. When we reach the place where the noise came from, find bones and remnants of meat and fur of a freshly killed animal. Shoot two baboons. With falling light find it safer to postpone search till tomorrow. Surrounded by a large number of baboons and with only two cartridges left we retreat from the gallery. Chief says he is happy we are doing something to chase the baboons away as they are destroying his vegetable garden.

Monday, April 23, 1951.

Move our equipment from Kiharo to Butetsi camp, which has been rehabilitated. On the way get stuck in deep mud. Are forced to unload everything and carry it 200 yards to a dry spot. Are then able to push the vehicle from the mudhole. Find one of the two baboons shot yesterday. Make blood smears. Organize new camp and leave Zaghi and Samson with work schedule for the next weeks until I return. Spend the night at Kiharo rest house. Leave the next day at eight to arrive back in Astrida at three in the afternoon. Several towns on the way are short of gasoline.

Three weeks later I was back in the Mosso, this time driving my personal car, a 1950 Chevrolet convertible. Mutima adored riding in that car, with the top down. Whenever we stopped for gasoline, hordes of shoppers, young and old, would stare at the vehicle, a very unusual model at that time in Africa. Mutima, pretending complete aloofness, mixed with a degree of complacency, sat quietly, staring before him or at times consenting to look at "the other people," a blasé look on his face.

Things had been going well at Butetsi: a total of 690 *G. morsitans* had been dissected and showed a high infection rate with trypanosomes. A platform had been built in a tall tree of the Mazimero forest gallery to observe the biting range of tsetse and to collect canopy-biting mosquitoes. We had acquired four goats to feed tsetse kept alive in "Bruce boxes" for later studies. An "inventory" had been made of mosquitoes found inside the huts of two villages, collections of biting mosquitoes had been started in three different biotopes, and mosquito larvae had been collected from five river systems and identified. Only one large *Glossina* had been found, however, indicating that the fly's habitat was not in the same areas where we found *G. morsitans*. I suspected that we might have better luck in the forest gallery of the Malagarasi River. We first tried to reach the river by foot, guided by a villager I suspected of being a leper, but we ended up bogged down in a marsh labyrinth, surrounded by resentful, snorting hippos. Suspecting less visible but more dangerous crocodiles, we scrambled to the safety of higher ground.

The next day I tried again, this time accompanied by half a dozen villagers armed with spears. Mapping a route that followed the 1200-foot contour line on the topographic chart, we arrived at the river two hours later at a very pleasant spot of tall *Ficus sp.* and *Diospyros mespiliformis* (African ebony). The river here was only about 130 yards wide, swift-flowing, between well-defined banks that, at this point, formed a U-shaped bend and a kind of bay which I called Kamubeye Bay on my working map, after the name of a nearby hill. The place felt comfortable and interesting, well located for the pursuit of our *G. morsitans* research in the savanna further inland. I also suspected that it was here that we would find and be able to study the large tsetse fly. Without further ado, I decided this would be the place to build our permanent camp. Referred to on my working map as "Malagarasi Camp," it was later "immortalized" on official Ruanda maps (1952) by the name "IRSAC Camp."

In its final form, Malagarasi Camp was a delightful place, about 400 yards from the river in a pleasantly shaded part of Brachystegia-Julbernardia woodland. An inner courtyard, 20 by

20 yards, was enclosed by a strong 10-foot-high post fence that protected both us and the experimental animals from the intrusion of lions, leopards, hyenas and other undesirable visitors. Inside the enclosure were the following mud-and-wattle structures: a laboratory, two huts for personnel, a kitchen, a shelter for the *zamu* (night watchman) and an animal pen covered with mosquito netting to exclude tsetse flies. My own hut was made from reeds, cool and breezy, and had a partitioned corner for occasional visitors.

A wide path, daily more marked by the passage of the water-carriers, led to the Malagarasi River. The path fanned out in the natural beach of Kamubeye Bay. The day I "discovered" the place, a small canoe made of bark was tied to a pole. I was shocked to find that *my* landing place had been discovered before. It seems that the canoe had been used a long time ago by "smugglers" from the Tanganyika side. What they smuggled, I had no idea. The population on the British side had been removed some time in the past as a measure against the spread of sleeping sickness. At this spot, the stream was swift, silent and, to me, somewhat mysterious and fearful, and at the same time romantic, the deep shade from the huge trees dancing a playful pattern on the surface. According to the season, the color of the water varied from light beige to dark brown. Beyond Kamubeye Bay, the river widened downstream, inundating a low-lying area during the rains. This was the playground for a large hippo population that could be heard daylong from our camp by its loud snorts as the animals surfaced or by a deep woh-woh-woh at other times. On rare occasions we saw crocodiles. Their resting places were probably somewhere upstream.

I decided that if I wanted to explore areas along the border more expediently, travel by river would be the easiest and most efficient means. So I asked the chief to make a dugout canoe. Unfortunately, his men were not traditional river people or canoe builders. The one they made was too narrow and, when launched, the craft looked rather unstable. I thought, however, that with a full load it might pass the flotation test. Planning to spend the night across the river in search of the habitat of the large tsetse, I loaded the canoe with equipment that included a movie camera and my 9.3 rifle, camp utensils and a small tent that I squeezed on top as a protection against splashes. Together with two fly-boys I set off. No sooner had we reached midstream when the canoe overturned and I found myself, once more, among the crocodiles. We all managed to swim the short distance ashore. I feared that all the equipment would be lost, but after we managed to haul the canoe to the bank (luckily it had drifted that way) and turned it back upside, everything was still in place held by the tent I had squeezed on top. Miracles do occur.

Persisting in my idea that a big canoe would be tremendously useful in our work, I started inquiring about finding a large, straight tree. One of the fly-boys said he knew exactly where to find one. We drove to a village and he showed us a gigantic *Chlorophora excelsa* (mvula in Swahili; iroko its commercial name.) The tree stood all by itself in the middle of abandoned fields. It was perhaps 100 feet tall and easily six feet in diameter and straight as a telephone pole—a superb tree. I asked the chief if he would allow me to cut down the tree for the construction of a canoe. I told him that the canoe would belong to him after we were through with our research and that I would pay for all the labor. He agreed. The tree was felled, but it took many weeks before a canoe was hollowed out from the massive trunk by means of adzes and fire. It was a magnificent craft. We had great pains, however, to haul it to the river. We had to cut a seven-mile long road and with one part of the canoe resting in the bed of the pickup truck we half carried, half towed the craft to the Malagarasi. The canoe floated well and straight.

A week later I was called to the director's office. He handed me a letter from the director of Agricultural Service, Ruanda-Urundi, denouncing my unpardonable act of felling the last remaining Chlorophora tree in the region. As luck would have it, he had received the visit of a high-ranking colonial official interested in forest conservation. Proud of his knowledge, the Agri director took the official to the distant Mosso to show him the last Chlorophora, remnant of a forest that had been destroyed gradually when agriculturalists had moved into the valley more than a hundred years ago. When our officials arrived at the place where the last of the giants once stood—one can imagine the proud smile on the director's face—nothing was left but the stump. The affair made quite a stink. I must confess that I felt awful and terribly embarrassed. I had acted on an impulse, not stopping to think that conservation had anything to do with my need for a canoe.

One of the questions when people, on rare occasions, ask me about our life in Africa is: "Did you ever kill a lion?" At times my mind wanders back to that night when I sat all by myself in my open convertible staring into the eyes of a male lion that, ten yards away, was staring back into the headlights, visibly annoyed. I had returned from an evening with the American missionaries at Kayero. Coming around a sharp bend of our new, self-made road, I had to brake suddenly as I saw a beautiful animal lying on the left of the road enjoying perhaps the remnant heat of the day against its belly. I turned off the engine and all was quiet. The animal did not move, hypnotized perhaps by the headlights. I pondered what to do. The lion and I kept looking into each other's eyes. I had my loaded 9.3 rifle lying on the back seat. At that distance I couldn't miss, so I thought. On the other hand, the distance was too short for comfort and even a mortally wounded lion might perhaps have enough instinctive energy to leap into the car (I remembered the "dead" crocodile). As I was debating with myself—all this may have taken only a minute or so—the lion seemed to be getting increasingly annoyed. It started shifting its front paws and that made me make my decision. Slowly, keeping my eyes looking into the lion's, I stretched my right arm behind me, groping for my rifle. It seemed an eternity before I had a good grip. As I lifted the heavy weapon inch by inch to bring it forward, the strap slipped off the barrel with a metallic click that sounded loud in the still of the night. I turned my eyes towards the gun and when I focused them again on the spot where the lion was supposed to be, it was gone. I could hear the rustling of grasses and then all was quiet. This was the closest I got to "killing a lion," although I had more encounters later.

I have in front of me a notebook that was in fact my "carnet de chasse," a "hunting record." The pages are yellowing at the edges; the cover is stained with brownish blobs of dried blood. Inside are notations about each of the animals I shot under cover of my scientific permit. Real hunters would give their souls for such a permit because it allows the killing of any kind of animal (except *Homo sapiens*) of any sex, in any numbers, of any age. Such a permit is very rarely issued, of course. Mine was obtained directly through the office of the vice-governor of the colony to assist in my research work on tsetse flies and trypanosomiasis. I never abused this privilege. If I had, it would have been taken away immediately and it might have been the end of my colonial career. The record in my notebook tells me that during my one-year stay in the Mosso I shot 42 animals: 3 baboons; 5 other non-human primates; 6 various antelopes; 2 warthogs; 2 snakes; 24 birds. The purpose of this hunting operation was first to collect blood from each mammalian animal that would later serve to inject rabbits for the production of antiserum, as I shall relate later. Blood smears from each animal were examined under the microscope for blood parasites, especially trypanosomes, our main research subject. Each animal was also inspected for intestinal parasites and ectoparasites that were collected and preserved for later study. None could say that I shot animals only "for the pot" although, of course, meat from some antelopes was welcome to my personnel and myself!

As could be expected, my hunting privileges were not always regarded with a friendly eye by ardent hunters who were restricted by number, species and sex of the animals they were allowed to shoot under their "resident hunting permit." In addition, some game wardens were on the alert when they knew that someone with a scientific permit was roaming their territory. One accused me of wholesale slaughter, while another denounced me for shooting a female topi. This was perfectly legal according to my permit, but when I met him one day, he brought the subject up. I asked him how he, from a distance of 200 yards, could distinguish between a male and female topi. Before he could reply, I said that I supposed he knew that both sexes of *Damaliscus korrigum* carry horns.

None of my hunting stories would grace the pages of *Life Magazine* under such a title as: "How I faced death reloading my 10.75 charged by a bull elephant." But as any hunter-at-heart will tell, to walk the early morning woodlands, a rifle swinging purposely on one's shoulder, one's eyes assessing distant shapes, aware of any unusual movement that could be interpreted as "game," is part of the fun. It tingles the ancestral hunting cord in no small way. Alone (Mutima was needed at home after our son was born) I felt like a mighty obligatory hunter in an unlimited domain that stretched to the horizon. I stopped occasionally under a tree and, without moving, turned my eyes in every direction hoping to catch a movement of an unsuspecting animal. Mostly it was the other way around: animals jumped out of cover before I had seen them, but not always.

Old Shinyanga

I had decided that the big tsetse fly was *Glossina brevipalpis*, not *Glossina fuscipleuris*, as I had thought at first. The species had not been reported previously from Urundi. The director decided that I should visit East Africa Tsetse and Trypanosomiasis Research Organization (E.A.T.T.R.O.) in Old Shinyanga, Tanganyika, to have the identification of the big tsetse checked. Furthermore, I was to discuss our work with the other glossinologists, as their territory bordered on the Mosso region. Comparing notes might be profitable to both sides while their long experience in tsetse research and methods of control would give us valuable information in planning our future surveys.

After my routine monthly Mosso safari, we, driver Budiaki, Zaghi and I, started the journey to Shinyanga the last week of October. We set off in the IRSAC Ford station wagon, the back well laden with all the paraphernalia Africans usually take along: food boxes, Primus stoves, complete kitchenware, Coleman lamps, camp beds and bedrolls, demijohns with drinking water. We also carried four jerry cans with extra gasoline, one gallon of engine oil, two spare tires and a complete set of leaf springs. We crossed into Tanganyika at the Muhinga border post and checked at the Ngara customs stations on the Tanganyika side. The road became narrower and more overgrown with tall grasses as we proceeded. Nowhere were there signposts, a matter that doesn't bother anyone unless one arrives at a (rare) crossroad or when the road turns out to be part of an alley system in a village, passing through several backyards. During daytime all this is taken rather lightly, but as night falls, as was the case one hour after we had crossed the border, things are no longer funny. And when, after passing one of those treacherous deep bridges, we heard a loud bang from underneath the car, the outlook was even less cheerful. My first fears were confirmed: we had broken the main leaf of the rear spring. We unloaded everything from the back of the car and by the light of a Coleman lamp, and by means of the two jacks we fortunately carried, we raised the vehicle, the second jack being used to shore up the spring support. In this way, Budiaki was able to insert a spare spring leaf under the broken one. The repairs were only a temporary solution to the problem. By driving carefully we hoped to reach the next small town, Nyakahura, where we might find a shop to help us replace the broken spring with the spare set we carried. In the dark night, only the reflection of the headlights on the tall grasses helped us to keep to the middle of the road. Budiaki stopped from time to time, shining a flashlight underneath the car to see if the extra spring leaf was still in place. All was well, so far—except at one of the stops. As Budiaki was kneeling beside the car, a lion slowly walked across the headlights from the right to the left side of the road. I looked at Zaghi, who sat next to me on the front seat, and Zaghi looked at me. We didn't utter a word, but I had an almost irrepressible urge to burst out laughing. We heard Budiaki stand up and walk to the front door. As he opened the door, he looked straight at the disappearing hind part of the lion. He quickly got in and slammed the door, and we all burst out laughing, a bit nervously perhaps. Tears of merriment and relief rolled from Zaghi's enormous cheeks. From then onwards Budiaki decided that there was really no need to check the repairs.

We reached Nyakahura around midnight without further adventures. Budiaki and Zaghi found a place to sleep with the help of a *zamu* and I stretched out along the front seat. We were lucky to find a mechanic shop the next morning and it didn't take too long to replace the broken spring with the spare set.

We arrived in Old Shinyanga during late afternoon.

Spearheaded by Major Bruce, who, at the end of the last century demonstrated that trypanososomes are transmitted by tsetse flies, the British have since thrown themselves wholeheartedly into tsetse research. Kaduna in West Africa, Shinyanga in East Africa and Tororo in Central Africa became THE centers of tsetse and trypanosomiasis research. They were followed later by similar institutions in Belgian, French and Portuguese colonies. Not only is trypanosomiasis of great public health importance and of enormous economic impact, but the study of tsetse flies and of the transmission of the disease have always fascinated scientists—to such an extent that the group of experts in this research has become a distinct "family" that includes parasitologists, entomologists, botanists, soil specialists, biologists, veterinarians, with medical doctors at the far end. The aim of all these passionate studies is to find the intricacies of the fly's ecology and biology that could be used to devise methods of control. The aim of the sophisticated research in microbiology laboratories is to probe the enigmatic genetic setup of trypanosomes that may lead to a successful vaccine.

The E.A.T.T.R.O. laboratories in Shinyanga are located in a *boma*, that is a fortified fort built in 1912 by the Germans when the country was still German East Africa. Its walls are 40 inches thick, the small, high windows are recessed, and the roof is of solid construction. In spite of the hot climate, the temperature inside is naturally kept fairly constant, ideal for the experiments going on inside. The center was pioneered and promoted by the late C. F. M. Swynnerton, after whom the local tsetse *Glossina swynnertoni* was named. Swynnerton died in an airplane crash in 1938, together with David Burtt, a botanist, while making an air survey of vegetation communities and game movement.

At the time I visited E.A.T.T.R.O., the chief entomologist, the late Dr. C. H. N. Jackson, one of Swynnerton's lieutenants, was director. He was an extremely likeable person and a marvelous scientist whose knowledge, good nature and wit I learned to value and esteem while I was a guest in his house during my week in Old Shinyanga. Members of the research center sentimentally insist on the "Old" before the name Shinyanga because the "boma" had been built at the site of the previous village of that name while the commercial center, added later, was along the new Tabora-Mwanza railroad line a few miles north.

The week I spent in Old Shinyanga was extremely valuable both to me and to Zaghi. My sessions with the various members of the research staff became the basis of my understanding of tsetse ecology and biology and the principles of tsetse control. It also greatly increased my knowledge and interest in vegetation communities and in the animals living therein. They made me strongly aware of the great need to understand the African environment and its inhabitants and the principles of land use. As for Zaghi, he learned not only finely tuned field collection methods by accompanying the fly-boy teams on their routine rounds, but also dissection techniques of tsetse flies for sites of infection and for age determination.

During our return trip to Astrida we teased Budiaki by reminding him to check the rear spring from time to time. "Only at night and while driving through lion country," he said.

After the pleasant Shinyanga intermezzo, research in the Mosso continued in earnest with our effort concentrated on unraveling the ecology of *G.brevipalpis* and of the trypanosomes they carried. I loved studying the fly's activities, which, we found out, were crepuscular. Around five in the afternoon I would walk along the path leading to the Malagarasi and observe the flies "sunning" themselves, their rear ends turned towards the sun. I was now skillful enough to capture them with a lightening-swift sweep of the hand. Strangely and interestingly, the "sunning" flies were all males—perhaps waiting for the females to saunter by at dusk. Very romantic. When disturbed, the males would resettle on the path, landing facing the sun and then turning about, heads away from the sun. These landings and turnabouts were observed again and again each time a fly was disturbed or flew off by itself. How fascinating all this was to me, a glossinologist in the making.

Because of the nature of their work which takes them to little-explored corners of Africa, tsetse ecologists have been known to make discoveries "far beyond their call of duty": unknown caves, unsuspected rock paintings, prehistoric artifacts, uncharted waterfalls, new botanical species and so on. Jackson once camped in a spot where, one week later, Williamson, another tsetse ecologist, found a 120-karat pure diamond embedded in a piece of rock he had used the night before as a stop under the wheel of his Land Rover.

Nothing of such magnitude happened to me in the Mosso. Yet it was still a great thrill one day to discover a deep gorge solely inhabited by baboons. I had followed the Kanka River upstream and, leaving the last village behind me, found myself in a narrow valley that penetrated far into the escarpment like a wedge-shaped cut in a cake. High above, I could see a two-step fall of the Kanka River—an unheralded scenic wonder. A well-marked path climbed the steep right-hand wall of the gorge. No human habitations or fields were to be seen.

"Kwa nini watu tembele hapa?" I asked the man who had proposed himself as guide in the last village. ("Why do people come here?")

"Hapana watu, bwana, iko makako. Iko mugini yake," was the reply. (Not people, sir, these are baboons. This is their village.)

The numerous paths that crisscrossed the valley were all made by the passage of baboons. Higher up I could spot two large rock shelters used, no doubt, as night quarters by the monkeys. I could see no movement, however. I supposed that they had left on their daily foraging on the lower slopes or perhaps on a raid in the chief's vegetable garden. I felt as if I was intruding in a forbidden sanctuary and that I would be challenged any moment for my indiscretion. Although I wanted very much to learn more about this unusual place, it was with relief that I followed my guide's suggestion that we turn back. I promised myself to return one day, but I never did.

While wandering in the forest around Pawa, I had always expected to see snakes. But in the Mosso I had far more encounters with snakes than I cared for. The one I remember best occurred when I almost stepped on a huge Gaboon adder *(Bitis gabonica)* on my way back to camp from a tsetse survey along the River Mazimero. My sideways jump would have rated well during an Olympic competition had such a sport been among the events. But the reflex of a hunter prevailed as I raised my rifle and put a 9.3 bullet behind its head at the moment the reptile started to slide into a hole in the ground. Do snakes make underground shelters? Or was it a tunnel made by some other animal? Anyway, the snake was rapidly disappearing in whoever's hole it was, in spite of its bullet wound. I took another shot at it, this time with a small-bore shotgun. Still it kept on sliding into the hole. I was not going to let the snake get away from me. Quickly I grabbed its tail end and started pulling. I might as well have tried to uproot a tree. It was a man-versus-snake contest and the snake was winning. I called my "gun bearer" to cut quickly a *kamba* (rope). When he finally arrived with a vine, only a foot of the snake was still outside the hole. Hastily we slipped a noose around it and tied the other end of the vine to an acacia tree. The small tree bent but held fast. So did the snake, nor did it show signs of weakening. Wounded by a 9.3 bullet and shotgun pellets, the reptile, I assumed, would not keep up this match forever, nor could it escape tied as it was to a tree. I decided to run back to camp, less than two miles away, and fetch reinforcements. When I returned, accompanied by five fly-boys, we managed to pull the snake out—dead. It measured almost 15 feet. At the autopsy, the stomach showed only unrecognizable debris (it must have been hungry) and a number of parasitic worms.

With research now well organized and on a routine schedule, I left the camp in charge of Zaghi and, accompanied by

Samson, started prospecting the region of Mutara, the extreme northeastern part of Ruanda. This region would become the location for my research like that of the Mosso in the following years. The preliminary surveys, I believed, would help in developing a plan to organize the coming long-term study.

My family and I, however, were due to begin a six-months' home leave on 23 March, a leave we had decided to spend entirely in the United States. Taking charge of the research in my absence would be M. Chardome, who accompanied me to the Mosso during my March trip. His main objective would be the identification of the trypanosome species infecting the local *G.morsitans* and *G.brevipalpis*.

As related earlier, M. C. (M. Chardome) had served in the "underground army" in occupied Belgium. At that time we were both laboratory assistants of Professor vanden Berghe at the Institute of Tropical Medicine. And we both ended up serving the same master in Africa, ten years later.

M. C. was far from being a modest man. He was constantly bragging about his incredulous—but true—adventures, which made them seem trumped up to most people. The stories about his hunting feats during his first years as a professional hunter in the Lake Albert region made the famous Selous look like a second-rank shot. I had bragged about the plentiful wildlife in the Mosso. But to him, nothing would ever compare with "his" Lake Albert. Zaghi had loyally confirmed my "lots of game" appraisal of the Mosso, but M C. just sniggered.

As luck would have it, his first morning walk around Malagarasi Camp was sterile as far as game was concerned, although he got plenty of tsetse bites. He came back disappointed, his gun unused, grumbling and venting his frustration at Zaghi as we stood talking outside the camp's fence.

"This region is bule (nothing)," was his verdict as he swept the horizon with a derisive gesture.

Zaghi gallantly defended "his" region in his stuttering French. Casting his eyes around in desperation on the surrounding woodland M. C. had so vehemently criticized, Zaghi suddenly meekly muttered:

"Par exemple, comme celui-ci, Monsieur Chardome" (For instance, like this one, Mr Chardome"), pointing to a superb specimen of waterbuck that walked stately across the meadow a hundred yards below the camp.

By the time Chardome had recovered from his astonishment over what seemed a magic trick on the part of Zaghi and from the reality that an actual animal was within easy shot, and fumbling to pull his rifle from his shoulder, the waterbuck had disappeared.

The joke remains forever attached to my memories of the Mosso and of M. Chardome.

A few weeks later we left on our six-months' home leave in the United States.

Part III

Return to the Forest

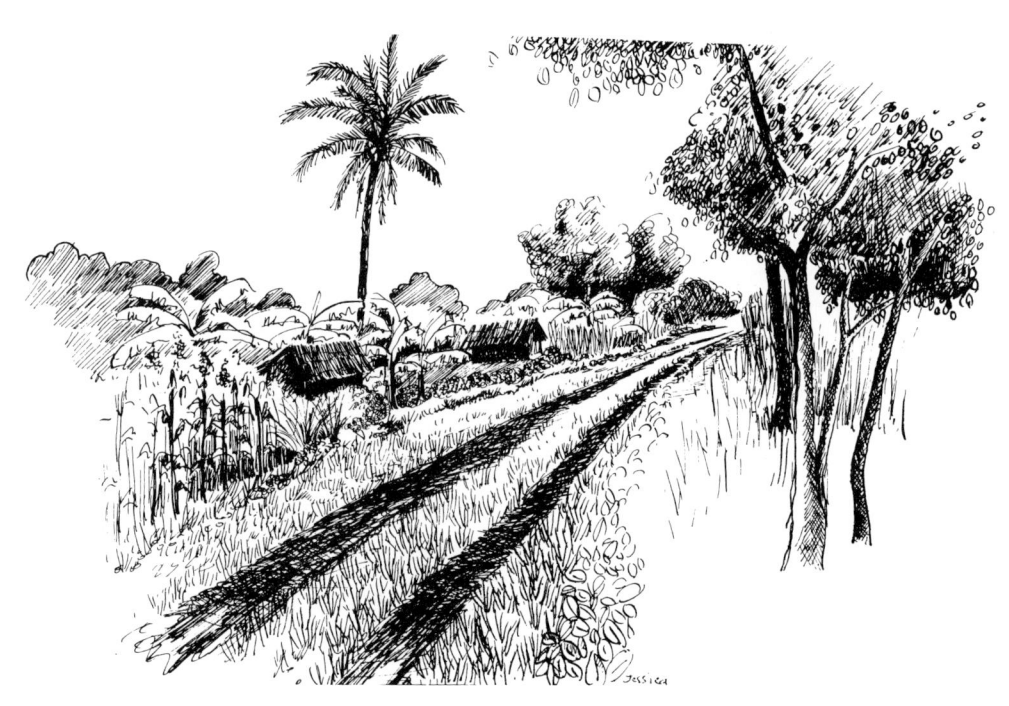

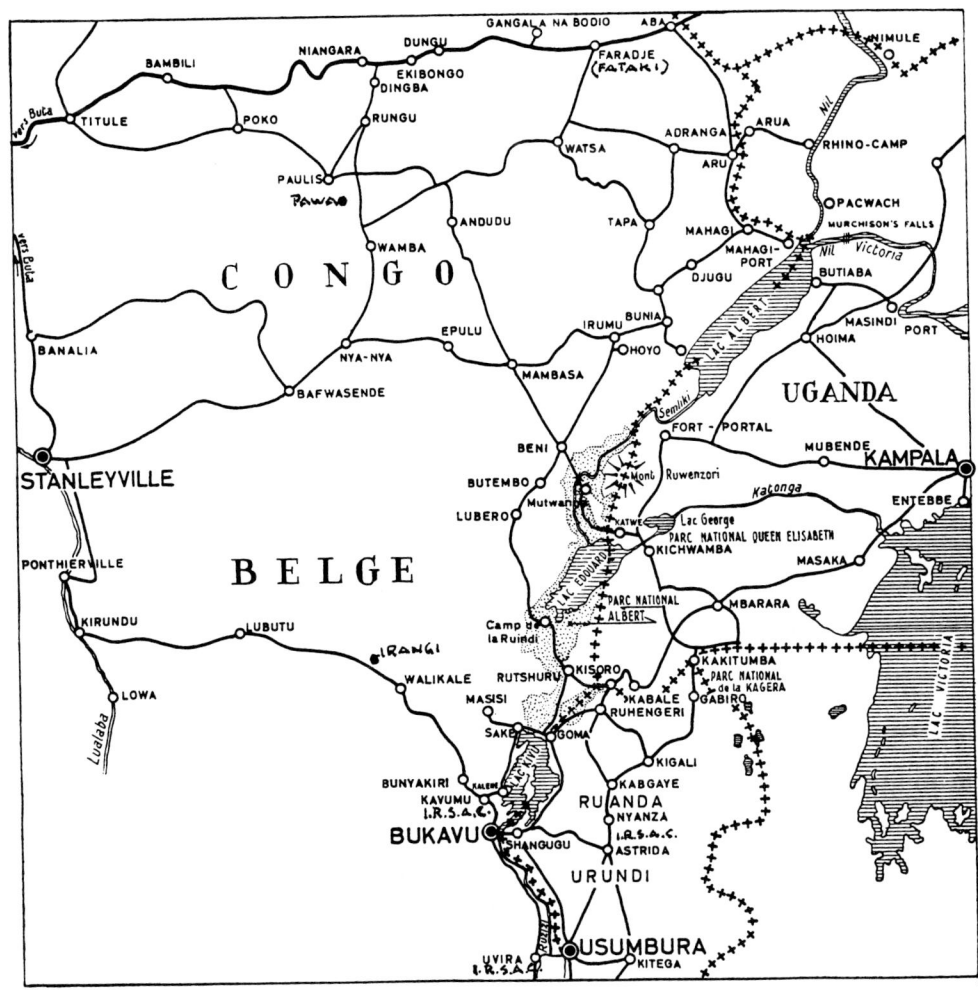

Map of areas mentioned in the text.

Return to Africa

By coincidence, we returned from America in the same ship that had taken us there six months earlier, the M.S. *Houffalize,* a 16,000-ton cargo ship that provided accommodations for twelve passengers. During our twenty-week trip we had toured forty-two states in a Plymouth station wagon bought for me by a friend. The car was waiting for us when we arrived in New York in April 1952. To the surprise of everyone in my friend's office, I managed to earn my U.S. driver's license at the first try. Our budget allowed us the modest expenditure of $20 a day to cover lodging, food, gasoline and extras for the whole family of four. Again to everyone's surprise, we had managed to stay within that budget, including an additional three-week stay in an apartment on Riverside in east Manhattan, while waiting for the return passage to Africa.

After an uneventful crossing, the *Houffalize* docked first at Lobito, Angola. Passengers and crew were allowed only a restricted visit of the quays. The visit wasn't worth the risk of being rowed across the docking area in a boat with only about an inch of freeboard in a choppy sea.

Twenty-four hours later the *Houffalize* arrived at Matadi, where we disembarked and waited for the unloading of the station wagon we had brought back from the States. Knowing about the rough handling of cargo in Matadi, we were saddened but not terribly surprised to find the rear window smashed when we went to collect the vehicle the next day. We lost several hours filling out insurance papers and looking for the person to sign them. Finding another window in Matadi was out of the question. I taped some plastic sheets across the window frame and took the road to Leopoldville, a 360-mile-long dirt road, but in good condition. The plastic sheets soon parted from air pressure because in the 95-plus-degree heat we could not keep the front windows closed. Sucked in by the vacuum effect of the open rear, clouds of red dust constantly circulated inside the vehicle. When we arrived in Leopoldville, no one could tell for certain to what ethnic group we belonged. At immigration I ran immediately into trouble because my British passport did not allow residence entrance without the required 50,000 Belgian francs caution money. A number of telegram exchanges with IRSAC headquarters solved the problem. Also helpful was a chance encounter with a member of the old hockey team who now worked at the Belgian Consulate.

We had reserved passage on the next river boat, the sternwheeler *Reine Astrid*—luckily because all cabins were booked when we sailed a few days later. This was my second, Dora's and the children's third trip on the Congo River. This time we were going upstream, which meant a journey of 11 to 13 days to Stanleyville.

To many travelers, anxious to "get home" or eager to rejoin their post, the journey is boring. Most of the time was spent in a deck chair in the steaming shade of a flapping tarpaulin strung across the stern deck except for the meal hours in the dining room where whirling ceiling fans tried in vain to dispel the overheated stale air. In spite of the many discomforts, *we* actually looked forward to a leisurely panoramic tour through the tropical forest with occasional moments of excitement when spotting monkeys, crocodiles or hippopotamuses. We enjoyed the thrill of arrivals and departures each day from the "postes-à-bois" (wood supply stations or wood yards) to take in a hold of wood that fed the wood-burning boilers of the ship.

Leaving Leopoldville soon after daybreak, the *Reine Astrid* heading north soon fought the silent but strong and treacherous swirls of the current inside the 15-mile-wide river, here known as "Stanley Pool." Twenty miles upriver, the "pool" narrows to a single channel formed by the steep banks between the foothills of the Crystal Mountains. Except for the changing vistas of the stream itself, the first day was of little interest; the surrounding bare country rather uninspiring. It took almost eight hours to cover the 130 miles of river, so we arrived at our first landing place, Kwamouth, around mid-afternoon. Except for a few places where regular docks and quays have been built, such as at Coquilhatville (now called Mbandaka), steamers make fast, bow upstream, by dropping the anchor some distance from the sandy beach. To avoid grounding, the maneuver is guided by two "depth-sounders" who, at the bow, measure the depth of the water by means of marked bamboo poles, calling out in Lingala "mai moke" (little water) or "mai mingi" (plenty of water). As soon as the anchor is dropped, four crewmen jump from bow and stern, swim ashore with cables to attach them around trees or posts. Willing hands haul the ship closer until gangplanks can reach the shore. Then all hell breaks loose when eager vendors, desperate shore-goers and nimble wood-carriers vie for gangplank space. After a while things calm down when the wood-carriers gain the right-of-way and start dumping their pile of wood inside the hold.

Besides a large group of hippopotamuses near one of the small midstream islands, the second day passed without much excitement until our arrival, during late afternoon, at Bolobo. All day we had been gliding on glassy water where one could sense rather than observe the swift current. Towering white cumulus cloud reflections, seemingly more real than those in the bleached sky, danced in the eddies. Doggedly, the *Reine Astrid* had been wandering across the river in search of the deepest channel, usually close to one of the banks and marked by means of white-painted boards nailed to a prominent tree. The two "depth-sounders" sat all day in the bow, swinging their long poles rhythmically in the water and calling out their findings to the bridge. The arrival at Bolobo rekindled the suspense. Informed of the arrival of the *Reine Astrid*, a throng of ivory carvers stood waiting along with their merchandise neatly displayed on a row of folding tables. [Still in its infancy at that time, the ivory work sold at Bolobo has since received international recognition and is currently mentioned in tourist pamphlets.] A lively trade soon developed as soon as the ship made fast, to continue well into the night by the light of hissing Coleman lamps and in the stench of burning insects attracted by the hot flames.

No sooner had the dumping of firewood in the hold ceased than we cast off the next day. It was close to five and only the faintest glow in the east indicated the birth of a new day. The reason for this early departure was our destination, Lukolela, 110 miles and 10 hours away. To us, the day promised new, interesting vistas because after Bolobo the river enters the dark canyons of the equatorial forest. We were not disappointed. All day we watched the somber walls of the forest, mysteriously aloof except for an occasional small group of huts shrouded in a blue haze from its wood fires. At times, the stillness of the forest was shattered by a cackle of alarm from red-tail or Colobus monkeys or by the raucous squeak of a panicking "bolicoco," followed by its cry: "co-co-co-co" that gave its name to this forest hornbill.

Lukolela came in sight just as the sun dipped behind the uncertain horizon. Lukolela used to be the stamping and hunting ground of the famous American ornithologist, James P. Chapin, who with his friend, Herbert Lang, collected most of the woodland bird species of western equatorial Africa right here in the forest surrounding Lukolela, between 1909 and 1914, and returned to the same spot in 1929 to complete the collection. I had met Jim just a few months earlier at the New York Museum of Natural History, where he was curator of the ornithology section. He still spoke with great enthusiasm about Lukulela. When he joined the IRSAC Institute as a visiting researcher three years later, we found ourselves at the same research center at Lwiro. We often recalled tender memories about Pawa areas where, as a young naturalist earlier in the century, he had known the great MaBudu and Mangbetu chiefs, Abiengama and Medje.

It was after the Lukolela overnight stop that the first signs of dramatic events began that would mar, psychologically, the rest of the journey. Rumors had it that the wife of a recently married A.T.A., the mother of a one-year-old child, had been taken ill with vague intestinal complaints. "Nothing serious," the young A.T.A. (Assistant District Officer) assured his friends. He was eager to join his "territory" at Nouvelle Anvers (Gangala) only four days away, where his wife would be able to receive proper medical attention. For the next couple of days, the matter rested, the interest in the matter confined to a polite: "How is Madam?"

The next overnight stop, Irebu, came and went. We crossed the equator. Then we arrived at Coquilhatville (Mbandaka), the capital city of the Equatorial Province. Had we known, we should have forced the young A.T.A. to leave the boat and take his wife to one of the several hospitals in town. Still in a hurry to join their post, now only two days away, the young couple decided to carry on.

Lulonga was our next port of call, only about 65 miles away in a straight line. This stretch, however, and farther north, is somewhat tricky, with rapidly shifting sandbanks and unchartered obstacles in the form of sudden build-ups of large vegetational debris from the surrounding permanently flooded lowlands. It was, therefore, only near sunset that we reached the overnight stop. A low overcast had threatened all day, making weird scenery of the inundated forest of ghoulish tree trunks draped with ghostlike vines sheathed in mosses and epiphytes—a most depressing sight. Rumors about Mrs. G.'s condition were equally disheartening, varying from "no change" to "worsening." With the lowering sky that robbed the day of the usually spectacular sunset, Lulonga looked lonesome and desolate. The ship's searchlights, switched on to load the firewood, illuminated a sharply defined circle of the wood yard beyond which nothing seemed to move. Indeed, Lulonga has only a small administrative office, a trading center and a rest house.

We left well before dawn the next day. It seemed clear that with the news of Mrs. G.'s worsening condition, which was confirmed by the agitation of the two Catholic Sisters who had nursed her since the beginning of her illness, the captain was frantically trying to gain time. Suddenly, the comfortable, complacent journey turned into a race against death. Reaching Nouvelle Anvers, our next overnight stop and the destination of Mr. & Mrs. G and their baby, now seemed of the highest priority, warranting the great risk of shortcut navigation. Mentally, we pushed the ship as hard as we could—we had no idea how the captain felt, aloof on the upper deck. Unfortunately, the distance Lulonga-Nouvelle Anvers was the longest of the journey: 140 miles as the crow flies, perhaps 250 as the *Reine Astrid* navigated, at least an eleven-hour trip. As the day proceeded, the desire to make more speed became unbearable. The reading of the breviary by the priest as he walked back and forth in front of Mrs. G's cabin seemed to gain in intensity, his attitude more ominous. As night fell, the rumor that Mrs. G had died was confirmed. A stunned silence descended upon the ship as the native crew and passengers heard the news. Only the murmur of the priest and the swishing sound of the sternwheel broke the dark silence. Everyone felt relief when we finally reached Nouvelle Anvers during the late afternoon. The captain went to inform the authorities; then the body of Mrs. G. was brought ashore. The last we saw of the tragedy was Mr. G. stepping ashore, holding his small baby in his arms and in an incongruous gesture, turning around and waving good-bye to the passengers. It took a few days before the impact of the tragedy was dispersed. The sight, two days later, of the beautiful station of Lisala, located on a plateau overlooking the river, eased somewhat the emotional tension on board.

And finally, after three more overnight stops at Bumba, Basoko and Yangambi, the *Reine Astrid* docked at Stanleyville, having covered 1,100 river miles in 13 days. Later in the day, the barge with our station wagon also arrived.

The day after our arrival I went to every garage and auto-dealer—and there are not a few in Stan—in search of a window for the rear door—but in vain. So, without further ado we left Stan the following morning for Bukavu, a distance of 920 miles, the first 500 miles through the splendid Ituri forest. Surprisingly, the road was dry this time, even rather dusty in places. Here, in 1945, on my way to Pawa, I felt for the first time the overwhelming closeness of the rain forest. It was on this same stretch of road that, in 1946, I drove to Stan in a crippled pickup truck on a piece of banana trunk, in replacement of a broken spring, to meet my family arriving in the *Berwin*.

Close to the equator and therefore within the zone of almost constant rainfall, the condition of the forest road is unpredictable. Muddy most of the time is a fair assessment. The day we left Stan, we traveled over fairly good stretches alternating with patches of deep mud where heavy lorries had torn up the roadbed. Luckily for travelers, a team of "cantonniers" (maintenance gang) is usually not far away or actually working to repair a bad spot so that when one gets stuck there are enough hands available to help one out of a mudpool.

Log of the voyage of the *Reine Astrid*, October 1952.			
	Miles	Total	Hours
Leopoldville (Kinshasa)			
Kwamouth	125	125	9
Bolobo	75	200	6
Lukolela	110	310	10
Irebu	60	370	5
			Equator
Coquilhatville (Mbandaka)	75	445	6
Lolonga	60	505	5
Nouvelle Anvers (Bangala)	140	645	11
Mobeka	60	705	5
Lisala	120	825	10
Bumba	75	900	6
Basoko	100	1000	9
Yangambi	60	1060	5
Stanleyville (Kisangani)	60	1120	5

At Nia-Nia, we branched off to the East. It was almost dark when we reached Camp Putnam. We continued to Mambasa, where we arrived near midnight. We woke the "zamu" of the small inn, who let us have the keys of a cabin and provided us with a bucket with water and a kerosene hurricane lamp. We divided the water between the four of us so that we could at least rinse our very dusty faces.

An 85-mile drive brought us out of the forest, the following day. We reached Beni where the road climbs and follows the ridge of the Rift Valley wall. We had a marvelous drive through patches of montane forest with spectacular vistas of the valley below. Auberge des Trois Canards, the overnight stop at the upper end of the Kabasha escarpment, was reached during early afternoon.

We left early the next morning and dropped down the escarpment into Albert National Park and, passing the range of the Virunga volcanoes in the East, reached the northern shore of Lake Kivu. A 170-mile drive along the western shores of the lake took us to Lwiro, the main IRSAC research center, our destination and our home for the next seven years.

Those seven years would prove to be the most enjoyable in Africa. M. Chardome, E. Peel, his wife, and I formed what became known as the Department of Medical Zoology, the only department under the direct supervision of Professor vanden Berghe, the general director of IRSAC. To Chardome and me, having been his research assistants at the Tropical Institute, this seemed only the continuation of a long association. And it worked well. Together we accomplished a tremendous amount of scientific work recorded in numerous scientific publications. Our mutual relationships remained intact and while Chardome would address the director as Mr. vanden Berghe, I would always call him "Prof." Among themselves, the rest of the IRSAC members would refer to him as the BM. BM stood for "Bwana Mkubwa," Swahili meaning "Big Master." It fitted both his official position as well as his height of 6'2". The initials BM became so common in our language that it was also used in official circles. It was also very convenient for use in telegrams or radio messages, for instance. I was amused but not surprised to hear Mr. Harroy, Governor of Ruanda-Urundi refer to a report he had received from "the BM." We were all one big family, occasional squabbles not withstanding.

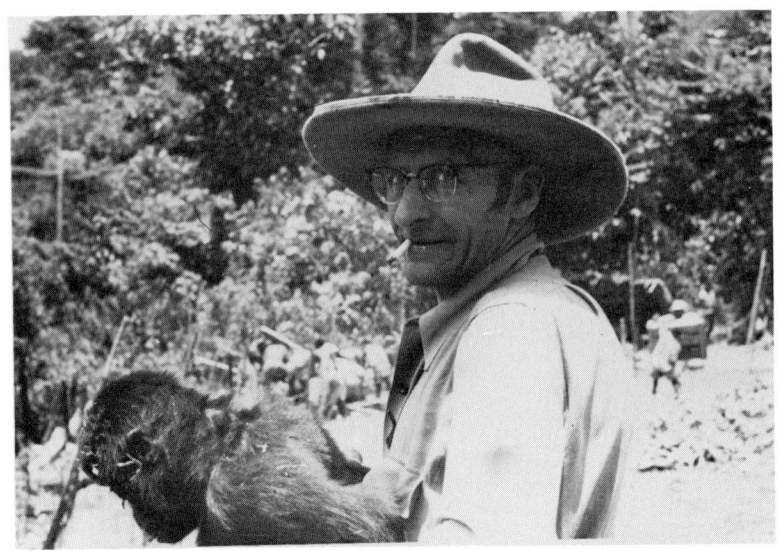
Marcel Chardome at Utu with young gorilla.

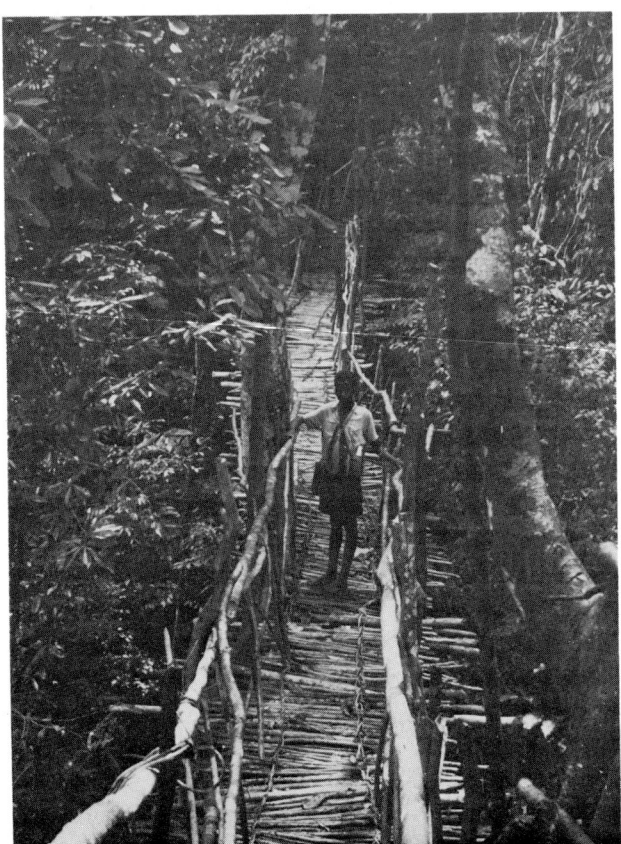
Swinging bridge spanning the Luo River naer Irangi.

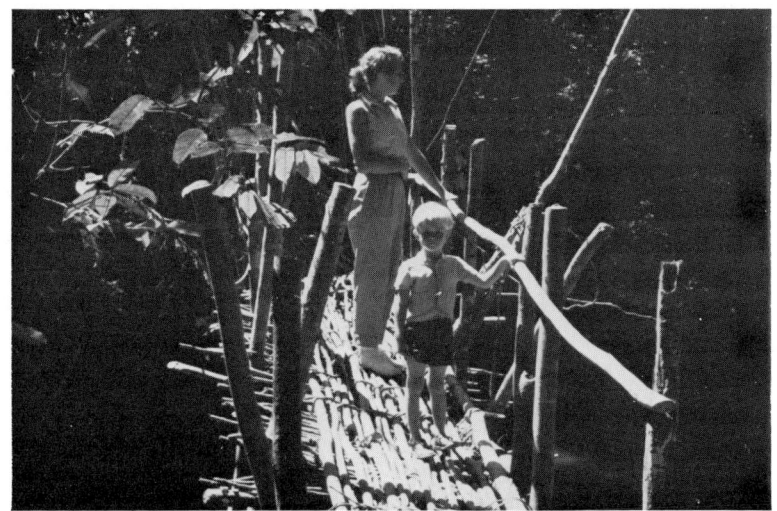
Dora and Richard (five) on the rope bridge at Irangi.

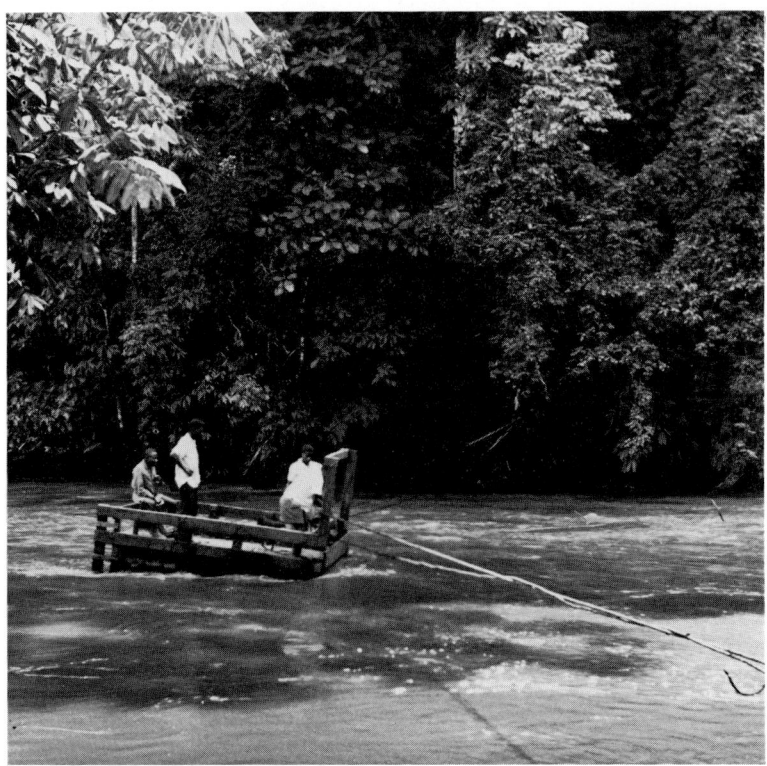
Our self-made ferry did not perform as well as hoped because the strong current tended to push the "bow" under. Samson, the captain, seems concerned. (Note one of the empty drums in the stern, part of the flotation device.)

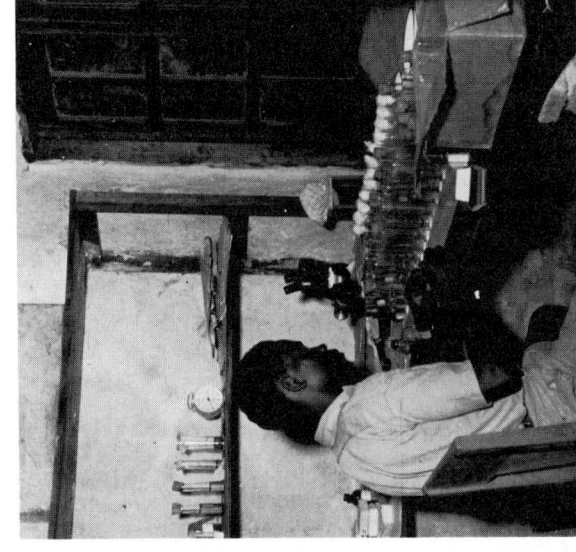

One of the mosquito boys is sorting live mosquitoes after a successful collecting night in Irangi forest.

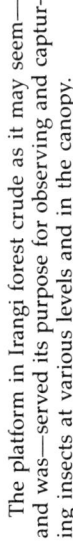

The platform in Irangi forest crude as it may seem—and was—served its purpose for observing and capturing insects at various levels and in the canopy.

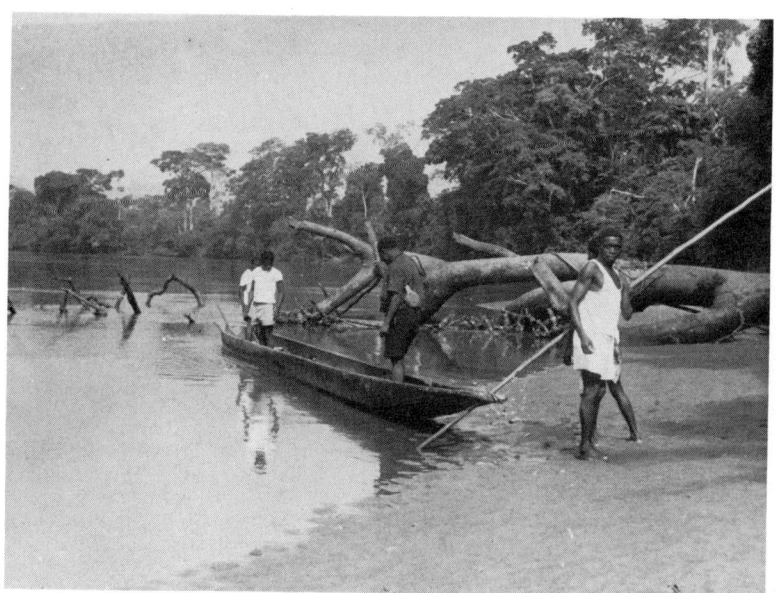
Tsestse search along the Oso River.

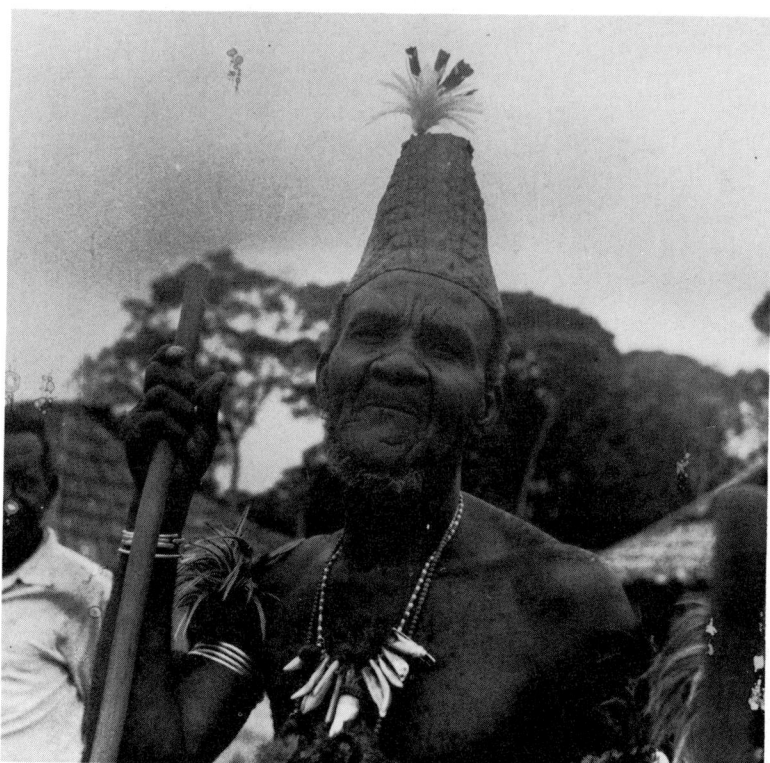
The witch doctor in Oso village.

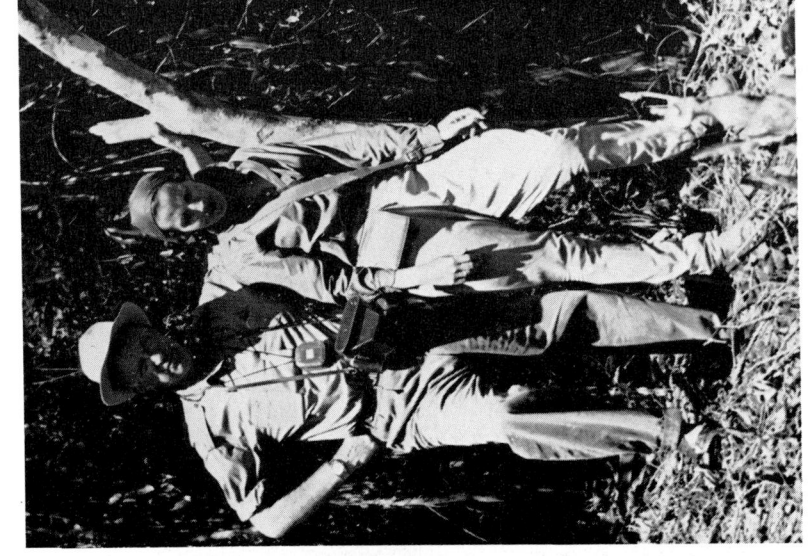

King Leopold and his wife, Princess Liliane, at Utu.

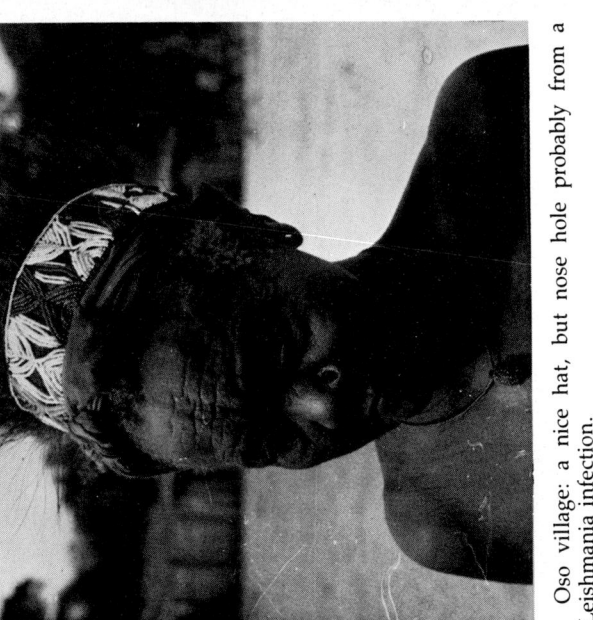

Oso village: a nice hat, but nose hole probably from a Leishmania infection.

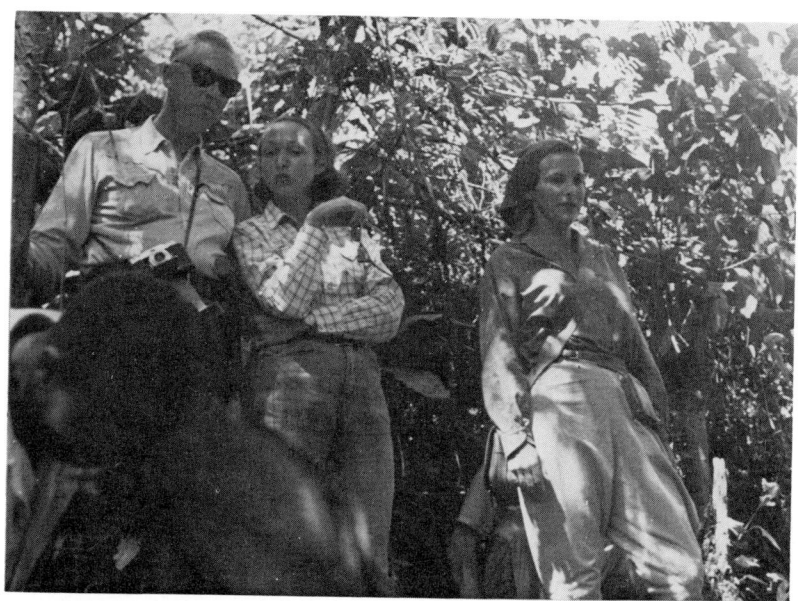

During the gorilla hunt: from right to left Princess Liliane, Mrs. vanden Berghe and Professor L. vanden Berghe, Director of the I.R.S.A.C. Institute.

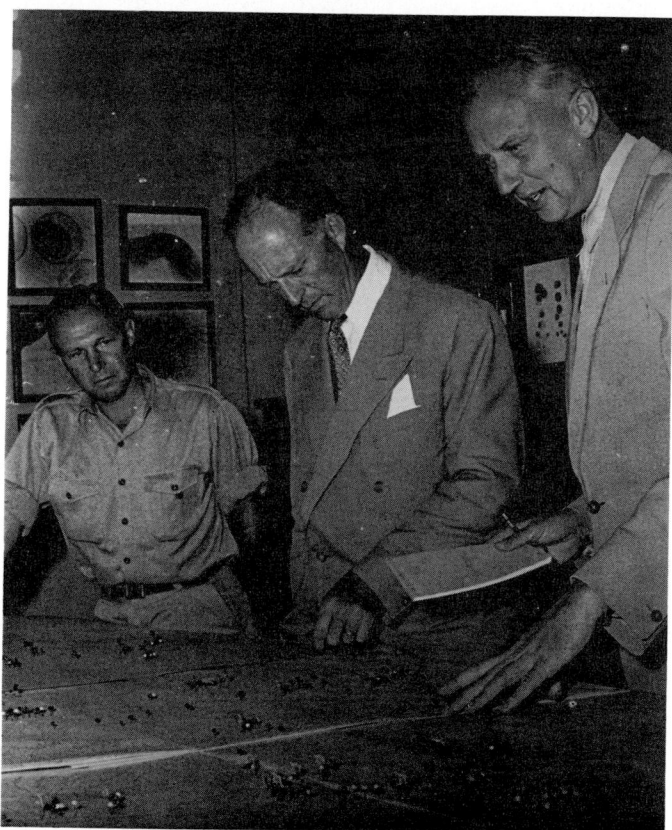

Visit of King Leopold to I.R.S.A.C. Institute: His majesty in the middle, Professor vanden Berghe, at right, explains the use of correlation maps on which the author, at left, has plotted the distributionn of tsetse flies.

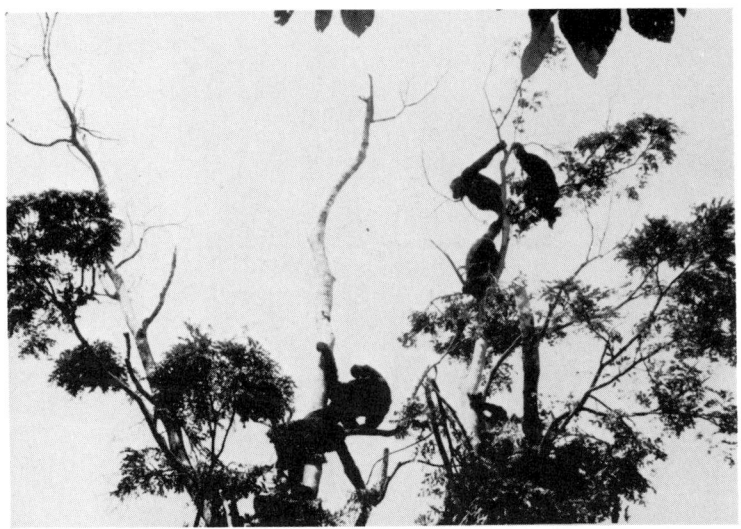
Gorillas "tree-ed" during an effort to capture them in Utu forest. Cutting the trees brought them down.

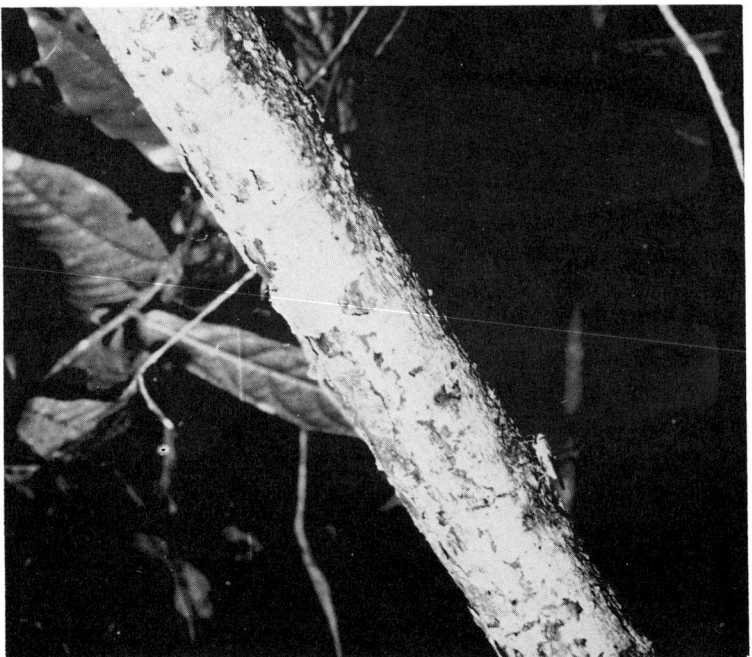
A nice picture of *Glossina vanhoofi* resting on a tree trunk; a thrilling discovery.

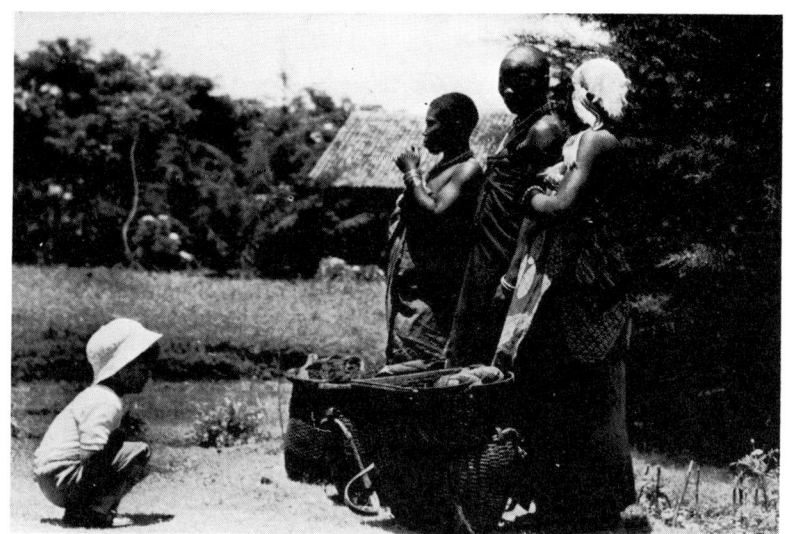
Richard at Lwiro inspecting vegetables sold by Bashi women.

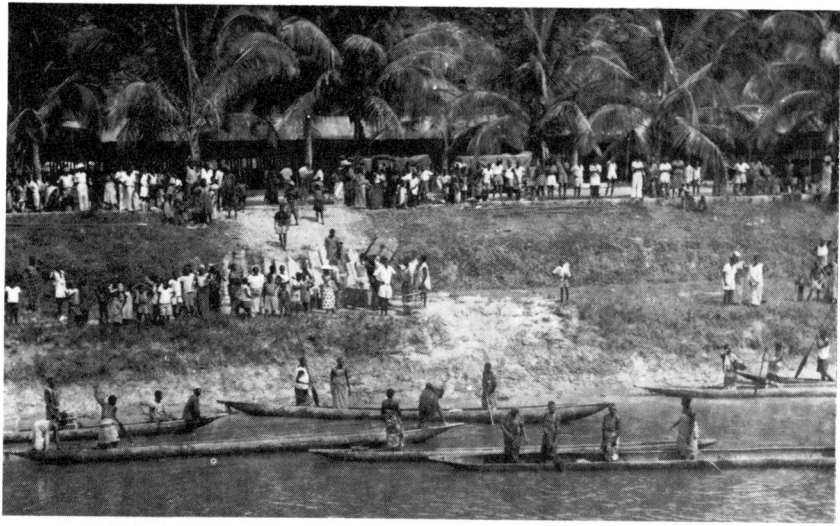
Halt at Bolobo village well known for its ivory carvers.

Seven Years in the Land of the Seven Volcanoes

The Kivu Province is the place where many colonials preferred to be stationed and perhaps, by the end of their career of 20 years and if luck would have it, buy or manage a small coffee plantation, own a bungalow with a view of the lake and of the seven volcanoes vaguely outlined in the distant haze. And if the heart longed for a bit of safari, there are three splendid Rift Valley lakes, the huge Albert Park with all its wildlife, the historical region of Maniema, the rough beauty of the western Ruwenzori slopes and, of course, the serene panorama of Lake Kivu itself.

As for me, I looked forward to being at the IRSAC center on Lake Kivu not with any desire of ending my colonial career there, (although eventually it worked out that way) but rather in anticipation of working at the institution's main center with all its advantages: good housing, a large complex of research facilities of the departments of geography, geophysics, biology, botany, cartography, zoology and nutrition. Moreover and for the first time, our daughters would be going to school only one hour's drive away and would be coming home every weekend by IRSAC school bus.

After a bit of a struggle to secure the house we liked—by now we had gotten used to fighting for it—we settled in happily. I resumed my research in the Mosso and Mutara, at last free from the administrative chores of station manager. So far, Dora had accompanied me on many of my field safaris, but soon after our return from home leave an event would interfere with her travel for some while: the birth of our son Richard.

Our lives had changed quite a bit since the "old" Pawa days, physically as well as socially. From the crude, but so dear, existence in a forest outpost of three families surrounded by villages inhabited by bark-cloth-clad Africans we had, by steps, "graduated" into increasingly sophisticated environments. At the IRSAC center of Lwiro we seemed to reach the maximum conditions of comfort one can expect from living in tropical Africa. We had a beautiful, cozy home built from natural stone, with an open fire, electric lights that worked 24 hours a day, cold and hot piped water, an electric refrigerator, nice hardwood furniture, an electric washing machine and an electric cooker. We had weekly movies at the beautiful guesthouse complex, and frequent social events and guest speakers.

Dora laid out an attractive garden, which in that climate and with the full collaboration of the fertile volcanic soil, was a constant joy of color and fragrance. A graceful volcanic rock outcrop in the front lawn, where a clever *Grevillea* had emerged to grow into a pleasing shade tree, was a favorite gathering place for the family. The tree became the mizzenmast of a square-rigger when our son Dick was old enough to climb to the top, where, as Captain Slocum, he surveyed the horizon which, from that point, happened to be the seven volcanoes of the Virunga range.

In spite of all that unaccustomed luxury and the lovely scenery, we kept remembering and talking about Pawa. My present research work, however, was far more interesting to me than the previous routine medical work at the Congo Red Cross. Another reason for talking about Pawa and its people was that Mutima had returned to his native village of Bafwagada after we had left on our six months' leave, and we were wondering how we would be able to get him back quickly. The solution came sooner than we thought, when a few weeks after our arrival at Lwiro I was asked to accompany a lorry with supplies for Chardome, then working on malarial parasites of chimpanzees in the forest around Andudu. Making a slight detour on the way back, I managed to "retrieve" Mutima and his family from their village. And as they and their voluminous belongings were loaded and the lorry sped on its way, cries of "Enawé! Enawé!" (expression of grief or astonishment such as "Great Scott" or "Good Heavens") and "Kwenda mzuri!" "Bakea mzuri!" ("Farewell!" "Stay well!") followed us until we were out of sight. And so Mutima returned to the family.

For our growing baby son, Mutima was, indeed, part of the family. Dick crawled or staggered around when Mutima was dusting or waxing the furniture or busy peeling potatoes. Mutima chased away the large rooster when it boldly picked the bread from Dick's hand or retrieved his football each time it landed in the bushes. Mutima helped moor the ship as directed by Dick—sorry, Captain Slocum—high in his tree, sorry, mizzen. The great emotion Mutima showed at the moment of our final adieu when we left Africa for the last time (so we thought) was the expression, I feel, of his great grief at the realization that he would never see Richard again.

But this was still several years away. After settling in, my work followed a sometimes erratic schedule. In principle, I devoted one third of my time, about 10 days each month, to my field research program on tsetse flies in Mutara and later Bugesera. The remaining 20 days were spent in laboratory work involving working out results from field research, microscopic examination of bloodsmears from people and animals, experimental work and production of antisera in laboratory animals, and insect taxonomy. Laboratory time, however, was often interrupted by unscheduled trips and, after 1956, to monthly short visits to our forest research station at Irangi. I also steadily drifted into establishing a mapping section and organizing a reference and correlation mapping service. All this kept me as busy as during the most hectic periods of my "chef-de-poste" times, but this was far more fun. Working under ideal conditions in laboratories equipped with the latest scientific tools and the availability of our well-stocked library helped tremendously. The almost constant presence of one or more visiting scientists from other parts of the world often sparked new interests and ideas. We boasted a magnificent large clubhouse, with pavilions for guests, perched on a slight rise that overlooked Lake Kivu and the volcanoes. Below was a kidney-shaped swimming pool fed by warm water from a nearby underground hot spring. Of course, I had been the instigator for the building of a tennis court, my second one in Africa.

The climate at this altitude of close to 5,000 feet was almost temperate. From the main plateau of the laboratories and houses complex, a twisting road led to a higher ridge at more than 6,000 feet, passing a natural fresh water spring that, captured in a reservoir, provided pure water for our community, averaging about twenty families, an African staff of about fifty families, for the research complex and a medical clinic. The road ended at a high plateau where cattle, buffaloes and a number of experimental animals were kept. Near the stables was a small building that held the director's own medical research laboratory. The bushland higher up had been converted into more pastures where later a huge enclosure of solid stone walls was constructed to hold a family of gorillas in an essentially natural environment, for observation and holding station until some were transported to zoological gardens. The same plateau held the house, a mansion, rather, of our director, Professor Louis vanden Berghe, and an annex guesthouse, for many years occupied by a guest scientist, Dr James P. Chapin, worldwide known ornithologist. Further, there was the house of George Gillis and his wife, who managed the farm, stables and the animals that included several horses owned by him and by the director.

It would be inexcusable not to say a few words about Dr. Chapin because he was one of the scientist-pioneers of the Congo. His first expedition to Africa, sponsored by the New York Museum took place in 1909 during which, and a second expedition, he took notes and made collections for the museum that later turned into the monumental *Birds of the Belgian Congo*, a five-volume publication that to this day remains the base of Central Africa's ornithology. I recall my first meeting with Chapin in his office at the New York Museum in 1952 when, hearing that I had been health officer in Pawa he started singing a song known from that area: "Uele, Uele malibali makasi." It was, indeed, in the region of Pawa that Chapin had made his first collections. He knew the old chiefs of the area and visited the enormous ceremonial halls made by the Mangbetu. He had hundreds of stories to tell. Chapin spent many more years in Africa and many other parts of the world constantly increasing his notes of the world distribution of birds. He spent several years at the Tervuren Museum near Brussels, Belgium, to work on his book. He became a friend of King Albert who, like Chapin, was a devoted admirer of the rich Congo flora and fauna. He received the Belgian "Ordre de la Couronne" in 1931 and "Officier de l'Etoile Africaine" in 1956. Chapin loved Africa and the Congolese people. He has always defended the work of the Belgians in the Congo against the severe criticism of the world, and the United States in particular, during the years following the disastrous Congo Independence. Some say that the pain he felt at that time might have hastened his death on 5 April 1964 at the age of 74.

Our director, Dr vanden Berghe, was an equally remarkable personality. With doctors' degrees in medicine and zoology, and an excellent draftsman of animals, he was also well acquainted with the arts: music, architecture, photography in addition to his extensive scientific knowledge about protozoology, haematology and tropical diseases. Tall, of noble bearing, casually but distinctively dressed, and an excellent *ad lib* speaker, he seemed to dominate any gathering, spiritually as well as physically. I became acquainted with vanden Berghe during the courses in tropical medicine at the Institute for Tropical Medicine in Antwerp, where he lectured in protozoology and haematology. I was immediately attracted to him although he was generally quite aloof and seemed to have more on his mind than explaining protozoology to a bunch of heteroclitic students varying in age from 25 to 45, including a black-bearded priest and a wheezing nun. I never talked to him during the course work. After I had graduated with a Diploma of Tropical Medicine and Hygiene (D.T.M.&.H.), I asked him if I could work as a volunteer in his laboratory, explaining my somewhat precarious position vis-à-vis the German occupation of Belgium because of my British passport. He immediately agreed and a day later I left one non-paid job in chemistry of the same institute and found myself in the laboratory of protozoology, proud as a peacock. Those were happy days in spite of occasional raids by the S.S. looking for undocumented personnel. The friendship between V. D. B. and me grew steadily although I always felt awkward and restrained. I was constantly aware of the social distance between director and staff even after many years of scientific collaboration.

At the end of the war, our paths, which had crossed in circumstances of war, divided temporarily: V. D. B. to devote all his efforts to the organization of the future IRSAC Institute, I to take up my appointment with the Congo Red Cross. It seemed a natural course of events when at the end of my CRC tour I should join the new IRSAC and become V. D. B.'s assistant.

As fate would have it, while I among all IRSAC members was the first to have known V. D. B., I was also the last to see him alive. Many years after we had left IRSAC to immigrate to the United States, we met V. D. B. and his wife again in Kenya, where they had established a stud farm in the Ngong Hills near Nairobi after they had left the Congo following the independence disaster. We visited them many times at their farm during our two years of tsetse research with I.C.I.P.E. (International Center for Insect Physiology and Ecology). It was during our stay in Kenya that V. D. B. died in South Africa, where he had gone for surgical treatment at the end of 1979. We had spent some happy hours together a few months earlier in his cozy second floor living room that overlooked the farm and the stables. Earlier that afternoon, we had witnessed the birth of a foal filly—a bit of a mess, but it had been wonderful to see the first attempt of the baby horse trying to stand on its unsteady legs, a bewildered look in its enormous eyes. Later that night we had talked about travel and revived memories of "the good, old days." We had even discussed the possibilities of putting together one more paper about . . . the world distribution of leprosy! Alas, two months later "Prof" was dead, leaving only the memories of "the good old days."

But to go back to Lwiro in the early fifties. We were a happy bunch of some 20 to 25 scientists, individualistic perhaps in taste and ideas, but dedicated to what we loved best: scientific research in Africa. Unavoidably, there were clans; there was gossip; and there was occasional friction. Gossip was called "petrol," meaning that whenever there was a spark or "faux-pas," the indiscretion would gain in degree by subsequent travel along the gossip vine—as petroleum on smoldering fire. Such things are not confined to the tropics, of course, although perhaps enhanced by circumstances of isolation. They are also rather typical of small villages where the number of inhabitants is too large for complete harmony, too small for rumors to dissipate. Once a year, however, we were brought together for an organized party. It all started one eighth of November when the "club," of which Dora had become president, decided to have a yearly event promoted by a committee and based upon a given theme or time period, etc. The first eighth of November theme was: "The Wild West," a kind of fancy dress ball requiring everyone to wear or represent something of that period. The preparation of the huge ballroom of the guest house alone was a lot of fun, but hard work for the "volunteers." Parts of the walls were covered by panels of cardboard appropriately painted in desert scenery, prairies and mesas. Pillars were transformed into totem poles by means of painted paper. The bar lights were turned off and replaced by storm lanterns. The floor was sprinkled with sawdust, supposed to convey additional feeling of the "dusty west." We drew the line when the newly arrived Swiss zoologist proposed to ride in on horseback. I was one of the barmen; Winnie and Jessie (14 and 15), in period dress, served drinks to the noisy and dusty horsemen just back from a rough cattle roundup. The evening was a huge success. Acquaintances became friends, friendships were reaffirmed, peace returned to the West. It was then and there that we committed ourselves to organize similar parties on every eighth of November, on whatever day of the week it might fall. We kept that vow, and the eighth of November will remain forever in the memories of many IRSAC members, wherever they may be.

The following eighth of Novembers were even better organized, the themes ever more sophisticated. Credit should go to the club's driving president, and the five-man committee members.

"Ancient Egypt" was the next theme. The guesthouse's main room was transformed into the formal courtyard of an Egyptian patriarch, and included a real fountain. Guests arrived and walked around in mock thoughtful conversation, dressed in shoulder-knotted white sheets and wearing garlands. Women were draped in "canonical" robes—clearly their most fancy nightgowns—ornamented with tassels, bangles, tiaras and other signs of their importance or great wealth. All was very stately until the band struck the first swing number. The guesthouse's African staff looked on as if we had all gone berserk.

The following year the theme was "Breughel and his time." The spirit and times of the great Flemish artist (sixteenth century) seemed to have stirred regional pride and interest in national heritage, judging from the great effort many had made to simulate those historical times, so colorfully depicted by the artist—and his son—in their canvasses of jolly folk festivals. The decoration of the guesthouse room had proven quite simple this time. In fact, the high, beamed ceiling and the massive open fireplace needed little improvement. Bales of hay had been thrown haphazardly in the corners. In one, a man in rags was drinking from a dusty wine bottle. A single long table and benches had been placed in the middle of the room, the lights had been dimmed or replaced by huge candles, the open fire crackled. Simple, rice-based food was brought in on wooden trays with long handles carried by two rather unsavory characters. At the end of the evening, many joined the man in the corner.

With so many ideas proposed after the Breughel episode, the committee suggested an evening of "variety show" during which everyone would be given a chance to display their talents. By the time of the fourth eighth of November, the organization of the event had become almost routine. Our technicians had by now constructed a preassembled stage that fitted against one of the guesthouse's walls—the same with the sound system, lights, and so on. Some members had managed to form a band, proudly named the "scientific six," composed of: piano (secretary of the director), drums (seismologist), base (biologist), guitar (ionospherist), trumpet (accountant) and clarinet (botanist). The band always started with a lively swing tune called "Coquette." The fun during the rehearsals alone would have been reason enough for having a band. The "variety show" was a tremendous success. Some of the highlights were a beautifully executed Japanese geisha dance, a Mardi gras party in New Orleans, and a women's fashion show of self-made dresses, Dora's "sack dress" of burlap stealing the show.

No one has ever contested that the funniest, most daring and most successful eighth of November was the last one, the circus. Getting bolder from previous successes, the desire to do greater things the next time and the audacity nurtured by the absence at that time of the director were contributing factors for the proposal by the committee. Of course, they could not have foreseen the unreserved enthusiasm, the inventive creativity or the lofty visions of the "technicians." It was like opening the symbolic Pandora's box: torrents of ideas, each more daring than the other, flowed unchecked. Before our very eyes a real circus unfolded inside the ballroom, complete with stands, trapeze rigging, the round arena area covered with a thick layer of sawdust (from our carpenter shop) and, to make things look even livelier, real elephant dung had been collected high above the Tshibati farm and judiciously arranged in the center of the arena. The evening opened with a tour of the band playing lively marches, greatly applauded by the spectators. Then followed all the special numbers and performances by gymnasts, clowns, knife-throwing, horse dressage, a gorilla hunt, and so on. Oh, for those memories to last for ever! So good and funny were most of the performances that they were played again the following afternoon for the children, including those of the African staff.

While from the above one gathers that life at Lwiro was far from dull and that we felt happier than we had been in Uvira or Astrida, we still missed that one element that had made Pawa so special: the feeling of integration in a "primitive" environment and native community. Of the Bashi, the local population of the Lwiro area, we saw little. We had only an occasional glimpse of a group of heavily laden women, carrying market products from their fields higher up the mountains in large baskets balanced on their backs and tied with a wide strap around the front of their load. On the way back, they carried heavy loads of firewood. They looked poor, scruffy and unkempt. Their once dark blue *kitembe* were knotted on one shoulder, Watutusi-like, unctuous goat skins tied over the other, serving as a baby sling when need be. Their territory comprises the fertile, volcanic slopes west of Lake Kivu, bordered in the north by the range of volcanoes, in the east by Lake Kivu and in the south by the strong, aggressive Warega. The leading families of the Bashi claim Hamite descent, which would explain the love, possession and wealth of cattle of certain Bashi groups. The tribe is vigorously organized with a strong sense of land tenure and clan leadership invested in the *Mwami* (Chief). More than other people of the mountains, I thought they were a morose-looking lot. It may be prejudice on my part. We were never in real contact with them as we had been with the MaBudu people in Pawa.

We did not like the climate of Lwiro too much: at its altitude of 5,000 feet, only the midday temperatures allowed for the wearing of short-sleeves. The mornings, evenings and nights were quite chilly, averaging about 63°F. The low temperatures were even more uncomfortable during the rainy season, from October to May. Of course, the combination of fertile volcanic soil and adequate precipitation was greatly praised by the "gardeners" among the European women.

Unlike most other Lwiro residents who did not seem to mind Lwiro's climate, even loved it, I was glad to "escape" each month to enjoy the "more clement" savanna regions of eastern Ruanda.

Besides the organized entertainment events marking the year with great flourish, we had many opportunities for recreation all around us, the most obvious being Lake Kivu, where we could go boating and sailing. Several local planters had small sailing boats and there were yearly regattas. Our seismologist had built his own twenty-footer, a handsome craft, on which my daughters and I went sailing once in a while. My acquaintance with the lake went further when the director put me in charge of the IRSAC motorboat. It gave me constant trouble because the high mineral content of the lake's water kept choking the pipes of the engine's cooling system. Swimming in the lake was risking infection with *Schistosoma mansoni,* causing a debilitating, even fatal disease called Bilharzia (or Schistosomiasis). The larvae of *S. mansoni,* a trematode worm, develop in fresh-water snails found in the lake. After development in the snail, infective larvae are released in the water, from where they can penetrate a human bather and further develop into mature worms. Eggs are constantly released by the female worm in an infected person's stools, from where the larva escapes to start its development cycle in the snail. There was a rumor that the former IRSAC accountant had acquired the disease in the bath of his Bukavu home. Apparently, the infective larvae had survived their journey through the city's water-supply system that drew its water from the lake.

For those willing to face the hazards of road travel, there was the drive southwards along the lake shore to the beaches at Goma or Kisenyi, a distance of about 100 miles or farther south to the Albert National Park, an additional 75 miles, with all its wildlife, the views of the majestic volcanoes and Lake Albert. For the more conventional, there was always the shopping spree to Bukavu, a 70-mile round trip. And finally, for those desiring a bit of physical exercise there was a dash up nearby Mount Biega or Kahuzi, both extinct volcanoes rising to about 10,000 feet.

Mount Kahuzi, at 3,317 meter ASL, is the highest peak of the Mitumba mountain range. It is a natural forest reserve and the home of the mountain gorilla. Its volcanic activity ceased by the end of the Pleistocene. Remnants of that activity were found right in our front garden, where a decorative volcanic outcrop was our favorite *al fresco* picnic place.

For many people a high mountain is a tantalizing challenge, an urge especially strong in those for whom mountaineering is a preferred sport in spite of unfavorable odds of freezing discomfort, broken bones or worse. Ask a mountaineer why he is so anxious to climb the vertical walls of a high cliff, dangling on a tenuous hook, and the classic reply will be: "Because it's there." For others, the fascination of mountain peaks may still be strong, but not an obsession, the innate impulse harnessed in the course of unhappy experiences during childhood.

De Reine, our librarian, was one of the former. He kept on looking at Mount Kahuzi until one day he said to no one in particular "Let's do it." Besides his wife, Anne, two others signed up. I was one of the two others.

From Lwiro, the mountain was perhaps seven miles away in a straight line, but it took a 20-mile drive along a tortuous one-way road to reach a place where an ill-traced path starts the climb. The climb, tough as it is, requires no special mountaineering skills. A good walker can reach the top in something under four hours and descend in less than three. The "Alpine Club of Bukavu" had installed a prefabricated aluminum hut at the top so that one could spend the night on the mountain, making the climb and the descent in the same day no longer essential.

The two De Reines, Christiaensen (botanist) and I would be the first IRSAC party to "attempt" the ascent. We chose a day at the end of May, the beginning of the dry season in that part of Africa. At that time chances of rain are slim, the dry season haze has not yet built up and the atmosphere is still clear.

The path up the mountain starts in a rather undignified way. A rusty sign-board, the Alpine Club's emblem barely visible, marks the beginning. Unbecoming as the signboard may be, without it the path would be hard to find, overgrown as it is with tall grasses. A bit blindly, one plunges into the green wall to find the first obstacle in the form of a shallow but wide rivulet with a creamy, slimy bottom into which a thoughtful soul has dumped a few logs. Not long thereafter, a second brook lurks, just in case you missed slipping into the first, this time filled with black mud. After tunneling through a few hundred yards of very wet vegetation, one emerges into a magnificent bamboo forest *(Arundinaria alpina)* through which a path runs pleasantly along the undergrowth-free shadow-dotted even floor.

A bamboo forest is very different from any other kind of forest. The evenly spaced, straight, hard-walled stems, fifty or more feet tall, somehow look artificial, resembling a painted theater stage background. There is no strangling underbrush so common in other types of forests. The sparse short grasses are covered with straw-colored leaves, slippery in dry as well as in wet weather. Alone and lost in a bamboo forest where every spot looks the same must be a frightful experience. Moreover, weird groaning sounds not unlike a swaying barn door, produced by the stalks that bend in the slightest breeze, enhance the fear. At times, stalks hit each other, making a sound as if someone is cutting firewood. Most nerve-racking and baffling, however, are the whistling noises created by the wind forced through cracks in the bamboo stalks.

Quite abruptly, the pure bamboo stands gave way to a Hagenia forest *(Hagenia abyssinica)*. Our botanist ponders whether the Hagenia is encroaching upon the bamboo or whether the bamboos are invading the Hagenia forest. Compared with the green gloom of the bamboo forest, the widely spaced hagenia trees give the impression of a parkland. If the bamboo trees with their delicate lanceolate foliage could be compared with a young girl dressed in a lacy dress, the Hagenia would be a stiff-shirted gentleman, a bit stand-offish. The purple flowers of the Hagenia form large clusters, the shape and size of a bunch of grapes. On the first days of bloom, these flowers are creamy white, turning purple as they age, and finally brown. In the later stages they stand out attractively against the background of the bright new green leaves. The Hagenia is typical of central African mountains at altitudes of between 6,500 and 7,500 feet.

We came to a swift river which we crossed by doing a balancing act across a single tree trunk that spanned the banks. The path ran for a while along the opposite bank, but we suspected that its direction would soon change. We guessed correctly. An abrupt turn to the left brought the path up a sixty percent slope and our climb was on in earnest. Soon my heart was pumping furiously in an effort to urge the blood to receive more oxygen from the rarefied air. One slips on loose gravel and momentum is broken. In spite of the cool mountain air, perspiration runs freely—blinding the eyes, and one stumbles more.

On and on we went, followed by three porters and proceeded by our official guide, the latter imposed by National Park regulations. After two hours of sustained effort, we reached a kind of platform. Here we had a wonderful view of the surrounding country and also of the summit which seemed still a far way off. The altitude meter read 8,550 feet, so we still had another 1,500 feet of climbing to do.

After a 20 minutes' rest we started off again. We crossed another bamboo forest, this time alternating with patches of tree heath (*Erica* sp.) and treelike *Philipea* sp., all draped with long green-gray filaments of "old man's beard" (*Usnea* sp.). We were dismayed to find that on three occasions the path descended into steep valleys—a waste of energy and momentum, especially since walking down these steep declines proved as tiresome as walking up. We came to a long narrow ridge of bare dark rock from where we had a hair-raising view, if one could take one's eyes off the narrow ledge cut out from the bare mountain slope that fell away to the right almost perpendicularly.

The final gradient near the summit was covered with deep mosses on soppy, muddy black soil. Very slippery, it added greatly to the difficulties of the steep last hundred yards' during which I had to rest four times. With an effort that seemed to require the last reserve of strength I finally stumbled to the top, where Charles was lying flat out, pumping air like a leaky compressor. The actual summit was very small with just enough room for a few meteorological instruments and a geodetic signal. The aluminum hut in which we would spend the night stood on a slight depression about fifty feet from the highest peak. Charles managed to get inside the hut through one of the windows. I joined him and together we succeeded in taking off the lock and opening the door by the time the others arrived. Ours was an unorthodox way of entry, but we had been unable to secure the keys in time. The hut was a mess: old newspapers everywhere, pieces of firewood, discarded tins and wrappers, bits of wire and some broken tools. There was no built floor other than the black, damp earth that covered the rest of the mountain top. The "furniture" consisted of a wooden box obviously meant as a table, a small cupboard, a sink, and two double bunks made from metal tubing and canvas. Against the wall, above the two windows, were single shelves with a few tins, one containing gasoline, one with kerosene, one with insecticides, and two dozen candles. A hurricane lamp dangled from a long wire attached to the center of the roof. We cleaned up some of the mess while we sent the porters to collect firewood. After their return, they were sent back below because it was against the rules to keep African personnel at the top during the night. There was no shelter for them at that time.

From two in the afternoon, the time when we arrived, till about four we had clear skies and marvelous views with a 360-

degree panorama. A storm was brewing in the west, but it stayed there. The whole of Lake Kivu could be seen from its southern end at Bukavu to well to the north, but haze in that direction prevented us from seeing the volcanoes. Directly below us was Idjwi, a large island, and smaller satellite islands that seemed to float above the water level. The Ruanda shore, on the far end of the lake, rose abruptly to a steep escarpment that sloped onwards to the Ruanda highlands.

A little after four-thirty a sudden gust of wind cooled the balmy atmosphere and brought moist air from the valley below. This condensed into flimsy white clouds right at our feet. It became bitterly cold. We sheltered in a narrow gully out of the icy wind, but after a while the sun disappeared behind the clouds while the wind stiffened to a full gale. In a matter of seconds, the blithe atmosphere changed into a world of gloomy grayness and of roaring winds. We retired hastily to the hut and made our first attempts to get the fire going. This was not easy. The stove smoked badly, the sides holed from rust. It took constant attention to keep the not too dry wood alight. The warmth emitted was purely illusory, entirely psychological. The stovepipe was barely warm to the touch. It took a long while before we had enough hot water to make tea. Showing a lot of patience, we managed to prepare a meal of macaroni and sausages. A can of what was thought to be tomato sauce proved to be a strange dish of rice, but no one complained. In fact, it was delicious. Keeping the fire going was a major undertaking. We also tried to keep warm by drinking cups of hot coffee, of which we luckily had a good supply. Outside the wind howled, blowing tons of water-saturated clouds against the windows, where they condensed into constant streams—a sort of horizontal rain. The icy wind seemed to streak right across the hut through the many openings between the roof and the walls. The main whirlwind, we discovered, came from underneath the door and between the door and the jamb. We plugged the smaller openings with newspapers—the presence of large stacks of them now became clear. The gap beneath the door was filled with earth from the hut's floor—the hollow in the floor of the hut also became obvious. After the repairs, climatic conditions inside the hut improved markedly and if the temperature increase was nothing to boast of, at least the wind velocity inside the hut had been reduced to something approaching a medium breeze. Even the candles stayed alight. We couldn't do a thing against the terrifying noise of the blizzard pounding the aluminum panels that rattled and creaked at each renewed effort to blow us off the top.

Cold and miserable, eyes smarting from the smoke, we went "to bed" at eight. We put on the clothes we had brought, crept into our sleeping bags and wrapped extra blankets around us. Even so, we all spent a very uncomfortable night, shivering with cold and kept awake by the unabating gale that shook the whole structure in sudden outbursts. After the fire went out, the temperature dropped to that of the outside, close to freezing point no doubt, the thin aluminum plates having no insulation value whatsoever. During the night I had an awful apprehension that if ever the door blew open, the wind pressure inside the hut would be such that we would be swept from the mountain top.

We were all mighty glad to see the first light of dawn and to find ourselves still anchored to the summit. The storm went on unrelentingly and now we began to worry whether the porters would be able to make it to the top in this weather. We had eaten all our provisions, the firewood was almost finished, and to spend another stormy night there—this time without food and fire—did not strike us as particularly amusing. Around eight the force of the wind seemed to decrease somewhat and from time to time we caught a flimsy glimpse of the sun's disk between gaps in the hurrying clouds. We were ever so thankful when exactly at nine our faithful porters arrived with the good news that farther down the sun was shining and the wind was less strong. We packed with haste, leaving the hut in a shameful state of shambles, just as those before us had done. We understood. Charles and I struggled in the beastly cold for about 20 minutes to fix the lock on the door. Then we descended in a hurry and caught up with the rest of the party as they were resting on the 8,550 feet platform. Here sun shone brightly and the wind was reduced to a strong breeze. We loitered for a while to let the sun sink in and soak away the bad memory of the night.

Camp on the Epulu River

Camp Putnam, May 11, 1953.

Dear,

Back again in the good, old Ituri forest! What a difference with "sloppy" vegetation of fallow fields around Lwiro! Life seems so different here among the high trees, bright sun, deep skies, dark shadows, dancing pygmies and a temperature where one can put on a short-sleeve shirt from early morning till late at night.

Our voyage was without incidents; we arrived at Camp Putnam Friday afternoon. De Medina, with his okapis and elephants, are at 15 km. from here. We would have liked to stay at his camp but as he has no room to put us up we are making our headquarters here at Putnam's place as first planned. Pat Putnam seems all right but he has to stay in bed most of the time because of his lung troubles; he is not permitted any kind of effort, even walking. Mrs. Putnam is very nice to us and with her help we arranged a small guesthouse that will serve both for lodging and as our lab.

Another guest at Putnam's is Schuyler Jones, a reporter-writer. He is a pleasant young (25-ish) fellow who lives in Paris but has traveled in Africa for the last two years. He pays his way by writing articles and filming. Of course, he is writing a book!

We haven't seen Pirlot yet. We have already a number of animals V. D. B. asked for so that it won't be long before we have completed his list. Caring for the animals keeps us quite busy and, of course, we take bloodsmears and have other laboratory work to keep us going all day.

Mutima is O.K. but I don't know whether we shall be able to fetch his wife on the way back. It is quite a detour to his village!

The director's arrangements with De Medina, Manager of the "Station d'Etude et de Captures" in the Ituri forest, led to my return to the forest in May 1953. When BM mentioned his correspondence with De Medina, our zoologist, Paul Pirlot, jumped on the occasion and proposed a survey of the monkeys of the Cercocebus-Colobus group along a 60-mile transect between Epulu (Camp Putnam) and Andudu, Chardome was given the assignment to study the blood parasites of chimpanzees in the Andudu area while I was to carry out an entomological study of forest blood-sucking insects of the Epulu area, especially of *Aedes* mosquitoes suspected of transmitting "jungle yellow fever" among monkeys.

The expedition was part of BM's plans for zoological studies of various lowland forest animals that—hopefully—could be kept in captivity and eventually could be bred for research on their physiology and other life functions. One animal of particular interest was the Okapi *(Okapia johnstoni)*, a rare animal found only in the deepest forest habitats of the Uele and Kibali-Ituri regions of the Congo. The existence of the timid Okapi became known to the western world only in the 1930s. Its dark-maroon and white striped camouflage is especially effective for this shy forest creature. It is closely related to the giraffe but, living among dense ground vegetation, does not require the long neck for browsing leaves. The Pygmies were well aware of the existence of the animal, which they hunted for its fine meat, long before it became known to the outside world.

Located along the lonely 400 miles stretch between Stanleyville and the Uganda border and the northern regions of the Province Orientale, Camp Putnam was more than just a beautiful rest spot, it was almost like a symbolic western haven in an alien environment. Not that Pat Putnam wanted it that way, I am sure, but his presence and reputation made it so.

Patrick Tracy Lowell Putnam was twenty-four when he came to live in the Ituri forest. He fell in love with the rain forest and the Pygmy inhabitants when, as member of the Belgian Congo Anthropological Expedition of Harvard University, he visited the area for the first time in 1926. After his participation in a second Harvard expedition to the Far East, he decided to return to the Ituri forest. To make a living while carrying out anthropological studies of the Pygmy populations, he took courses in tropical medicine in Belgium that would allow him a steady salary as health officer and to run a field medical dispensary. It was during a foot safari—there were no roads at that time in that part of the forest—that Pat discovered that extraordinary stretch of the Epulu River where it cascades across a boulder-strewn barrier and allows a rare view of the rain forest's edge.

He built himself a wattle-and-thatch hut and another for his dispensary and added other structures as need indicated. Later he built the large living room which he called the "Palace," and four guest rooms. The main room had a concrete floor, measuring about 20 by 40 feet. Prominent was the central raised fireplace that always held a few big logs, often smoldering even during daytime, to be re-kindled into a low burning fire at night. The walls were decorated with simple native hunting tools and various native implements. A large dresser and a number of locally made easy chairs were the only furniture. When entering the room, no matter how many times, the strongest attraction, however, was the view through the wide rectangular opening in the wall that framed the Epulu River as a living painting not only in sparkling colors but also with the sound of cascading waters.

Hidden among the tall trees, the Palace was cool and peaceful. Four doors gave passage to the forest beyond. Narrow paths linked the Palace to Pat's living quarters: two rondavels, the kitchen and a guesthouse. Deeper inside the forest were the dispensary and the huts of people taking part in Pat's activities.

We had written Putnam about our plan for a 2–3 weeks zoological and entomological study. We received a reply from Anne Putnam that Pat was not well, actually bed-ridden, but that he welcomed us to use the Epulu facilities for any amount of time. When we arrived Mrs. Putnam kindly offered the use of one of the large rondavels but apologized that her husband would be unable to see us unless he felt better and would send us a note. Indeed, two days later we received a message that he wished to see us. I had met Pat several years earlier but I was shocked to see him looking so tired and thin. I am sure that only his scientific interest in our forest survey made him want to see us at all. After we had briefly outlined our project, to which he nodded in approval, we left feeling that even the brief conversation had made him very tired. We did not see him again during our stay. Pat Putnam died six months later at the age of 49, having lived for 25 years in the Ituri forest among "his" Pygmies.

We went to work the day after our interview with Pat. Chardome left for Andudu to start his chimpanzee survey. I made arrangements, through Anne Putnam, with a team of six Pygmies to help me in capturing insects. Another team was set to work trapping animals.

As I walked to the Pygmy village the next morning, I was truly thrilled to see and smell the lowland rain forest of the Ituri again; its mixture of strange odors of wet vegetation and crushed fire-ants; the brightly lit clearings with yellow mud huts; the rhythmic pounding of manioc in mortars; the sudden rushing noise of swaying branches as monkeys leapt from tree to tree; the precise pattern of the musanga-tree leaves against the blue sky.

The village where my six Pygmy "assistants" lived was a short distance from the main road on the opposite side of Putnam's camp. Siafu was the brightest of the team and as he spoke some Swahili it was through him that I organized the task for each of the team members.

The Epulu Pygmies, locally known as Bambuti, belong to the large clan of the Efè Pygmies—other large groups in the Province Orientale are the Aka, the Basua and the Bakango. Smaller groups, the Batwa, are found in widely dispersed areas along the eastern Congo highlands and Rwanda. The word "pygmy" was first used by the Greek poet Homer. However, "the people of the forest" were known well before Homer's time by the Egyptians in the fifth century B.C. as recorded in Herodotus' writings. After these early historical annotations, the Pygmies disappeared from narrations, literally swallowed by the "impenetrable" forest. They were "rediscovered" by Du Chaillu in 1863, who in his book, *The Country of the Dwarfs*," describes his first encounter:

> How strange the houses of the Dwarfs seemed! The length of each house was about that of a man, and the height was just enough to keep the head of a man from touching the roof when he was seated. The material used in building were the branches of trees bent in the form of a bow, the ends put into the ground, and the middle branches being the highest. The shape of each house was very much like that of an orange cut in two. The frame-work was covered with large leaves, and there were little doors which did not seem more than eighteen inches high, and about twelve or fifteen inches broad.

Du Chaillu and his Ashango companions tried several times to catch the inhabitants while in their village but each time the Pygmies heard them coming and fled to the neighboring forest—until one day when he thought he had seen a figure hastily crawling inside one of the huts:

> It was so dark inside that, coming from the light, I could not see, so I extended my arm in order to feel if there was any one within. Sweeping my arm from left to right, at first I touched an empty bed. I

moved my arm gradually to the right, when—hallo!, what do I feel. A leg! which I immediately grabbed above the ankle, and a piercing shriek startled me. It was the leg of a human being, and that human being a Dwarf!

"A Dwarf!" I shouted, as the little creature came out. "A woman!" I shouted again—"a pigmy!"

How queer the little old woman looked! How frightened she was! she trembled all over. She was neither white nor black; she was of a yellow, or mullato color. The hair grew on the head in little tufts apart from each other, and the face was wrinkled as a baked apple. I can not tell you how delighted I was at my discovery.

I told Siafu that I wished to find out what kind of insects bite on the ground, half-up the trees and in the canopy and asked him how it could be done. He gave an order to one of the team who disappeared for a while then came back with a string of short-cut vines. We walked to a nearby tall tree. Our "mountaineer" tied one end of one of the vines with a loop to the ankle of his left leg. The other end was tied likewise to his right ankle after the vine had been crossed around the other side of the tree's trunk. With his arms around the trunk he worked his way up alternately shifting legs and arms. In a few seconds he was at the fist major branch fifteen feet above ground. This was the traditional method of getting honey from wild bee-hives high up trees, Siafu explained. They all laughed when I showed my amazement. Even Mutima expressed his astonishment by uttering repeated "enaweee! enaweee's!"

We choose an appropriate tree some distance inside the forest with major branches conveniently located at about 20 and 50 feet above ground. Siafu appointed three of his team to "man" the collecting station: one at ground level, the two others respectively at 20 and 50 feet. Together they quickly built a comfortable platform from twigs in the fork of the branches. Each spent three hours catching biting insects and putting each in one of the twenty tubes I had given them. They collected from six in the morning till six in the evening, changing places with each other every three hours. The same arrangement was made in a tree near a group of huts six miles down the road. In addition to these set-ups we also had a collector near an open manioc field and one inside the village itself.

This type of work became soon very popular and news about this unique opportunity of receiving money while just sitting in a tree soon spread throughout the forest. Recruiting eager "mosquito-boys" became easy. I stopped at twelve which was all Siafu, promoted head mosquito-boy, could handle.

While all this was going on I roamed the area in search of mosquito larvae breeding places in all kinds of water collections and again found how very specific some mosquito species were in the choice of their breeding sites. For instance, it was with great satisfaction that I found larvae of *Aedes simpsoni*—a potential yellow fever vector—inside the U-shaped stems of banana leaves. At their junction with the main trunk, the leaf-stems always contained sufficient water, gathered, no doubt, from dew that runs from the large leaves during the night and early morning. Banana groves are a classic example of a potential "jungle yellow fever" transmission sequence: the breeding of *Ae. simpsoni* in the leaf-stems/monkeys (carrying perhaps the yellow fever virus) raiding the plantation for food/the presence of people in the same location.

Searching for larvae in the forest gave me the opportunity to bag a few monkeys needed for our serological studies, besides making routine bloodsmears for blood parasites. The eight monkeys shot belonged to four species: *Cercopithecus ascanius, C. mitis, C. mona denti* and *Colobus badius*. They were all infected with a malarial parasite, *Hepatocystis kochi*. Other parasitological material came from animals captured by the pygmy hunters but which had died later during captivity. We had the rare opportunity of examining the blood from a dead Okapi at De Medina's camp. Chardome, who had returned from Andudu, and I had our hands full processing all this material at night by the light of a Coleman lamp. During less hectic evenings, it was pleasant to walk along the dirt road—still warm from the afternoon sunshine—and climb onto the rocks bordering the rushing waters of the Epulu River that made the air vibrate with cool breezes.

One day Pirlot came back from his survey with a number of caged animals. Together with the animals brought in by the Pygmies we now had our "quota." While Pirlot and Chardome left the same day to return to Lwiro with some of the animals and the trapping equipment, I needed another three days to finish my work and prepare the lorry for the return home with the rest of the animals and the remaining equipment.

I left during early evening so that I could travel during the coolness of the night. I said goodbye to Anne Putnam and gave her my best wishes for Pat. Schuyler Jones decided to come with me. He was more than willing to make a detour to the village of Chief Karume where I had decided we would fetch Mutima's wife. Two days later we were back in Lwiro.

The expedition ended with my letter to Pat:

Lwiro, 30 May, 1953

Dear Mr. Putnam,

First of all I should like to thank you and Mrs. Putnam for the hospitality you have shown me and my colleagues during our survey in the Epulu area. We arrived safely at Lwiro Friday at three o'clock in the morning, making Beni-Lwiro in a single trip, driving 21 hours without stopping except for feeding the animals. Unfortunately, we lost the small "Boloko" antelope and its baby. The Pangolin also died on the way. All the other animals survived and are doing well.

It is possible that we shall return to your corner in the forest on another occasion. In the meanwhile I should like to ask your help in the following: as you know, we caught some tsetse flies but they were all females. Female flies are more difficult to identify accurately than male flies where the morphology of the genitalia are characteristic and species specific. Would it be possible to ask some of your men to collect as many tsetses as possible and to send the flies in a small box by mail to Lwiro?

There were two species: (1) Glossina palpalis along the river and (2) Glossina fusca (large species) in the forest. It is possible that both species can be found closer to the river during the dry season than during the rains. The large species is probably easier to find during early morning and at dusk. Thank you in advance.

Please give my best regards to Mrs. Putnam.

Years of Adventure

Why call this chapter "Years of Adventure" when our entire colonial life seemed to be nothing else but. True enough, but the mid-fifties brought more than the average quota.

For instance my trip in 1954 to East Africa was certainly more exciting than a casual routine visit to that fine country. It promised elements of potential hazards from the start, mainly because it would take me to Mau Mau country at the height of the uprising of the secret sect of the Kikuyu tribe against the British settlers and the colonial occupants in general. The plight of the white farmers in the Kikuyu Highlands has been dramatized in Ruark's *Something of Value*. In spite of the horrid mutilations and killings, not only of white farmers but also of Africans working for them who refused to join the bloody revolt, most farmers stuck it out during the more than five years the blood bath lasted, planting and harvesting while protecting themselves with guns day and night, carrying on the pioneer spirit of their forebears.

"Life goes on", as the saying goes, and it was therefore not surprising when our director received one day an interesting price quotation from Carr Hartley, the well-known Kenya wildlife farmer, for two prime buffaloes raised at his Rumuruti ranch. Our director had been wrangling about the price for the two animals for some time. He intended to use them for observation and breeding experimentation at our IRSAC-Tshibati animal farm. Now Carr Hartley, feeling the pressure from the highly volatile political situation and the direct threat to his ranch, smack in the middle of Mau Mau country, was more forthcoming in meeting the BM's offer.

"Of course," BM was quoting to me from Hartley's letter, "You have to make your arrangements to transport the animals from my farm in Rumuruti to your place in the Congo."

BM was looking at me. I looked around the lab hoping to find other persons included in the conversation. There were none.

"You mean," I said.

"Yes, everything has been arranged for the transaction. All paper work is being prepared. The purchase has been approved. The accountant has managed (big deal!) to buy 25,000 shillings cash from the exchange bank. You can leave with Budiaki and the big lorry when it is ready."

Under normal circumstances, the opportunity of a free trip to Kenya would have drawn any number of "volunteers." Apparently, there had been no takers, this time, not even the most obvious candidate, Gillis the farm manager, a great fancier of East Africa where he had his wife had spent many years. Through elimination, and as BM's assistant, I was the next in line. Chardome, in the midst of important trypanosome transmission experiments, was not mentioned.

"How is the Mau Mau situation," I asked as casually as possible although this was my major concern, of course.

"Oh, rather calm these days" BM assured me, equally casually. "Of course, you never know," he added as an afterthought. "Therefore you can borrow my personal Smith-Wesson revolver."

He handed me the handgun.

"Now be careful," he warned, "I had no time to get a license for the weapon, so don't show it to anyone."

I wondered how I was to keep would-be attackers at bay saying:

"I have a gun but I can't show it to you," adding perhaps, "but I travel."

I opened the chamber: it was empty.

"Here is some ammunition," BM said, stuffing my hand full of snub-nosed bullets. "Very expensive," he added.

I promised not to waste any if I could avoid it. The whole scenario sounded by the minute more like a Humphrey Bogart film.

"Reyntiens has made adjustment to the body of the lorry to accommodate the buffaloes," BM went into details. "Don't forget to take a couple of buckets and some hay so that animals can be watered and fed on the way."

Desperately, I wondered whether I could come up with some valuable excuse such as break-through trypanosome experiments like Chardome; sick horses to be tended like Gillis; or desperately behind production of furniture like Reyntiens. But none came to my mind. I had my marching orders.

I went to see Reyntiens, the mechanic shops manager, about the changes of the lorry and to make sure it had been properly serviced and with extra fuel, spare parts and all the other things BM had mentioned.

"Some people have all the luck," he sighed, "I've never been in Kenya."

"Great country," I said "you should visit it sometime."

I left one day in September with Budiaki, the driver. I stayed the first night at the Mbarara Inn, Uganda, where I arrived late at night, securing a room from grumbling Blanche, the owner. The next day we reached Tororo on the Uganda-Kenya border, after another long drive of over 300 miles and put up at the Rock Hotel. So far, so good. We left Tororo early the next morning so that, barring Mau Mau or other incidents, we might be expected to reach Rumuruti before nightfall. As we left Tororo, we entered Kenya and into the "danger zone" although the main road to Nairobi was probably fairly safe.

After Broderick Falls the road reached the highlands with wonderful views of mountains, including Mount Elgon, vast fields of wheat and farms. In spite of my apprehension I admired those enormous expanses of wild country enhanced, strangely enough, by, so it seemed, judicious cultivation of the flat parts. Beyond Eldoret the road was completely void of any traffic—not a very encouraging sign I thought.

When we turned off from the main road at Nakuru onto the road leading deeper into the highlands, we entered Mau Mau country. We stopped at one of the Nakuru ndukas to buy gasoline. The owner, noticing our CB license plate, came out to chat. "They just found an African on the road with his tongue cut out," he said when he learned that we were on our way to Rumuruti. "Was loyal to his master, you know. I knew him well. Was a good bloke. A real shame, but that's the way they operate."

As I paid, he added encouragingly: "Well, good luck. Nothing has happened on the Rumuruti road yesterday or today, as far as we know. Don't stop for anyone or anything and you'll be all right. But keep going."

To keep going with a three-ton lorry along a twisting mountain road was a tall order, but Budiaki, a really good driver, and greatly spurred on by the shopkeeper's advice, did his very best. We reached Thomson's Falls in good time. And we had no trouble during the following 22 miles to Carr Hartley's place although the road, now only a track, made it more difficult to maintain good speed. So far, we hadn't passed a single vehicle when suddenly a man with a spear appeared next to the road. We passed in great hurry fearing he was the advance scout for a large ambush higher up.

The last miles seemed very long ones, but at last we pulled up to Carr Hartley's without incident. It was still early enough to make a quick tour of Hartley's enclosures with various captured wild animals peacefully grazing the lush pasture grasses, including a rhino so friendly that one could take it by the horn and even ride on its back—if it were in a good mood. The African guard warned: "lakini kama siku ingini iko nyama mbuya" ("however, other days it can be a bad animal").

Hartley's living room was exactly as I had imagined a rich planter's home to be: big, solid wooden walls, stylish furniture (from the old country, he proudly pointed out), deep comfortable chairs, the wooden floor covered with various animal skins, a crackling open fire guarded by two Dalmatians. Another family was sharing the Hartley's home after their own farm had been burned down and the cattle destroyed a few weeks before. They were thankful to have escaped with their lives. The conversation was not about loss, however, but rather centered around speculations about the future of the colony and their fear that Britain, that is, the Colonial Office, would give up, in which case there was serious talk about the need to defend "their" lands, in some cases owned for three or four generations, till the bitter end.

Anxious to get off early the next day, I was up at sunrise, but before we got the two buffaloes rounded up and into the truck, it was nearly noon. Then payment for the animals ran into a snag. That is to say, Mr. Hartley would not accept the cash money, an amount of 18,000 shillings, first because he did not want that amount of cash in the house and would have preferred a bank transfer; second, he was afraid that under the present circumstances it was against international regulations to bring in large amounts of cash, which he would have difficulty depositing without official approval. We hadn't thought of that. Anyway, he categorically refused the money, saying that he would get it from his friend, Dr. V. D. B., later on by some other means—not to worry about it. But I *was* worried. I was disconcerted that I should have to carry all that money once more strapped to my side in the paltry army sack.

"All is calm, for the moment," was Hartley's farewell. "You won't have any trouble to Thomson's Falls." He didn't seem willing to guarantee the rest of the way.

The lorry, now heavily laden with two live buffaloes, could not make the speed we had wanted. I actually did not want more speed, being afraid that over the rough roads the animals would get hurt or crushed while going too fast around a sharp bend. It was already late afternoon when we reached Nakuru and out of the number one danger zone. We had filled our tank at Thomson's Falls. It always felt good to have a full tank, in addition to our reserve 50-gallon drum, as the next station might be out of fuel.

Not wanting to risk driving in the dark to reach Eldoret, the next possibility for an overnight stay, I decided to stay in Nakuru. I put up at the Staggs Hotel, after having offered a bucket of water and hay to the buffaloes who seemed too carsick to bother. Carr Hartley was well known in Nakuru so that neither the hotel manager nor the servants thought too much of it when we parked the lorry and its live cargo in the courtyard.

We left the following morning, hoping to reach and stay the night in Kampala, Uganda. Then we would be out of the curfew zone and only one day away from our IRSAC-Astrida station. The buffaloes seemed in better spirits and were kicking each other. One incident that could have had nasty consequences marked the otherwise smooth progress. At one of our stops to water the buffaloes, Budiaki dropped the bucket between the buffaloes' legs. Of course, we just couldn't go in and retrieve the bucket without annoying them—and I hate to deal with annoyed buffaloes.

So, we agreed on the following plan: I would shunt the animals into the back of the truck while Budiaki, leaning across the sideboards and holding fast to my hand would, with the other hand, try to retrieve the bucket. It almost worked except that at the last moment one of the buffaloes suddenly moved up within an inch of crushing Budiaki's head against the headboard. He had barely time to grab my arm and pull himself up, but in the process he released the bucket which, once more, crashed between the buffaloes' legs. A bit shaken, we repeated the performance, the second time with success. The buffaloes eyed us with great disdain.

On the way up to Rumuruti, we reported to the custom's officer at the Tororo Uganda-Kenya border. I wanted to report my return and was greatly annoyed to find the custom's office closed. Not daring to wait perhaps several hours for his return, and being caught on the road during curfew—Kampala was still

130 miles away—we pushed off, planning to report to the Kampala authorities.

It was near sunset as we drove into Kampala. Anxious to get official matters over so that we could start early the next day, I asked Budiaki to stop at the first police station, which was near the town's center. I was introduced to the officer in charge, Lt. Swan, a severe but not unfriendly looking chap, young, fair, his freshly starched uniform lending him an appearance of great efficiency. I presented my passport and explained my business. The mentioning of the two buffaloes seemed to amuse him. As he looked at my passport, a sergeant who had stood by and looked at me rather intently for the last minutes, bent over Swan's shoulder and whispered something in his ear. I was able to catch the word "Mombasa." As if the sergeant had stabbed Swan with a long needle or applied a mild electric shock, the lieutenant suddenly sat up, glared at me, his smile all at once gone, his mouth fixed in, what I thought, a sinister twist. Even before Lt. Swan spoke I knew that something was terribly wrong. It seemed as if the lights dimmed, turning an unhealthy green hue, and a cold stream of air swept the stark room. It felt as if a cozy room with an open fire and two Dalmatians had suddenly turned into an ice box, the fire out and the two Dalmatians replaced by the same number of hungry wolves.

"Tell me, Mr. Lambrecht," Swan began his interrogation, "Where were you last night?"

I was so taken aback that my fumbling to answer and my hesitations could only confirm my interrogator's cherished suspicions, whatever they were. "Why, I spent the night at the Staggs Hotel in Nakuru," I replied after a while.

"From what time to what time?", was the next question. "Please remember that we shall verify your reply." He didn't say "statement"—yet.

"Oh, I hope so," I said in sudden defiance. "I arrived from Carr Hartley's place in Rumuruti at about five o'clock in the afternoon and left the hotel this morning at about six." "May I ask you why all this questioning?" I added, now terribly afraid and at the same time annoyed.

"This is a serious affair, Mr. Lambrecht." Lt. Swan suddenly took the bull by the horn, so to speak, "I have to ask your permission to search your belongings before we proceed," and gave a sign to the sergeant, who took my army bag and handed it over to Swan.

The room suddenly turned hot once more, but the lights grew dimmer. I shuddered because I knew what was to follow and that I would be put in an even more precarious position, than I was in at that point. Up to now, I thought that the whole procedure had perhaps something to do with the Mau Mau; perhaps something that had taken place on the road we had traveled.

"Ah, ah," came the triumphant voice of Swan, fishing out delicately the Smith-Wesson revolver. An even more triumphant, "Oh, oh," followed when he retrieved the bundle of 100 shilling notes. "Now this is very interesting."

I was stunned, as if the two buffaloes had suddenly crushed my head against the headboard, which I would have preferred at this point.

"Do you have a license or permit for this gun?" It sounded like a rather inoffensive question, but Swan's cutting voice promised more was to come.

"No," I said, "the gun is not mine; it belongs to a friend who gave it to me for my protection in Mau Mau territory."

"And who might this friend be?" Another slash.

"I cannot tell. I do not want to cause him trouble. He gave it in good faith," meekly from me.

Lt. Swan emitted a dry laugh that could have shaved inches from a soft-wood board.

"You are in far more trouble than your friend. You see, Mr. Lambrecht (I began to hate my name), you see, Mr. Lambrecht, a rich merchant was murdered early yesterday in Mombasa, killed with a gun like yours. The murderer escaped with roughly 25,000 shillings, the same sum we find in your possession. The assassin was dressed in khaki, as you are, and carried an army bag just like yours. The rest of the assassin's description couldn't fit you better," he added with the final flourish of a successful prosecutor.

The ground under my chair collapsed. I was falling in a deep, dark shaft. My vision became blurred. I could not think straight. My brain was frozen. Surely, this was a dream. I would wake up soon. But I didn't. It was real.

"The name of the owner of the gun, Mr. Lambrecht. The name of the owner of the gun, Mr. Lambrecht," echoed Swan's voice from high up the shaft. I was still falling, the head of

Swan outlined far away against the ghastly greenish bare electric light. I struggled to get my voice back. When I did, there was nothing else for me to do but to confess that the gun belonged to Dr. V. D. B., director of the IRSAC Institute and that I had no permit to carry it. That was bad enough, but it was still better than to face a murder charge, although I could not figure out whether my confession was for the better or worse.

"Thank you, Mr. Lambrecht," came Swan's voice, now suddenly close as I seemed to have resurfaced from my hole in the floor, "that will help." He didn't elaborate in which way. "Now let us go over your story again, and see if you want to add or change anything. Of course, we shall check your statement with third persons."

Since I had confessed about the ownership of the gun, things seemed to clear in my mind. At least I had nothing more to hide, and as Lt. Swan began reading my statement, I began to tote up the scoreboard inside my head: "Swan versus Lambrecht" as follows: Swan had all the evidence: the gun, the 18,000 shillings, the army bag, my description and clothing. Lambrecht had all the alibis: my stay with Carr Hartley, the night spent at Staggs Hotel, a possible statement from Budiaki who, I supposed, would be or had already been interrogated, and, of course, the two buffaloes. No assassin or burglar travels with two buffaloes as far as I could remember from Agatha Christie's novels. Of course, it could be argued that the animals were cover-ups. Hardly. Even Swan must have thought that I would not go to that extent unless—suddenly my heart shrank again—unless I had also murdered the chap who was the owner of both the lorry and the buffaloes. I could read in Lt. Swan't mind, as they say in detective books, and I didn't like what I read. How would this thing end, I wondered. But then again, why should I be so impertinent as to go to the police station to have my passport checked *if I had done something wrong* when I could have slipped out of town quietly and driven out of Uganda without seeing any Swans? All these things whirled inside my head, but I could not as yet sort them out reasonably and evaluate them.

"Right," Swan said as I was still trying to sort things out, "I shall have to ask you to spend the night in Kampala. I suggest the Victoria Hotel (exactly my plan, I thought, relieved that I was not going to be locked up, at least not immediately) and to report to me tomorrow, let's say nine, shall we?" "I shall have to keep your bag and contents in custody until then," he added, obviously expecting no objection on my part.

I nodded, not sure whether to thank him. Outside, the night, although dark and cold, felt lovely. Budiaki was waiting for me by the truck. The buffaloes were quiet and silent as if asleep. For them it had been a long day too. We drove to the Victoria Hotel, THE HOTEL in Kampala, with its stately rooms, its solid English furniture and respectable atmosphere. The smell of dinner met me as I registered at the desk. The Hindu clerk looked up as I wrote my name and—was I growing super-sensitive?—with a twinkle in his eyes that made me believe that I had been expected, no doubt informed by Swan.

Anyway, I got a nice room on the second floor where I was more than happy to shower away the grit of truck travel and some of my blackest thoughts. As I left my room, I noticed someone in the corridor ostensibly reading a newspaper—at this time of the day? An excellent dinner restored some of my confidence and even the presence of the chap in the hallway, now without doubt my "guard," could not dampen my spirits. I hadn't done it, had I? Worn out by the long exciting day, I slept profoundly and without interruption.

In broad daylight, Lt. Swan looked less sinister than the previous evening—very matter of fact. "You can go now, Mr. Lambrecht," he said without preliminaries. "Here is your bag and the money. Please verify and sign this form of repossession. I shall have to keep the gun, however, as it was brought illegally into this country." "A serious offense," he added with returning aggressiveness.

I made a faint attempt at arguing for the gun, but was willing to let that go before the stony stare of Swan. I was only too glad to leave the police station and to put many, many miles between Kampala and me.

My story swept through Lwiro like wildfire. Everybody thought my encounter with the Uganda police hilarious. No one congratulated me for having brought two live buffaloes a thousand miles out of Mau Mau country. BM was very annoyed at the loss of his handgun.

Many times I felt the urge to write Lt. Swan asking whether they had caught the real murderer. But what if they hadn't? Wouldn't my curiosity seem suspicious? I never did write him. Perhaps he will read these lines and let me know.

Irangi

The forest: the cradle of the primates, among them the precursors of Man; warm and hostile, beloved and feared, a climax of maximum condition for growth and diversity.

The first forest communities appeared during the Carboniferous, 350 million years ago. They have since evolved into present primeval forests as found in the Congo, where they cover the whole of the Congo River watershed as they once had the whole of Africa and the other continents. Man and the forest have always enjoyed an ambivalent relationship. Man, the hunter, dwelled in the forest for food and shelter. But man, the agriculturalist, as he later became, cut the forest to plant his crops. The larger the human population grew and the more efficient its implements, the bigger the areas of deforestation became. In Britain, for instance, a country once entirely covered by forests, now only five percent is still under trees.

The largest, unbroken, unspoiled remaining areas of rain forest are the tropical forests of Southeast Asia, South America and Africa, occupying the high rain zones straddling the equator.

The great diversity of ecological niches in the tropical rain forests accounts for the equally great variety in other life forms. Examining in detail a patch of forest is like opening a book on natural history. Not surprisingly, therefore, several IRSAC researchers proposed to establish a permanent field station in the forest west of Lwiro—the more so because a motorable road crosses the "shoulder" of the Biega-Kahuzi range and descended along the western flank of the Itumbo range and the valley of the River Luhoho, where the mountain forest dominated by *Hagenia abyssinica* changes to give way to rain forest tree species. Here the high mountain ridges and flanks have been scarred by eons of erosion into repeated deep gullies, each carrying its load of the high rainfall towards the bottom of the main valley, forming so many tributaries of the Congo River, 200 miles to the west. The overall panorama resembles a great sheet of crushed cardboard. The road drops gradually from its highest point of near 6,000 ft. to below 2,000 ft., with correlated climatic changes and corresponding faunal and floral life zones. The succession of the life zones and their extension into the lowland forest were the major attractions of our interest in this area.

It is a sunny, bright day in July 1953. A large, green stationwagon cautiously negotiates the first downgrade of the Walikale road from its highest point into the Luhoho River valley. The passengers are BM, director; James Chapin, ornithologist; Paul Pirlot, zoologist; and I, driver.

Exclaims BM: "What a view." I: "Road very slippery." Pirlot: "Many people get carsick on this road." Chapin: "Stop, I have seen a white-breasted, fan-tailed hornbill."

BM, after the hornbill is lost in the foliage: "This is a most wonderful spot, but we should go farther down, lower into the valley where the lowland forest begins. I can see it, a nice log cabin in the middle of a clearing at the bank of a clear stream."

"There are no tsetse here, too cold, but there should be lower down," I say, catching BM's enthusiasm for the log cabin in the rain forest.

"They must be most difficult to find, I'm sure," enjoins Pirlot, "but monkeys are probably abundant."

"This reminds me," dreams Chapin, "back in 1927, we had a camp along the Ituri River. . . ."

On the way down we pass several spots that seem suitable for a permanent forest station, the object of our journey, but one of us comes up with an objection, and we need 100 percent approval. We drive past Bunyakiri. We do another 20 miles and keep in mind two locations that seem to meet approval of all.

"No use going any farther," BM says. "We must decide upon one of the two suitable places we passed on the way up." "Turn around at the next opportunity," he adds for my benefit.

I find a place a few miles farther along near a group of huts with room to turn around in a clearing. Driving into the open space I am about to back into the road when Chapin shouts "Wait, I want to have a look at all those birds across the river."

The river, the Luo, is indeed only about 30 yards away. "Look!" cries Pirlot excitedly, "a band of Colobus monkeys is crossing the canopy above the river!"

"And why," asks BM, "should we not adopt this spot?" in a style probably similar to that of Christopher Columbus when he spoke to his ship's company on that historical day and declared, "This, my friends, is India."

"Splendid spot," agrees Chapin, talking through his binoculars and his pipe.

"Absolutely marvelous," affirms Pirlot, eyeing the disappearing monkeys with regret.

"First class," I express my uninvited opinion. "The forest looks super; the river is a beauty; I wonder if tsetse flies. . . ."

And so IRSAC's Irangi Field Research Station is born.

I spent many lonely days and nights at Irangi Field Station—lonely simply because I was alone, not because I felt so. Just observing the forest wall across the river was entertainment. At the first light I could see the mist generated by the damp forest inwards, rising slowly in the warming air. I lay on my back, comfortably tucked in sheets and blankets on my camp bed, gazing through the mosquito net at the spectacle of a day being born. Since the first days, I never slept in the rather confined sleeping quarters of the narrow wooden cabin, but had my camp bed moved outside on the porch, despite the rumors of prowling leopards. I never slept so well but on the few occasions when raging thunderstorms chased me inside.

In a way, Irangi was a bit like Pawa. The same smell of close vegetation, the vibrant silence, the agitations of the bolikoko, the sudden cackle of monkeys or the mysterious snap and fall of a branch.

The evenings were long, however, and I did a lot of letter writing; copies of these helped reconstitute this autobiography. One very long letter to my friend in Australia is a fair description of the field station and its activities at that time. It reads thus:

It is Sunday morning. The Luo River murmurs peacefully past the walls of trees at the edge of the forest. Whiffs of tattered morning mist escape from the tree-clad hills. The sound of wood chopping. The laboratory, the center of bustling activity during the week, stands silent. The camp is full of paradoxes, the latest scientific apparatus to be seen in the same line of vision as implements from the stone age. Two calabashes used to fill our water tank from the river below rest against the pole of a self-registering rain gauge. Dawili is filling the kerosene lantern near the tree stump onto which we have fixed our dome-shaped actinometer that measures sun intensities on a revolving drum. Samson, the wood-cutter, wields a nasty-looking machete with the hand that only yesterday manipulated the tiny scalpel to remove the salivary glands from a mosquito.

The station is built on the left bank of the river. The first structure, a prefabricated aluminum hut, has been replaced by a permanent wooden hut, containing, reading from left to right, a barza (porch), a dining room, a bedroom and a small bathroom, all in a row like a Pullman carriage. The bedroom, for instance, has superimposed bunks, a pair on each side with a narrow passage in the middle. From the barza we have a superb view of the river. My camp bed occupies the side parallel with the river. In front of the barza is the old laboratory. The mud-and-wattle structure now serves as a botanical specimen storeroom, while a new laboratory has been installed in what used to be the garage. The camp has seen many changes over the three years since it was built. From the start, a series of new discoveries and the accumulation of puzzle-generating facts has kept us all spellbound. Popularity of the station has grown, not only among naturalists but also picnickers from Lwiro, for whom a 60-mile drive enables them to spend a weekend in the real forest.

Behind our hut, on the river side, we have two rows of self-made cages made from sticks and covered with fencing wire. In them we have an average of about 20 monkeys of the three species found in the nearby forest. Besides their study by the zoologist they also serve as bait animals in a certain type of mosquito trap. Other animals are kept because we know they are infected with a blood parasite we want to study. For instance, at the moment we keep several *Atherurus africanus centralis*, in which I discovered recently a new rodent *Plasmodium*. But the mind of a biologist/naturalist works in a devious way. Not content with the discoveries of the new malarial parasite, we are now looking into where it comes from. As all mammal plasmodia are transmitted by *Anopheles* mosquitoes, we have been collecting mosquitoes in and near porcupine holes and rock shelters. We have found an *Anopheles* mosquito, also perhaps a new species, and feel sure that our dissections of its salivary glands will show infections with *our* malaria parasite. Fascinating, what!

In the same quarter of the camp with the animal cages are three huts for the animal caretakers. In the other half of the station are ten huts for our regular African personnel. One big hut, grandiose in proportion compared with the others is a house, fenced all around, built by our African laboratory assistant and general supervisor. It looks a bit like the town hall of a small village. These buildings border a kind of central plaza in which I had young oil palms planted three years ago. Half of their number has fallen victim to the unending soccer games of the small children running around in the "African Quarter." The other half is growing beautifully, now commanding respect from the soccer players. I look at the survivors with pride, imagining how, when I shall long be gone, people may still reap the fruits and press the oil to make the delicious native "moambe" dish.

Some parts of our mosquito research program require daily observations, including Sundays. So today you may find a chap climbing one of the trees in the compound to a lower branch where an 8-inch-high bamboo section has been attached. The tree climber inserts a long glass tube into the bamboo cup and, by means of a rubber bulb attached to one end of the tube, removes water from the bottom. This is transferred to a glass jar until the bamboo section is empty. The jar is then lowered with a string to another chap waiting below. He pours the cloudy water into a white enamel bowl. If you look carefully, you will see any number of wriggling creatures: mosquito larvae. We have dozens of such artificial larvae traps on both sides of the river and farther inside the forest. They inform us about some of the mosquito species present, their breeding dynamics and seasonal fluctuations, activities all very innocent and quite routine to us, but often baffling to occasional layman visitors.

One day a traveler stopped at the camp and, as he was talking to me, he noticed one of the fly-boys collecting something bulky from underneath the large monkey cage.

"What is he doing?" he asked.

"Collecting excrement of the monkeys," I said with an apologetic smile. "It is going to be put at the base of a tree in the forest," I tried to explain.

"Oh," he said, looking at me in a certain way.

"Just an experiment." I desperately wanted to close the subject.

"Ah," he wanted to continue, a suspicious gleam in his eyes.

"To attract tsetse flies," I had to admit, feeling like an idiot.

"Eh," he said, and I could see that he had made up his mind. "How far did you say Walikale is from here?"

The description of Irangi Station is now complete but for one last structure that looks very much like any kind of small mud-and-wattle hut. It contains what the botanist cares to call the botanical specimens drying oven.

Past the botanical contraption a path leads towards the river. When we first established the camp, a hanging "bridge" connected the two banks. It was a lovingly, romantic affair of intricate liana-work, precariously hung from vines that naturally descended from the canopy above. Unfortunately, repairs could not keep up with deterioration. Also we feared that the flimsy structure would not be able to support the heavy equipment we had to take across into the forest. So we resorted to the traditional "bac" (ferry), common on all Congo rivers.

Our ferry consisted of a wooden platform, about 8 by 8 feet, rigged onto six empty 50-gallon gasoline drums welded together on a steel frame. A sturdy handrail enclosed the platform on all four sides, two of which could be unhinged when loading bulky materials. I hoped we were better biologists than engineers because the navigational characteristic of the contraption was one of the worst invented by man. On a smooth lake the ferry might have worked satisfactorily. Pulled across the turbulent Luo River, the craft developed submergible tendencies, the swift current forcing one side under water. Trying to counterbalance the effect by scurrying to the other side seemed to make things worse. At first we navigated the ferry across by pulling along a single vine strung across the stream. The picture that developed in our minds the day the vine would break made us decide to seek a safer solution. The botanist said he didn't want to see himself carried all the way down the Lowa and into the Congo River and out into the Atlantic Ocean. This we assured him would never happen as the crocodiles would get him long before that.

Now the ferry is hooked onto two trolleys running along a steel cable attached to a big tree on opposite banks. The vine is still used for pulling. The support of the trolleys helps to make crossing somewhat smoother—and a lot safer.

During early morning when shadows are still deep, the view during the crossing is quite spectacular. Kingfishers may be seen darting about and the first insects begin to buzz, their wings like transparent gold against the sun. Low-hanging leaves are gently rocked playfully by the stream, their shadows floating up and down on the glittering surface. The wall of tropical vegetation looks invitingly cool, but seemingly inpenetrable. But as one lands, the wall opens up, revealing a three-dimensional Walt Disney decor. The giant *Macrolobium* trees stand strong, silent and straight. Undergrowth is surprisingly scarce while the sky is blotted out by the kaleidoscopic view of the canopy some 100 feet above. Notice the almost complete absence of grasses. This is explained, of course, by the lack of sunlight. Absence of humus is typical of tropical forests and accounts for the low fertility of its soils. The reason for the lack of humus is related to the climatic conditions which consume the fallen leaves almost immediately as a result of an accelerated process of chemical decomposition. In the temperate climates the leaves falling at the beginning of winter have time to be buried and undergo a slow, latent rotting process, releasing, as it were, measured dose amounts of life-sustaining materials ready to be absorbed at the time when spring spurs growth again.

Under the twilight of the giants' canopy grows a population of small saplings, erect, evenly spaced it seems waiting—waiting for the giant to fall one day and to die, so that they can get a place in the sun and a chance to grow and push their own crown towards the life-giving sunlight.

From the landing stage of the ferry, a path leads to the ridge of a steep hill, 55 meters above the Luo River. Representative of similar terrain in every other direction, the hill is the site of bustling scientific activity. The path was laid down during our own first days of exploration when we decided upon a program of research. The path soon became a kind of mud slide that, going down, needs occasional checking of speed by grabbing vegetation along the way before one meets the river. Improvements have been made by cutting out steps reinforced by sticks. Along this path you will see a number of things normally not encountered in virgin forests, such as wooden signs with numbers, black on white, one every 60 meters. These are "catching stations" for tsetse flies. At each of them, three "fly-boys" stop, three times a day every day, to search for tsetse flies. The catch is recorded for each "catching station" noting the insect's sex, hunger stage, the vegetation on which they were resting and height. The flies are then marked by means of color oil paint and released. This is the routine "fly-round."

Other trees are marked with numbers, this time white on black, as part of a botanical survey. They mark transects, called "Catenas," in which vegetation species and communities are recorded.

At certain points along the path, the soil has been hoed and raked smooth as if someone were going to plant radishes. Not at all. More activity of the tsetse people. It is supposed to help find out how many times and what kinds of animals live near the places where we catch tsetse flies and, therefore, could serve as potential host animals on which they feed.

The open drum you see lying carelessly on its side is not a sign of sloppiness. It is supposed to provide a shelter for *Anopheles* mosquitoes. This is in connection with our search for the carriers of our new *Plasmodium*. They are collected daily and have their salivary glands removed in the lab for signs of plasmodium infection.

We arrive at a tree on which a number of steps have been built. It leads to an artificial mosquito breeding place, that is a bamboo section as explained above.

Why do you stop so brusquely? Oh, yes, I forgot to warn you; the small Trojan horse without a head in the middle of the path is called a Morris trap. It is supposed to catch tsetse flies through a slot in its belly while one is reading the *London Times* or other informative literature in camp. The form, suggesting to the fly the shape of an animal, is, to quote an authority in this matter, "more appreciated by the entomologist than by the tsetse fly." Unquote. But our hopes are high.

And now I want you to stand back and take off your hat. So far, you have been led from small, if strange things, to more complicated methods of research. We have built up to a climax, so to speak. As you round the top of the hill, you see IT. Like Manhattan around the bend of the Hudson River. THE PLATFORM. We have this structure close to our heart maybe because it was such a major undertaking with so many unknowns. It is, in fact, an intrusion into the privacy of the forest canopy because that is where the highest ladder of this contraption leads. It is an intricate structure of poles and sticks and vines seemingly defying laws of gravity and rationale. Making use of the steep slope of the hill, first a kind of bridge was built that linked it to a huge limbali tree. The bridge forms a first-level platform as it reaches the tree at about 40 feet above the forest floor. From here, a complicated array of ladders to conform with the shape of the tree, leads to a second landing platform, and then a third, where the level of the canopy itself is reached. At each of the three platforms, and at ground level, catches are made of insects and other observations carried out including metereological recordings. The first platform looks somewhat like the local pub, a tank of carbon dioxide standing next to a table with a series of glasses above which a round "light-trap" swings in the wind. The botanist suggested that we attach a poster: "Guiness Is Good For You." Carbon dioxide is fed into the modified "light-trap" on the theory that it will improve attraction of mosquitoes. The tray with the glasses is our day's collection of mosquito larvae from the various artificial and natural breeding places. At other times, the platforms look like a zoo with all kinds of caged animals underneath small-sized mosquito nets hung again with the intention of attracting bloodsucking insects. Watch out not to get your hair caught in the several rolls of flypaper I have hung in various places. At the moment, the upper level is occupied by one of the Trojan horses.

Our path, known as "fly-round I," goes down the other side of the hill. Halfway down the slope a mosquito net is hanging between the trees. The site is *not* the camp of one of those hard-boiled Congo pioneers roughing it. Its purpose is to catch mosquitoes which, attracted by the bright white patch against the dark forest, will investigate and, flying inside the net from the lower open edge, try to escape by flying upwards where they can be collected at any time. I was delighted when the device also caught a few tsetse flies.

We go down and reach a small stream called Nyamutalo. Its crystal-clear water runs along a quartzite-sand bottom between flat rocks, convenient stepping stones for crossing, but watch out. Oh, I *am* sorry. I should have warned you, the rocks are treacherously slippery. Not to worry, though. Farther on a patch of dark mud, to be crossed on wet tree trunks among entangled creepers, will probably get you anyway. By now, excitement, provocation and sheer folly suppress your usually prudent nature. Wet from perspiration—the ambient humidity 90 percent—bothered by flies, you swab, sweep and get hooked by a thorn; you slip in the mud, a fire ant stings you in the neck and you swear and you fight and crash through the entanglement without further regard for your best pair of shorts. You scratch your neck and now you have mud there too. But you have almost made it. Terra firma is in sight: a hill higher and steeper still. On this one you work with both feet and hands to get to the top. As you stand panting and gaze into the next valley, a roaring sound meets you: the rapids and falls of the Lutunguru River. Down near the edge of the bank the noise and sight of the rushing waters are hypnotizing. Watch your step because the roots on which we stand are the only support. Underneath the earth has been washed away. The river tumbles high from the rocks, forcing its way down natural steps and steeper cascades, past huge boulders in a perpetual rush towards the sea. You have to shout if you want to say something. Spray is everywhere, refreshing and drenching. The trees lining the banks are twisted in crazy shapes, their trunks padded with spongy mosses. "Old man's beard" epiphytes, glistening with moisture, wave in the wind like shredded curtains. It is a strange world.

At this point, the river is about 50 feet wide. Undermined by the current, a middle-aged tree has fallen across. My courage whipped up by sound and sight, I once walked across on this tree until I reached halfway. Then I sat down gingerly, hypnotized and terribly frightened. For many minutes I did not dare to move. It took all my will power to do something to get to the other side. I did not dare to stand up, but completed the other half of the journey, not step by step, but "behind-by-behind."

A visiting Dutch biologist who was making a sketch map of the area in which he was to make a one-year research project was kind enough to mark his map: "Lambrecht Falls." This was a return courtesy as some weeks earlier I had shown him an almost as lovely waterfall in another valley which I had christened "Laarman Falls." I doubt very much that in these times the names will become official! But they serve the purpose of landmarks and our ego as well!

You are now aware of Irangi's many attractions. I wish I could add the sounds and smells.

Yours aye,

More About Irangi

Among many other papers, reports and old letters at the bottom of a trunk, I found, one day, part of a diary related to the period before King Leopold III's first visit. Among the letters was one dated 22 June 1955, which describes the visit of the reigning Belgian King, King Boudewijn I (Flemish spelling), to our research center at Lwiro. The letter seems a good introduction to the period of great activity that would follow.

Dear J & J,
Things here have been rather lively lately. The main event of last week was the visit of the king to Lwiro. It was a lovely morning at the start of the dry season, when the air is still clear enough to see the distant volcanoes. The king arrived in an open convertible, a black De Soto, accompanied by the Governor General, Mr. Petillon, and the Governor of the Kivu Province, Mr. Brasseur. Our station was bulging with press photographers and amateur cineastes. The grounds were so overstocked with them that in any picture the rate of photographers/king was about twelve to one. The sound of whirling movie cameras was like that of the furious activity of a beehive on a fine spring morning. This was the setting when the car bearing the royal license plate 1 stopped in front of the laboratories, and the king, with a large smile, stepped out and was met by our director, Professor vanden Berghe. From the start, the king seemed to inspire a sense of informality which persisted throughout his visit. The relaxed atmosphere made everyone feel at ease. He was led to the new wing of the library and asked to sign the "livre d'or." We were astonished at the apparent total absence of security guards and the lack of formality. Arriving in the Prof's private office, the king sat down on the first low table, mopping his brow with a sigh, giving the impression that he thought not very highly about the job of being king. Having signed the visitors' book, he was led into the various laboratories, where he was introduced to staff in charge. I had the honor of being presented as the one in charge of tsetse fly research. Our work in the Mutara region was explained. He peeped down into a microscope to look at a tsetse fly, one of the very few flies to receive that honor, no doubt. Everywhere he showed keen, genuine interest in what was going on. The party then proceeded to the guesthouse where the wives of staff were assembled. Eyes flashed modestly, eyelashes quivered prudishly; you could have knocked the ladies down with a feather. The king is very good-looking and very friendly. He was a big hit! At noon, he had lunch at the

Prof's house at Tshibati, in the company of James Chapin, the ornithologist who has been with us for the last two years studying bird migrations. Dr. VDB later told us that the lunch had been a complete success, again because of the king's relaxed manners. Most of the conversation centered around Chapin's present and previous work in the Congo—he worked in the Pawa area in 1904–07! In the heat of the conversation Chapin, who otherwise speaks excellent French, kept forgetting that the king is always to be addressed in the third person. Thus: "Votre Altesse," or "Votre Majesté." The king didn't bat an eye. Informality reached new heights when Chapin brought in a tray with a selection of brightly colored stuffed birds. The scene, as described by VDB, was, reading from left to right: the king down on one knee, bending over the tray with stuffed birds, the governor general on both knees examining same birds, while lesser subjects such as the Prof and Chapin were comfortably sipping their after-lunch coffee in easy chairs. The *Grand Maréchal* of the Court stood stiffly by the chimney, a monocle in his left eye, wondering, no doubt, what had become of royal protocol. Chapin then offered one of the birds to the king, a bird with feathers the colors of the Belgian flag: red, yellow and black. The *Grand Maréchal* was visibly shocked when the king happily accepted, asking Chapin to send the bird *personally* to his palace in Brussels. So the next day a parcel left the Bukavu post office labeled: A Sa Majesté le Roi Baudoin, Palais Royal, Bruxelles.

For me the king's visit was just an episode in a very hectic month. It had been quite inconvenient for me to be absent from my work in the Mutara, where I was about to wind up my research to begin a similar project in the Bugesera region, and it was possible for me to be in Lwiro only when the date of the king's visit was changed from 29 May to 4 June.

Immediately after the king's visit I was on safari once more—this time with Dora and Dick. I had to see people at the tsetse research center in Tororo, Uganda, and it was an occasion for Dora to make one more safari before her departure for Europe on 3 July. After a one night stopover in my camp in Mutara, we reached Tororo the next afternoon. The Uganda roads are quite good, long stretches even paved! This may sound funny to you people who don't know an unpaved road! We stayed a couple of days in Nairobi, Kenya, the busy business center of British East Africa. We visited Entebbe, on the shores of Lake Victoria, headquarters of the Virus Research Laboratory. Dick behaved rather well and seems to like travel, although the Land Rover is far from comfortable! The travel gene must be a dominant trait in the family, I suppose.

The next important event will be the departure of the family for Europe. Dora, Winnie, Jessie and Dick will leave Bukavu by plane on 3

July. With stopovers at Karthoum, Cairo and Athens, they arrive the following day in Brussels. After a few weeks at the seaside, it will be school for Winnie and Jessie. I shall leave Lwiro about February in 1956 for my regular home leave.

Hope to get a line from you. Best wishes and cheerio.

Your brother,

The period covered by the following diary extracts was one of great personal activity in Irangi. I had planned and started a complete mosquito inventory of the forest bordering the Luo River, a one square mile area. Furthermore, I was aware of the presence of at least two tsetse fly species, *Glossina palpalis*-group and a *fusca*-group fly, several of which had been occasionally captured. It was especially the large *fusca*-group fly that intrigued me. The more so when it proved to be *Glossina vanhoofi*, known only from the Congo forest and described only once in 1939. Nothing was known about its biology. What was particularly perplexing was its great elusiveness and its reluctance to attack man. The few specimens had been caught almost casually while walking along the road—hardly a forest fly habitat! Probably they were stray flies on a binge.

Another reason for spending many days in Irangi during this period was that Dora and family had left on an extended home leave. Under the circumstances, I did not mind taking up a long and lonely vigil looking for the shy *G. vanhoofi* while also working on my project of cataloging the mosquito fauna.

I was not always alone. Besides myself, others had come under Irangi's spell: Christiaensen, a botanist; Laarman, a visiting scientist from Holland; and occasional other IRSAC members or foreign researchers.

Wednesday, July 13, 1955
Leave Lwiro at 9; arrive at Irangi at noon. Install mosquito light-trap along the Fulongo River. Search for adult mosquitoes not fruitful. Join C. (Christiaensen) at the slope of Nyamitalo Hill. Decide to build an observation platform in the canopy. Select a huge *Gilbertiodendron dewevrei*, a dominant rain forest tree species in this part of the Congo Basin. Leave the capita and eight men to prepare the materials and to start the lower landing. As the tree is standing on a steep slope, this will not be too

difficult. Murebwa has captured two *G. palpalis*, but failed to find pupae sites. Back to camp at 13:30. Various activities during the afternoon. L. (Laarman) returns from Lwiro at 18:00 with a supply of CO_2 tanks to be used as bait for his mosquito traps.

Our evening meal is interrupted by the arrival of the D.C. and the Bukavu urbanist, whose vehicle (clutch) broke down a few miles away. We lend them our IRSAC car so that they can return to Walikale and, hopefully, find a mechanic.

Thursday, July 14, 1955

Into the forest with L. and his CO_2 tanks. My light-traps have caught only one *Anopheles* and two *Culex* mosquitoes. This may be because the lamp was out due to lack of kerosene, one of the men say. Install the CO_2 tanks and walk back to Nyamitalo Hill to inspect work on the platform. Back to camp at 13:30. Find C. in conversation with the D.C., who had returned our station wagon. Back to the forest with L. at 16:00 to prepare our mosquito traps for the night. A dark menacing sky soon transforms into a drizzle that gradually takes heart and joyfully turns into a downpour, leaving us just enough time to set the traps. Our descent from the hill is toboggan style. I divide my army "anti-gas" cape into two pieces so that each of us may have some kind of protection. Back in camp at 17:30. The D.C. is still there but when he wants to borrow our vehicle, we find that the battery is dead. At that moment, another visitor pops in, a geologist from Bukavu. This gives the D.C. the opportunity to return to Walikale, and leaves the three of us once more to ourselves with a dead battery. The rain has stopped.

Friday, July 15, 1955

I have hurt my ankle during the slide down the hill the previous day and decided to stay in camp. L. and C. go to check the traps and the progress of the platform. In the meanwhile, I paint two signboards to be placed a mile or so on either side of the camp entrance warning travelers of two-way traffic over this part of the road. (I have failed to mention that over most parts the road is one-way traffic, the direction alternating with every day of the week with the exception of Sundays when traffic is allowed in both directions.)

Ankle feels better, so go to check on the work on the platform. Stay there until 13:30. Work is progressing well. Catch one *G. vanhoofi* and a Chrysops fly. On the way back meet C. back from a botanical specimens collection. In camp at 14:10. L. returns at 15:10 and leaves again at 17:30 to check his traps. My trap has caught two *Anopheles* and 5 Culex mosquitoes, but the lamp, once more, was out of kerosene. The workers come back with seven more Chrysops flies.

Saturday, July 16, 1955

The small field clinic started for our workers and families attracts more and more people from surrounding villages that we were not aware existed. Today is no exception and a long line of patients awaits me. Another reason for today's popularity is that it is Saturday, when many people are traveling and take the opportunity to air their complaints "en passant." Among the patients is an eight-year-old girl with a large, ugly tropical ulcer near her ankle. From experience I know that it will take weeks, months even, to heal and only through constant cleaning, disinfecting and frequent dressing of the wound. So I advise her mother to stay at Irangi until the next transport can take them to Lwiro hospital.

Travel by road to Km. 104 where a small self-help ferry allows the crossing of the Luo near the village of Makwe. The ferry being on the other side, Mutembezi, one of the mosquito boys, climbs along the cable to fetch the ferry from the other bank. A one-and-a-half hour walk brings us to the village of Mai. Most villagers are away at a distant market. A survey of a few inhabited huts reveals no Anopheles mosquitoes. We collect several larvae of this mosquito tribe, however, along the banks of a small stream. I also observe Simulium larvae and pupae attached to rocks beneath the water surface—a classical Simulium site. The adult of this tiny fly is the vector of the dreaded disease onchocerciasis, better known as "river blindness." I also catch a very dark Chrysops fly. This fly is the vector of another filaria worm, *Loa loa*, that also causes eye problems.

Sunday, July 17, 1955

Today is Sunday. It is the second birthday of our son Richard.

L. leaves for Lwiro, returning with his wife and another IRSAC member who came for a visit. My intention to visit the platform is cut short by a steady, heavy rain lasting till sunset. Everything is miserably dripping and soggy wet.

Monday, July 18, 1955

In the forest at eight. Change mosquito light-trap from the bank of the Fulongo to the top of the hill. Then join C. to supervise the construction of the platform. During the evening I go to check to see if the light-traps are still in place and alight. Starts to rain as I return.

During the night I am wakened by someone bringing mail from Lwiro—early morning service.

Tuesday, July 19, 1955

I drive C. to Makwe, the western limit of our IRSAC forest reserve. C. intends to survey in order to start a botanical map. I take the occasion to do a bit of exploring myself and climb Makondo, a prominent hill south of Irangi. A path to the top starts at the village of Kalaho. The incline is rather steep and the path has made no compromising hairpin turns that would make the ascent easier. The compensation at the top is a marvelous panoramic view with the valleys of the Luhoho and Lutunguru rivers prominent features. A slight depression leads to the source of a small tributary called Kalalo. Collect some Anopheles and Culex larvae.

Back in camp at 13:10. C. not yet back. At 17:00 go into the forest to light the light-trap lamps. Coming back, meet C. returning from his botanical inspection.

Pass a miserable night because of a sore throat.

Wednesday, July 20, 1955

Drive C. to Makwe, where he is to resume his survey. After my return to camp, go inspecting the work on the platform. The "bridge" connecting the slope of the hill to about one quarter way up the huge Gilbertiodendron tree is finished and the men are now fashioning the ladder that will take us higher up to a massive branch and a second "landing." I use the word "fashioning" because the way the ladder is being constructed resembles more an elaborate lattice than a purely functional ladder. All the extra ties, supports, transoms and rungs will make the structure stronger, I am told. The two empty tins I had previously attached to a tree prove to be very successful artificial breeding places for mosquitos.

Back to Makwe to "retrieve" C. At 18:00, the mosquito boys leave for a night collection of biting-mosquitoes. They "misunderstood" me, they later explained, and spent a cozy evening in the village of Bukanjo. As arranged before they left, I fire my shotgun at midnight to call them back. C., not knowing about this arrangement, gets entangled in his mosquito net and rips it jumping out of bed to investigate and prepare himself to repulse the "attackers."

Thursday, July 21, 1955
I shall always remember this 21st of July, [so my diary starts the record of the day.] After last evening's "misunderstanding" I decide to supervise the night-catching of mosquitos myself. Leave camp at 20:00 and arrive at the catching site by the light of a Coleman lantern about an hour later. At that moment, a severe thunderstorm unleashed its full fury, opening all of heaven's available watergates. There was nothing we could do but return, feverishly hoping we would be spared falling branches and the flashing bolts that seemed to crash all around us. No mosquito would be foolish enough to forage in this kind of weather. The inevitable mud-slide down the hill by the light of a hissing and steaming Coleman lamp that, by some sort of unexplainable miracle, kept on burning, was a scene of high drama that would have warmed the heart of a film producer specializing in horror films. But the stage reached its dramatic climax, and so did the storm, at the moment of crossing the wildly swaying liana bridge across the swollen, thunderous Luo, the whole scene illuminated by blinding flashes of continuous lighting.

"Daȓaja karibu kukatika bwana," warned one of the mosquito boys as we reached midpoint. (The bridge is close to breaking). I could have bashed his head with a blunt instrument. But we reached the other side safely, and all thoughts of violence disappeared as we thankfully dripped into camp.

Friday, July 22, 1955
A good part of the morning "licking our wounds" from yesterday's wet adventure: cleaning equipment and drying clothes. L. arrives with Dr. Vincke, discoverer of the famous

Plasmodium berghei, a rodent malaria parasite now used worldwide in malaria research. We show him around and he seems agreeably impressed with our platform and plans for mosquito work. He complains, however, about the stiff climb up the hill to reach the spot.

With the three of us sharing the narrow bunk-type bedroom, preparing for the night becomes a bit of a hassle. L. particularly seems cumbersome. He is one of those persons who, just by standing there, seems to fill every nook of a small room. True, he is a good-sized bloke, but that doesn't give him the right to be in the way whenever one reaches for something. When he sits down, it will be precisely on the trunk that contains one's much needed socks; when he stands up, chances are that it will be in front of the cupboard where you keep the teakettle; and when he starts deploying his mosquito catches of the day on the table, it will be just about time for the evening meal. If, somehow, they could use this kind of competency in the army, half of the boys could be discharged and the army would still be better off. While L. caused exasperation during the day hours, his role was taken over at night by Vincke who, during the first night, started reading by flashlight which shone directly in my face from his bunk opposite mine. He obviously had some difficulties in adjusting the beam at a proper angle and the light wavered in all directions as he tried to support the flashlight against the wall or steadying it by means of various objects, including respectively a bottle, a pair of shoes and finally the water kettle. It felt like sleeping in front of the revolving beam of a lighthouse.

Sunday, July 23, 1955

With Vincke on a mosquito survey. It was the second time that I was part of his field research methods, which consisted of dashing into unknown waters in complete contempt of the hazards such an approach entails. The first time was during our mosquito survey in the Ruzizi Valley, when he decided to "explore" a mile-wide inundated marshland alongside the Ruzizi River. With complete disregard for the strong possibility of crocodiles in the murky lagoon fed by the Ruzizi River, he resolutely started walking into the water that reached to his thighs (Vincke was a small man). As for me, his assistant, it seemed that I could do nothing else but follow suit. Till this very day I cannot explain how we eluded the crocodiles and missed walking into deep pits. As dusk fell, we reached, miraculously I thought, the other side of the swamp, and the road. Two more miles took us to Vincke's convertible. In the open car, covered with mud and swamp vegetation, we must have offered a sorry sight.

The adventure at Irangi was, in many ways, similar. Having climbed for a while along the torrential river Heke within deep forest, we suddenly came to a level plateau where the stream collected in a 300-yard-wide basin, from where it resumed its downward rush across a rocky natural dam. The expanse of water, though small in comparison with Vincke's usual standard, was irresistible to him. Without pause, Vincke stepped inside the pool. The water was crystal clear, but the bottom consisted of highly polished and very slippery cannonball-size stones. The pool was only about one to two feet deep, but the actual depth didn't matter. It could have been twice that depth because, by the time we had waded a distance of 20 yards and stumbled that many times into the icy waters, we were drenched through. In spite of the cold temperature, trying to keep an even keel on the slippery bottom soon had us perspiring like workhorses. I thought we were lucky when we reached the other side of the pool without broken bones and found a nice open, sunny spot where we collapsed onto a lovely huge warm boulder, trying to catch our breath.

"Water too clear and cold for Anopheles," said Vincke as he got his speech back, referring to our "survey." I could have told him the same thing before fording the pool.

We all returned to Lwiro, I after a two weeks' stay. I returned for another fortnight two months later.

Wednesday, September 21, 1955

Find that the villagers have moved to the opposite side of the road and a bit farther north. Reason: a few days ago, an antelope crossed the village during the first light of day, a sign for the Batembo and Warega people that many people are going to die soon in this spot. The antelope was easily killed because, the villagers explained, it is not really a true antelope, but a spirit. We met the chief who had come to investigate the matter and who had recommended and approved the move to the new place.

Quite independently of this story, I too made a decision to move. From now on, I placed my camp bed under the open barza instead of sleeping in the narrow and stuffy "Pullman" bunk inside the hut, in spite of warnings from the staff about prowling leopards.

It is so delightfully cool outside. Every morning I wake with the first light and the first stirrings of the forest, seeing a new day being born with the unveiling of solemn tall trees as the mist slowly dissipates and the first movements of monkeys agitate the large leaves, causing the heavy dew drops to splatter to the ground with an exaggerated sound in the quietness of the still slumbering forest.

Thursday, September 22, 1955

This is one of those days when my diary looks as if it is describing the activities of a dozen people. Up at 6:45. Run clinic for children till 8:00. Have argument with the man who sold me a civet cat yesterday. Animal caretaker accuses wife of the cook of having left open the door of the monkey cage, and one of the red-tails has escaped. Have to arrange to buy rice for the chimp. Put one monkey, a *Cercopithecus mitis,* in a cage I made for capturing mosquitoes, a contraption invented by L. and myself. Decide to partition the garage, keeping one part for a storeroom. The cook accused Murebwa of being absent from work, which explains why his wife had to take care of feeding the monkeys and inadvertently left the cage open.

Escape with L. and try our new "ferry" made basically from empty 50-gallon drums across the Luo. The strong current tends to push the "bow" under. When the three of us move to the other end, the ride is somewhat improved, but we still have difficulty pulling the contraption along the vine we have tied across the river.

I place the mosquito trap with the monkey in it on the lower landing of the "observation tower."

After checking the artificial (bamboo) mosquito breeding places, return to camp where I have a word with the carpenter regarding the modification of the "hull" of the ferry so that it would be lifted, rather than pushed under.

Samson, to be the new "camp commander," complains about the poor state of the hut he was assigned. I decide to allow him the use of the aluminum hut, and instruct the workers to clear a space to put up the hut. Carpenter is given measurements for making proper doors for the workers' quarters. The house first allocated to Samson now given to Mutembezi (head mosquito boy) and Alphonso (head tsetse boy). Have a well-prepared moambe chicken for lunch. Back in the forest at 14:30 to increase the number of artificial mosquito breeding places. A slight rain falls. Return to camp to do some laboratory work. As the rain stops, I go back to the forest to check on the monkey/mosquito trap. Everything O.K., but no mosquitoes yet. Cross with the ferry with great difficulty. The carpenter should work on it first thing tomorrow.

Sunday, September 25, 1955

Dull morning (feels like Sunday) everyone seems to move in slow motion. Lorry leaves early with our men to buy food at a market some miles up the road. Work from nine till noon putting up the prefabricated aluminum hut for Samson and family. Briefly check our different capturing stations across the river. Lupao has to swim along the vine to fetch the ferry. Noise of wood-chopping from the forest sounds nostalgic and cordial. Reminds me of the book *Southseaman*, describing the woes and joys of the construction of a sailboat by noncarpenters.

Work most of the day in the lab identifying mosquito larvae and examining blood smears from various animals. Find *Trypanosoma lewisi* in several squirrels and one Plasmodium. Dream up a method of determining egg-laying habits of various forest mosquitoes by using a series of bamboo traps, glass jars or other artificial breeding places to be opened or closed at different times of the day or night.

While working with L. under the barza, two bees suddenly divebomb from the sky and score direct hits: one on L.'s underlip, one above my right eye. When dust settles over the commotion of slapping slippers and threshing towels, we find ourselves with greatly swollen and painful facial features.

In the course of examining a squirrel L. let it escape and the animal is in a tree in a flash. I bring it down with a well-directed 12-gauge shotgun. I make blood smears while L. collects ectoparasites.

A discussion about the biology of mosquito larvae goes on till midnight!

Tuesday, September 27, 1955

My eye is swollen from the bee sting and I look like a shady Chinese character on the dust jacket of *Peking after Midnight*. The capita of the village of Mai arrives to tell me that the villagers refuse to come to the camp to have their blood taken for a malaria survey. Since I am not an "official," there is nothing official I can do to summon them. In retaliation, I tell the capita that I won't buy any more animals from the Mai people in the future. Ha!

With increased time required for tsetse research and surveys in the Mutara and Bugesera regions of eastern Ruanda from 1957 onwards, my visits to Irangi inevitably became more spaced and each of shorter duration. But my work there never really stopped—especially the project I had just started of a quantitative and qualitative inventory of forest mosquitoes based upon breeding activity over the 24-hour period, a study I intended to continue for at least a full year. One could spend a lifetime at Irangi and still come up with new scientific data. It was actually during the period of "reduced activity" that I enjoyed some very gratifying findings, as my diary during that period shows.

Wednesday, October 31, 1956

There comes a day in the life of even the dullest biologist that makes him feel like shouting "Eureka," "Holy smokes," "I'll be darned," "Great Scott" or whatever his or her favorite expression of jubilation he or she may fancy at a moment of great rejoicing. Days of soaking rain, clinging mud, torn flesh and grueling heat in the marshes are flushed out from memory with the excitement of a new scientific discovery.

Today, the victory bell tolled for me. Left early this morning with two men for the small river Lianga, where we had encountered *G. vanhoofi* and *G. palpalis* on previous occasions. The river, a small mountain stream tumbling from a scenic series of low waterfalls, produces a constant billow of fine mist. It is rather a damp place for tsetse, in my opinion, but since we have found flies there before, we comb the area for several hours without success.

Resume search after lunch, this time along the path leading to the platform where a few *G. vanhoofi* are occasionally caught inside a mosquito net strung between trees. Crawling on my hands and feet in underbrush and small saplings, my heart misses a beat when suddenly I see the unmistakable silhouette of a large tsetse along one of the saplings, head down. I freeze for a while, imaginatively rubbing my eyes, making sure they are functioning properly. But it is no imagination nor a single occurrence. With the newly gained knowledge of where to look, Kisele sees another tsetse in exactly the same position, and I discover one on a large tree, perfectly blending with the background of the rough bark. Frantically, I prepare my camera and flash which—would you believe it?—does not work and I am also running out of film. I change film, but by the time flash and camera are ready, "my" fly decides it has posed long enough and takes off. Soon we find others and I finally manage to get some good shots, used later to illustrate a scientific paper: "The Discovery and Ecology of *Glossina vanhoofi*."

Meet L. on his way back from his mosquito traps and tell him the stupendous news. Together we find three more *G. vanhoofi*, all resting on small saplings where they are easier to see than on the larger trees where they blend with the background. Finally, we have seen more than a dozen flies all resting head down, a position typical for hungry flies.

Back to camp as light fails (I could have stayed for hours) concluding one of my best days at Irangi. L. works on his mosquito collection till midnight while we discuss the newly found information on the *G. vanhoofi* resting places.

Sunday, November 4, 1956

Start unloading the lorry with rice L. bought yesterday at Homo, and store it in empty 50-gallon drums. This is the staple food for our animals. We now have a dozen monkeys of four species: *Cercopithecus ascanius*, *Cercopithecus mitis*, *Colobus badius* and *Cercocebus aterrimus*, several brushtail porcupines: *Atherurus africanus centralis*, a pangolin: *Manis tricupis*, and several litters of guinea pigs to be used for feeding mosquitoes and tsetse flies.

Mostly busy during the morning making and staining blood smears from the porcupines on which we have fed *G. vanhoofi*, hoping that, if infected, they would pass trypanosomes to the porcupines. The slides turn out to be unusable because the stain has precipitated, most probably from the use of river water for dilution instead of distilled water. I refrain from throwing the slides away, but put them aside with the vague intention of restaining them at some other time.

After lunch I cross the river with difficulty because of the very strong current caused by the swollen waters. Can hear a violent thunderstorm in the distance, so I hastily install the artificial tsetse "breeding sites." On my precipitous way back I have a bad fall coming down the hill, my feet simply slipping away from under me. I hear a cracking noise and for a moment believe that I have broken my arm. But I feel no pain and hurry on to the ferry. Cross the menacing waters, again with difficulty, just as the thunderstorm strikes.

A steady rain keeps me inside the laboratory for the rest of the day. A good time to have a look at those badly stained slides. They are too darned dark to see anything. Having nothing to lose (so I think) I wash two of the slides with soap and water—an extremely unorthodox way to treat a blood smear! However, the treatment seems to have cleared most of the dark muck and when I put one of the slides under the microscope, the blood picture is that of a normally stained preparation. I scan the slides for trypanosomes: nothing. But wait! What is this!? By jove, I rediscover a plasmodium (malarial parasite) I had seen for the first time two years ago and which our parasitologist has been searching for—in vain, so far—in all the brushtail porcupines coming his way. What a stroke of luck to find the parasite again in a badly stained smear I was about to throw out! I am now in an awkward position. Of course, the parasite never described or seen before except by me should be described in a scientific publication. But I cannot do this on my own without telling the parasitologist, who is only too eager to pounce on the discovery himself. Oh, well. [The parasite, indeed a new species, was eventually described as *Plasmodium atheruri*, in two separate papers in which I figure as co-author, thank you.]

A *G. palpalis* comes flying into the lab. It is immediately captured and dissected. No trypanosomes.

Near nine o'clock that night, a thick column of army ants starts moving in the direction of our hut, dislodged, no doubt, by the rising waters of the river. It veers off in another direction just as we are about to pour kerosene on it and stop the ants from invading our quarters. We hope that they will not invade the cages and kill the animals. We keep a sharp vigil although there is little we can do for the moment. Nothing else, however, disturbs the evening except the rumbling retreat of the thunderstorm and the sound of dripping, rain-soaked trees.

The next days were spent in organizing a program of quantitative assessment of the *G. vanhoofi* population. I measure a path that runs over the top of two hills till it reaches the Lutunguru River. The distance is divided into eight sections, each of 60 meters. A team of fly-boys will walk along the path twice a day, three times a week, from eight to ten in the morning, and from three to five in the afternoon to observe and, if possible, capture all tsetse flies on vegetation or attacking them. We hope this will provide us with enough flies for experimental work and at the same time give us some idea of the fly population and its fluctuations over the seasons. One drawback will be the daily presence of people who will disturb and chase away the host animal(s)—*G. vanhoofi* probably feeds on forest hog—this will also have an effect on fly densities. We shall see after a few weeks.

My next Irangi diary tells me that on Monday, 7 January 1957, I left on a special forest safari with two German scientists, Spaatz and Stephan, who had come out to study and collect certain animals from the Congo lowland forest, more particularly *Elephantulus* shrews. That day I ran a high fever from an oncoming cold. I had gone to bed at two in the morning, but had not slept the rest of the night because of the cold—a combination that made me carsick three times while coming down the twisting Kahuzi road. I felt much better the next day, but my morale had suffered a serious setback. Still there was plenty of work to be done and activities were at a high pitch when two entomologists returned to Lwiro after four days, while the German zoologists and I resumed our safari to the lower altitudes of the forest where we hoped to find the animals in which the zoologists were interested.

Saturday, January 12, 1957

We arrived yesterday and occupied the rest house on the left bank of the River Oso, at a place called Muhulu. The heat and the smell of guano have prompted us to sleep outside under the barza. Now, as the mist is lifting, we have a wonderful view of the still steaming river. Distorted, hollow voices drift from the village across the water, and there is an occasional clanging, metallic sound of smithing. After a hasty breakfast, a canoe takes us across the river, where we meet Chief Useni. A Moslem, he has seven wives who bore him 27 children, a rather splendid performance. The chief bombastically avows that we shall be able to find all the animals we need in his territory. A long discussion follows with half a dozen of his men with whom we try to describe the animals we are looking for. We are much amused when, during the discussion, some of the men try to characterize some of the animals through mimicking their walk, sound, cry and general behavior. Others supply details about their diet and places where they sleep and eat. A remarkable mimicry act!

Strolling through the village, I meet the same witch doctor I met two years ago. He tells a long story of failing crops and hard times. A generous gift of tobacco seems to restore his faith in life and he departs with a bouncing gait.

Having nothing else to do but await the efforts of the chief's "hunters," we spend the rest of the day at the rest house, leisurely performing small tasks, but mostly gazing across the river where the village, stunned by the hot afternoon sun, has fallen into deep silence. The ocher-colored huts, blurred by the tremors of heated air, seem to have become part of the dark olive forest background as if perspective has suddenly disappeared. Unheeding, the waters of the Oso River glide by with sluggish might, an occasional whirlpool denouncing its hidden vitality. A colorless, depthless sky covers all like an inverted clammy drinking glass. Gazing dreamingly into the shimmering horizon, I imagine being back at some European seaside resort. This makes me sentimentally sad and, once more, I realize how inescapably my heart is torn between two continents; how much I regret leaving one while declaring my love for the other. Resuming my reading of Beverly Nichols's *Sunlight on the Lawn*, is no remedy for changing my mood.

As the glowing sun sinks behind the forest canopy, painting the river in shimmering gold, the fly-boy team returns, Fukenye with three *Culex* mosquitoes taken from a brush tail porcupine hole, Amisi with two *G. palpalis*, and Dawili limps in with two *Cercopithecus ascanius* monkeys.

Sunday, January 13, 1957

Early sunshine promises another hot day. Everything indicates that the dry season is asserting itself. It will last about three months in this region and I wish that Irangi would have a similar seasonal dry spell. We drive a while along the road and enter the forest at a village where we inform the capita of our wish to buy animals. We see a band of red-tail monkeys and one of Cercocebus monkeys, but none are hurt by Stephan's and Spaatz's barrage of Hornet bullets. We return empty-handed.

In the evening we pay a visit to the chief to remind him of his promise for animals. A lively dance is in progress in front of his hut. The women, sticks in their right hands, dance in a circle around a couple of drummers who are giving their all with a swinging beat that would make Gene Krupa feel like a beginner. Two of the chief's wives are in front of the dancing chain, singing a leading strophe repeated by the rest of the dancers. According to a translation by several villagers and mosquito boys, the lead strophe seems to be something like: "Tonight our men are going to make love and how joyful this will be."

Monday, January 14, 1957

A misty morning. At 8:30 a dugout canoe and four boatmen arrive to take Dawili and me upriver. Always mindful of my previous unhappy experiences with canoes, I am rather apprehensive, especially when Dawili, who is grossly overweight, upsets the delicate balance of the craft more than once. But soon we are off, and the easy rhythm of the paddling boatmen keeps the canoe on an even keel.

How lovely the early morning on the river is! We pass the village clearing, the forest drapes the riverbanks with overhanging branches and vines that form a cool shade under which the canoe glides with grace. Now close to the bank, the boatman in front uses a pole to propel the craft. This makes it rock with unpleasant jerking movements. My confidence in the pole man is severely clipped when once he nearly falls overboard when his pole slips from an underwater obstacle and later as he loses the pole altogether when it gets stuck in the mud. Luckily, the pole is retrieved by one of the stern boatmen as the canoe glides by.

We land at a sandy cove. Large *Ficus* trees and underbrush make a pleasant shady pattern that feels like typical *G. palpalis* habitat. And indeed, soon we capture several of this tsetse species. I miss a red-tail monkey as it jumps from an overhanging branch. More monkeys are seen on the other bank. They are Cercocebus and as Stephan and Spaatz are anxious to collect this species, we cross and make fast underneath a large ficus in which the monkeys are nervously scurrying about, having spotted us. Dawili steps ashore with the 12-gauge shotgun while I remain in the canoe ready with the 22-Hornet. One of the monkeys walks in full view on the highest branch of the tree, about 40 meters away. Taking careful aim, I know I have hit it, but the animal keeps dangling with one arm around a branch. After a while it drops to the ground. A good shot, the small bullet having gone through the left side of the chest, just missing the heart. We hear the explosion of Dawili's 12-gauge and he too comes back with a Cercocebus. Stepping into the canoe from a branch, the wood breaks under his weight and Dawili, once more, nearly capsizes the canoe. With the strong downstream current we make good speed on our return journey, reaching camp just before noon.

I resume the river survey in the afternoon, now going downstream and accompanied by Mutembezi. Here the natural vegetation has been highly altered leaving only secondary growth and signs of old shambas (fields). We return without animals, but have collected eight *G. palpalis* while paddling along the banks.

We stay at Muhulu for a whole week. Chief Useni's promises turned into more promises each day and finally we gathered most of our animal collection through our own efforts and through village headmen outside Useni's territory. I kept busy mostly making blood smears of the animals, looking for Atherurus rockholes and, hopefully, mosquitoes associated with them. I surveyed the riverbanks for tsetse flies, but near the end of the week felt that I was wasting my time. I was glad, therefore, when on Friday Stephan and Spaatz declared that they had apparently exhausted the range of "available" animals and that of their food supply. I decided to leave early the next day in an attempt to reach Lwiro the same day.

Saturday, January 19, 1957

A record day in hardship traveling. Left Muhulu at five in the morning, with me driving the GMC truck. Road very muddy at places. Slip from the roadbed into a shallow ditch, but manage to get the vehicle back on the road. Reach the camp of famous Swiss animal collector Cordier. Intend to stop only long enough to fill our tank, but Stephan and Spaatz want to stay for breakfast and so do the African staff, clamoring that they will die if they cannot eat now. I am upset when Cordier tells me that BM has promised him that I shall return for three months in order to help supervise the construction of a bungalow that will serve as a temporary residence during the visit of King Leopold III and Princess de Rethy, his wife—a visit still treated as a great secret. Finally, I manage to drag everyone away, reluctant no doubt to face more grueling hours on the muddy road to Irangi and Lwiro. Up and down, swerves and turns, slips and slides, too heavily loaded. The boys want to stop. Stephan wants to buy bananas. Spaatz has spotted a pangolin skin for sale. Boys want to borrow money. It is hot and very humid. The road seems endless.

As we arrive at Irangi it starts raining as if to reinforce my worst fears. It takes a while before we have all reorganized our belongings, especially for Stephan and Spaatz, who have to repack everything as they will move on from Lwiro to other regions to complete their animal collection. Off finally at 15:00. After the new rain the road is in a terrible mess. Pure determination and the prospect of reaching Lwiro with a bit of luck the same day keep me alert and tense. Arrive at Lwiro in good form at exactly 20:00. I am out, done for, a heap of tired bones and flesh, but with the spirit of a racer ready to collapse after winning the "Grand Prix." The whole distance from Muhulu is only about 200 miles, but, except for the half an hour breakfast at Utu and the one and a half hour repacking at Irangi, I have been behind the wheel for 15 hours.

Royal Hunting Party

I had been only a few days in my March 1957 stay at my camp in the Mutara when an IRSAC stationwagon arrived at the entrance in a bellowing cloud of dust. Out jumped François, BM's personal driver, handing me a letter—a far cry from the old split stick days. I have BM's letter before me. It reads:

Dear Frank, I am leaving in a hurry for FIS camp with my car and a lorry Monday morning till Saturday (gorilla capture.) I *need* you badly so come immediately. I had to prepare everything myself in a hurry. Ch. and Zaghi will also be coming. Return with François and take your tent. Bring all the 12-gauge shotguns. Hope this reaches you Saturday so that you can leave immediately or Sunday at the last. I have to leave FIS camp this Monday at 8 a.m.

It was the start of a hectic time that began with the visit of King Leopold III of Belgium, a week earlier. As in all his travels, the king was accompanied by Princess de Rethy, his second wife. His first wife, beautiful, popular and well-loved Queen Astrid, lost her life in a car accident—the King was the driver—during a vacation trip in Switzerland in 1935. Only a few years earlier, King Albert I, Prince Leopold's father, died in a fatal fall while mountaineering. And then King Leopold was thrown into World War II when the German army swept through the Lowlands and France in May 1940, forcing the king to surrender unconditionally. Political debates during and after the war, criticizing the king's action, led to his abdication in favor of his son Boudewijn, the present king.

King Leopold's visit was directly related to the making of a scientific film to be produced by F.I.S. (Foundation Internationale Scientifique,) of which the king was the president, inspiration and sponsor. The king wanted to witness the filming of animals living in the rain forest. A main theme of the production was about the "secret life" of forest animals—animals rarely seen, many of nocturnal activity—in their deep forest habitats. That King Leopold became involved in such a project did not surprise those who knew about the king's passion for science, travel and photography.

When the FIS film director and technicians selected the Irangi area as a base of operation for several film sequences, our

Irangi forest station proved, once more, to be an outstanding location, especially for the filming of gorillas, which was to be one of the highlights. The proximity of the many facilities at our research center at Lwiro and the presence of a large scientific staff versed in many disciplines were an additional bonus. No doubt, the king's personal house staff also approved of the marvelous site of Lwiro, with lodgings "fit for a King." From what I saw later on, the king couldn't have cared less about "dignified" lodgings. His Majesty seemed quite happy in the bush!

But to return to BM's urgent message delivered on a Friday at ten in the morning at my Mutara camp. Dropping everything, I hastened to Lwiro, arriving around midnight. BM had already left, but I found ample instructions and a long list of items to be gathered and added to the lorry already loaded with furniture for the king's bungalow at Utu camp, where His Majesty planned to remain for a week. I was to proceed with all haste to Utu, collect Zaghi—stationed at Irangi at the time—organize a temporary laboratory at the Utu-FIS camp and get busy making a quickly constructed bungalow fit to receive the royal visitors. By the time all the items had been gathered and loaded, and the soda water for His Highness had arrived from Bukavu, it was Saturday 19:00 hours. I left immediately and arrived at Irangi around midnight. On the way, the driver had almost killed us by falling asleep at the wheel, admittedly at a convenient place where the ditch was shallow. He was very much shaken and for the rest of the way drove with his face outside the window so that the icy breeze would keep him awake. He nearly froze to death. I had some difficulty first getting Zaghi out of his mansion and second making him take me seriously about packing and making it snappy. He groaned, but by then I had snuggled into the corner of the front seat, trying to keep warm and snatch 40 winks. At three in the morning I was told that Zaghi was ready to load his gear. Tumbling from seat into the black night, I nearly broke a leg over an array of beds, buckets, mattresses, armchairs, pots and babies and less identifiable objects faintly silhouetted against the light of a kerosene lamp. I felt cold and miserable. It took another half hour trying to load the essentials of Zaghi's household, hoping that the king's coffee table or icebox would not be crushed during the swaying of the lorry along the rough road. We left Irangi at three-thirty of a very black night. Zaghi insisted on traveling in his own car, which caused us no small amount of trouble. Luckily, I had him drive ahead of the lorry. Difficulties arose at the first two steep hills, where we had to push his car, an old Studebaker. For a while everything was fine until we came to a long escarpment which his car refused to tackle. As I was under strict orders to reach Utu, whatever the circumstances, I had to leave Zaghi behind, but loaded up his wife and children.

We arrived at FIS camp at seven-thirty that morning. I immediately got busy setting up a resemblance of an active field laboratory inside an empty storeroom. I pitched my tent near a cluster of wooden bungalows since there was no other lodging available. In the afternoon we unloaded and put the furniture in the king's bungalow, a fine wooden structure built some way from the center of the camp, surrounded on all sides by dense forest. It had a large high roof made from local materials and thatches, as traditional in this region, with large forest leaves that formed a cool and watertight bond. This high roof protected a platform supported by gradually increased lengths of poles alongside the slope of a steep valley. The bungalow itself occupied about half the space of the platform and consisted of only a small bedroom and three annexes: a shower, a toilet and a large closet. The rest of the platform was completely enclosed in mosquito-proof screening and divided into two parts, one arranged as a dining room with heavy log cabin style furniture made of local wood; the other designed for a living room with a low coffee table made from the buttress of one of the forest trees, and eight simple "Morris" armchairs. The bungalow gave one the feeling of living inside the forest.

The next day, Sunday, was dull with rain and low-hanging clouds. I took it easy, lying inside my tent reading *Take These Men*, about desert warfare in North Africa. We had a heavy shower during the night. On Monday morning the weather improved and the sun came out. Mrs. V. D. B. arrived with the king's food, cutlery and dinnerware, marked with the IRSAC emblem, and odds and ends for decoration. We, that is Mrs. V. D. B., a FIS technician and I spent a very busy afternoon putting the bungalow in order, sweeping the floors, making the kerosene refrigerator work, stowing the food, and so forth. I made up the beds. Fancy me making the bed of a king and a princess! During the Middle Ages, one was knighted for doing that kind of thing! By four o'clock the bungalow had been turned into lovely living quarters with soft lights, simple grace and restful charm, set off against the dark background of the primeval forest. The day lingered on and turned into soft dusk when the cars arrived. First a blue Ford with Leopold III and Prof. V. D. B. Next a gray Ford with princess Liliane and the Vicomte du Parc. Then three more cars with the aide-de-camp, the chambermaid and Dr. Schaffer, the scientific director of the project. Most of the technical staff was gathered in the mess hall and so was I, talking to Siehlman, the head camera operator. As we had been told there would be no official reception, we all stayed inside until Dr. Schaffer came bursting in, very angry, telling us how ill-mannered we were not to come outside and greet the royal visitors. So we filed out one by one, extremely embarrassed. I was the first to be introduced to the king, and then to the princess. The king looked rather older than I remembered from official portraits, and had put on weight. He had a low, husky voice and a slow speech as if he pondered every word. This was perhaps because most of the conversation among the group was conducted in English, a language that, in one form or another, was understood and spoken by most of the film crew and the scientists who represented half a dozen different nationalities. Leopold was dressed as we all were in the Congo: khaki trousers and short-sleeved shirt. The princess looked very beautiful in khaki jodhpurs, a colored shirt and a ribbon to hold her brown hair. I never saw her without this "hair-dress." She had a clear voice, rather low, a kind face, a winning smile, very white teeth—somewhat separated—and prominent cheekbones. Her dark brown eyes were vivacious, casting a sparkle of wit and humor—features that make people feel at ease. The king was far more distant, perhaps not so much on purpose but because of a crown prince's education. I thought that his face showed signs of the heavy burdens in the past and the marks of the many tragic moments of his reign.

Dusk had settled for good when the royal couple were led to their quarters. I had collected my Leica camera that I had left on the mess window sill and got dressed for supper at Cordier's. We were still at the table when one of the FIS staff popped in asking if we had seen the princess's camera that she had left somewhere. None of us had. He moved off to pop in a short time later with a Leica camera the princess said was *not* hers.

"Certainly not," I said after examining the camera. "It is mine. Thank you. Where did you find it because I am sure that I had put it away in my tent?"

"It was found in the mess," he replied.

I could have sworn that I had put my camera in my tent. End second act.

The curtains rose once more for the third and final act when the FIS man popped in again—we were about to invite him to stay the rest of the evening, saving him traveling time—when he asked me: "Are you sure the camera you said you left in your tent wasn't that of princess?"

I felt the floor sinking underneath my feet and only wished it would do so more quickly and swallow me up entirely. Sure enough, when I checked the camera in the tent, I found it wasn't mine, so it must be that of the princess. After that I spent a bad night dreaming about the consequences of stealing a princess's belongings, which, again during the Middle Ages, would be punished by beheading.

The day started clear and sunny; the birds were joyfully active both in flight as well as in voice, and the forest smelled good. After attending to details in our field laboratory, I became absorbed in the filming operations in the large aviary enclosing a small stream. Then I saw, up on a high platform the king and princess busy taking photographs. After a while they left and the princess came to me, held out her hand and said: "Ah, Mister Lambrecht." I did not like the tone of the "ah," but she smiled, remarked that it was a beautiful day. I felt pardoned for stealing her camera, sure that I would finish the day with my head still on my shoulders.

The days passed by, each with sunny weather and clear, blue skies, rather unusual in the forest regions. I saw the king and the princess every day as they stood watching the various filming activities. When, one day, the local chief came to greet His Majesty, I also had a good excuse to do some photography myself. Wednesday night, V. D. B., who had dined every night at the "Royal Bungalow," came back with news. The king and the princess had insisted that they would participate in the gorilla capture operation scheduled for the next morning. The officer responsible for the king's safety had refused flatly to allow His Majesty to do so. But the royal couple were equally determined that they would. Whereupon the officer stated that he could not stop the king from doing what he pleased, but that in that case he, the officer, would not accompany the king and, therefore, be relieved of all responsibilities during that time period, and the king agreed. It followed that V. D. B. and I, were "invited" to accompany the expedition and to provide first aid medical equipment and care, thus a good deal of responsibilities would fall on us.

We left early the following morning and reached a place along a narrow forest road some 50 miles from Utu. We were told by the African hunters that Cordier had captured a young gorilla, and the animal was confined within a net surrounding a small area in a narrow valley. We unloaded our supplies and after a while the king and princess arrived. The team finally consisted of: the king, the princess, Vicomte du Parc (the king's personal valet), Dr. Schaffer, Dr. V. D. B., Mme. V. D. B. and myself. We plunged into the jungle and followed a small stream for a while. It was rough on shoes and trousers:—not that I was worried about mine because I was wearing my well-proven jungle outfit: walking shorts, lightweight jungle boots and canvas leggings. The king's black-and-white fancy shoes looked ruined, however. It was an old pair, I guess. After a three quarters of an hour struggle, we arrived at a partial clearing, fenced off by a double net about two meters high. The fenced-in area measured something like 40 by 60 meters. A young gorilla was trapped inside. Cordier was directing operations at the other end of the enclosure. The idea was to drive the animal near the periphery of the net, where it would be immobilized temporarily with tear gas. Eight Africans with tear gas guns had been posed at various places outside the net. In the confusion of the tear gas release (I wondered who would be confused most) the animal would be tied with strong ropes. (To break the unbearable spell of excitement, I can already concede that it didn't work and that at the end of the day, after twelve hours of effort, the gorilla jumped the net and got away.)

But to go back to details. The morning wore away rapidly. The king was, most of the time, at the other side of the enclosure with Cordier. For his safety, V. D. B. had asked me to lend the king my Smith-Wesson .38 (a new one, the one confiscated by L. Swan was never returned), and I had explained how it worked. Dr. Schaffer was at the far end of the net after cries from the hunters had indicated the whereabouts of the gorilla.

Our group, watching the eastern side of the net, consisted of: the Princess, Dr. and Mrs. V. D. B., the Vicomte and myself. In the cool of the forest we enjoyed a good time and a lively conversation which, for a while, went from music to Hungary, where the royal couple had spent a recent holiday. The princess admired Hungarian music and the flat, wide-horizon landscape that reminded her of the Flemish countryside. We touched even upon the tragic moments during the first days of the German invasion of Belgium when Leopold III, then reigning king, had to make decisions under great pressure, some of them criticized by many. As the sun reached its zenith, we unpacked our sandwich box and sat down to a very informal "royal" meal on the forest floor. A little later, the king and Cordier joined us. I mention here, in case you forgot, that one never addresses the king in the second person form, but in the third form. Thus, do not say: "Voudriez-vous . . . ," but: le Roi veut-il. . . . "Not: "Pensez-vous . . . ," but: "le Roi croit-il . . . ," and so on. Awkward to having a flowing conversation, what? It is difficult to observe the rules, for instance, when the king asks a question such as "Where is the gorilla?" You can't say "over there," but something like: "If the king would kindly cast His Majesty's eyes to the NWN near the foot of the tall *Gibertiodendron* over there, chances are that. . . ." Under the circumstances and with no protocol around, things worked out a little less formally, however. But even then it seemed strange to hear the princess refer to the king as "my husband," such as: "Mon mari trouve que notre fils Alexandre resemble a son père." During this lunch break I had many opportunities of taking photographs. A dedicated photographer himself, the king did not seem to mind.

Strategy was discussed and after lunch the gorilla's territory was halved by drawing in the net, leaving an area of only about 30 by 30 meters encircling the small stream at the bottom of the valley, where the gorilla was hiding in the dense riverine vegetation. Pressed by shouts and pieces of wood thrown in its direction, the gorilla would dash out from cover and when it approached the net, one of the hunters would let him have it with a tear gas blast. Though this threw the animal to the ground for a couple of seconds, the effect was never long enough so that it could be approached and tied up. This happened a couple of times until one of the hunters, by mistake, fired a cartridge of birdshot at the ape. The animal was certainly wounded—how badly we did not know as from then onwards it stayed mostly in dense cover, to lick its wounds, no doubt. So far having taken the operation in good, sporty spirits, the gorilla now began to take things seriously and showed signs of bad temper. It stamped both feet in rapid succession: pam-pam . . . pam-pam. It drummed with its fists on its chest, Tarzan style. Growls were not uncommon. It was a splendid performance. From time to time a dark body would be seen moving about at the edge of the trees and dashing back again. No doubt, the gorilla wanted to know how we were taking his bad temper and if, per chance, we had crawled away to safety. All this we watched from our grandstand on the slope overlooking the valley. And so the day wore on. At one point Cordier had stepped inside the net and had not been seen for a while. The king wanted to know what he was up to. V. D. B. asked me to investigate, that is, to look for Cordier inside the enclosure. "Good luck, Mr. Lambrecht," were the parting words of the princess as I left. "Thank you," I replied politely. Arriving at the far end of the enclosure, I told the hunters to let me in. They looked at me reproachfully as if they did not approve of this kind of suicide and later would perhaps be blamed for it. I reached a clump of trees inside of which I saw Cordier calmly sitting on a stump, his "gas-gun" between his knees. He looked and acted as if he were very tired and I didn't blame him. He had been playing this game since five in the morning. He was wondering whether or not he should shoot the animal—not knowing how seriously it had been wounded by the birdshot—and get it over with. I reported the situation back to the king. Finally, Cordier decided to make a last attempt to capture the animal by shortening the net further, confining it in a smaller area. This meant cutting a number of trees inside the enclosure so that the net could be drawn in. When the order was given to a dozen Africans, they, weary and afraid, just stared sulkily in a vague direction. Feeling that things had reached an impasse, I grabbed a machete and stepped inside the enclosure for a second time. It felt almost like home. I began slashing away at the smaller trees, anxiously watching the dark foliage in the center where the gorilla was hiding. I was only a short while inside the enclosure when I was joined by an African driver in army uniform who, stoked by half a bottle of brandy (I found out later), started cutting trees with great "elan" as if in a hurry to plant sorghum the next day. He was soon followed by half a dozen or so other Africans who had caught our spirit and zeal. No sooner had we cleared all obstacles up to Cordier's vantage point than a dark shape streaked past us towards the far end of the net. Suddenly the air was ripped by a loud report from one of the guns, followed by a long shout that could be interpreted as coming from Schaffer or from the gorilla. I jumped outside the net, past the king and the princess, and glided down the valley from where the inhuman sound had come. I found Schaffer. He was very excited, but he was not hurt. Neither was the gorilla. Schaffer had shot a gas cartridge at the animal, but the effect had not lasted long enough to be of practical value. Wearily, I climbed back on the slope. On the way, I stopped to attend to a number of Africans who had suffered minor cuts during the day. No sooner had I finished dressing the wounds than a big commotion was heard. By the time I reached the enclosure resolution had come by the gorilla. With sunset near, the gorilla decided that the performance was over and it was time to go back to the family for the evening meal. It simply jumped the net, which easily bent under the weight and disappeared with a jaunty fast walk. If the gorilla had worn a hat, it would surely have tipped it to one side of its head and shifted a cigar to the other side of its mouth, provided it also had the cigar. Well, that was that. Though we all felt very disappointed over this escape after Cordier's long preparations and hard work, I felt that we all were relieved that the issue was resolved without accidents and that we had learned a lesson. The gorilla had more than earned its freedom after such a gallant stand against more than 50 humans with eight guns!

    The sun was behind the trees and dusk fell. Everyone was thirsty. I happened to be standing near the king and the princess and they both were eyeing the unopened bottle of soda in my hand—but no bottle opener. I began prying off the cap with the point of my hunting knife. The king said I would break the bottle. I mentioned that I had opened bottles that way many times, which was true. Unfortunately, because I was nervous and wanted to open it quickly, my demonstration failed miserably when, instead of prying the cap further apart, as I should have done, I tapped it with the blunt edge of my knife. The cap came off, but with it an inch of bottle neck. "You see," said the king, "I knew you would break it." At that moment, I would not have minded sharing the inside of the enclosure with a threatening gorilla in order to be somewhere else.

With that incident, the adventures of the day were over. We marched back along the narrow forest path, through the small stream, now a dark tunnel, and reached the cars as the last light faded.

I know of few people who have been on a gorilla hunt, even fewer who shared the hunt with a king, and none who smashed the king's soda bottle. Not to mention stealing the princess's camera.

I left FIS camp the following Saturday morning, arriving late at night in Lwiro. The royal visitors arrived the next day. The king toured the IRSAC laboratories for two days. In our section he was particularly interested in our project of mapping the distribution of insect vectors of diseases and in our collection and work on tsetse flies. The royal visit terminated with a cocktail reception at the guesthouse, where Their Highnesses were presented to the entire IRSAC staff and spouses. So ended a memorable fortnight.

The end of the royal visit did not mean the end of my very busy time. I had to prepare for an interregional meeting at Lwiro, a few weeks later, about "Vectors of Diseases" during which I was to present a paper called: "Factors important to the distribution of *Glossina* in the Belgian Congo and Ruanda-Urundi." It was the first time such a meeting was held in Africa. With twenty-five representatives of various colonial territories, it was a significant achievement of interregional collaboration and mutual interests. The meetings lasted a week. An important outcome was the resolution of an interregional agreement to produce detailed maps of the distribution of vectors of diseases, all of them on transparent basic maps on the same scale, imprinted only with the quarter degree coordinates and watercourses or other major physical features. The collection of such maps would be available at one or two centers where they could be studied or copied. Other basic maps would show major environmental factors so that the distribution of vectors or disease patterns could be compared with climatic characteristics, population density, types of habitation, migration patterns, and so forth. The system became known as "correlation maps." Dr. V. D. B. was their prime promoter. Alas, by the time the undertaking got under way, the project collapsed following the independence of the colonial territories.

At the end of May I left for a fortnight's safari to Mutara and Bugesera, the latter a relatively new region for me. It had received high government priority because of an outbreak of human sleeping sickness there, starting in 1954, requiring investigation to seek its source and to find methods of containment. I was looking forward to this new challenge.

Part IV
In the Shade of an Acacia Tree

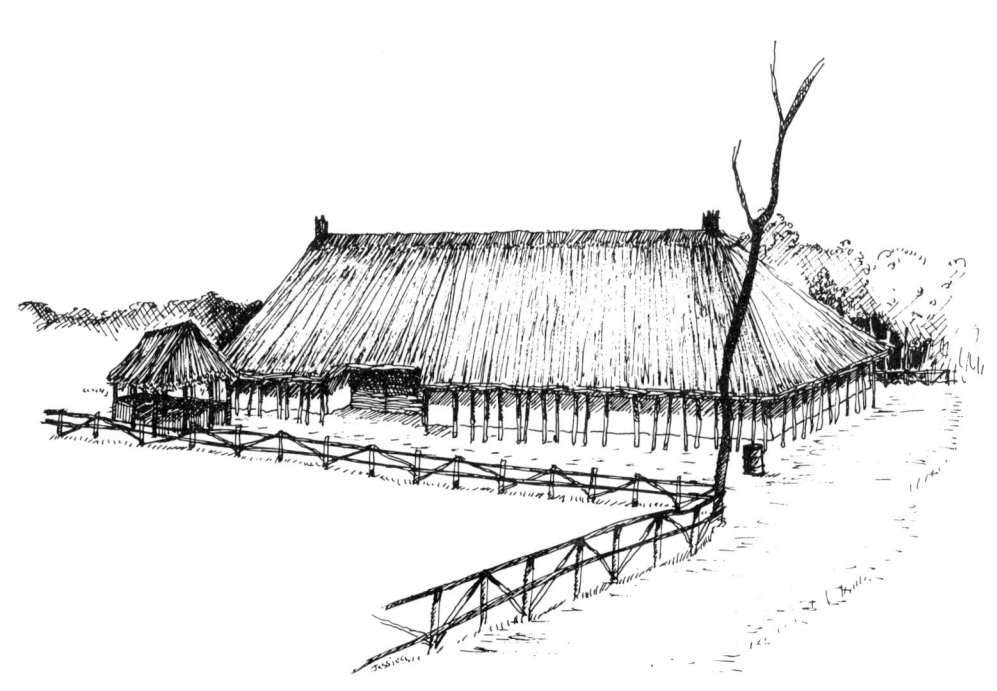

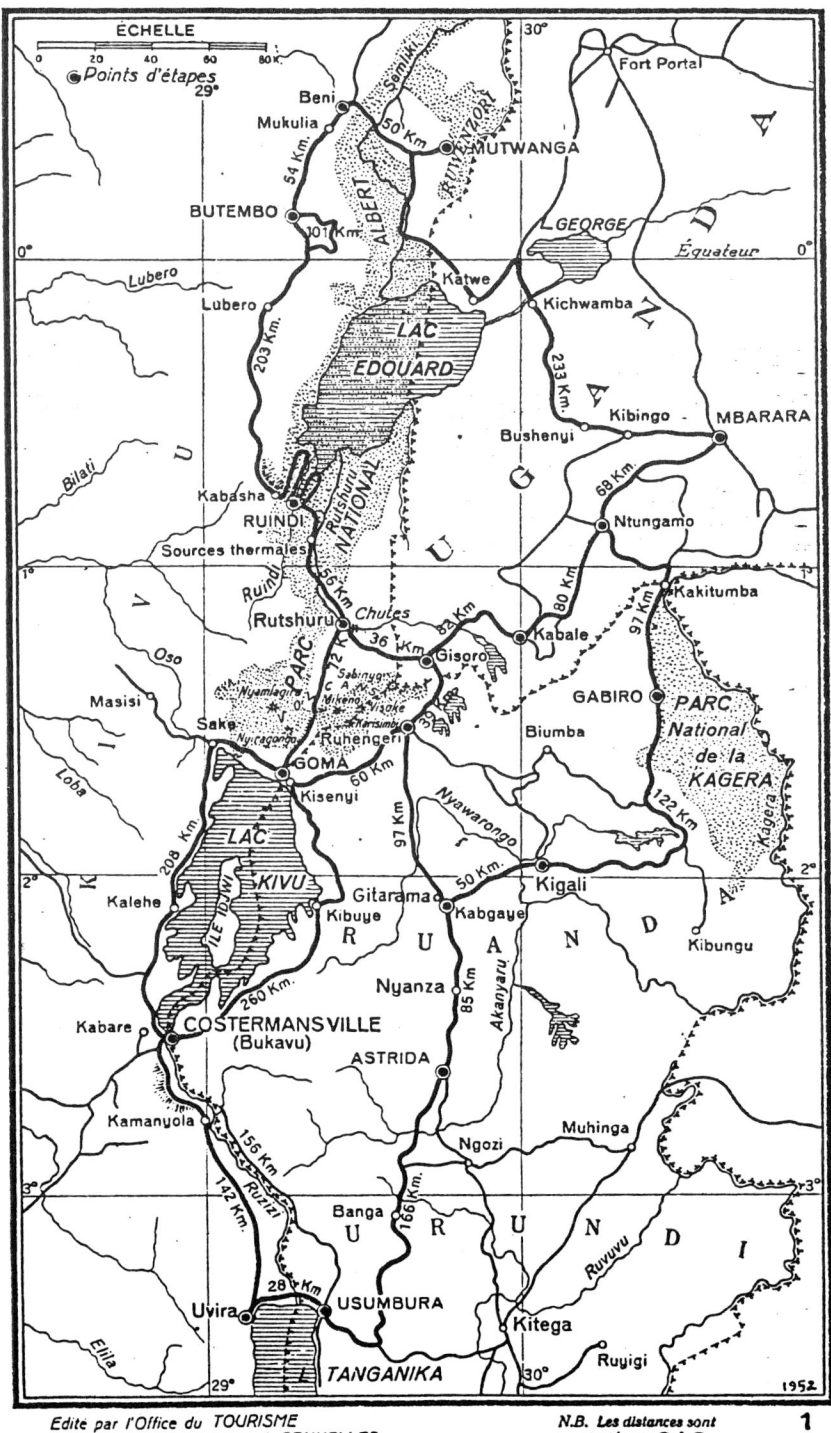

CIRCUIT TOURISTIQUE DU KIVU - RUANDA-URUNDI

Edité par l'Office du TOURISME
87, Rue de la Loi.- BRUXELLES

N.B. Les distances sont calculées de ⊙ à ⊙

① Mutara
② Bugesera
③ Mosso

Where the Antelopes Roam

I sit in my Plymouth station wagon, license number NY-114530. NY stands for New York. We bought the car when we arrived in the United States in early 1952 to tour the country during our six-month home leave. Right now it is early 1954 and the same vehicle that has taken us across 41 U.S. states now stands at the foot of Kakole Hills about 500 yards from the river Kagera that separates the Belgian Protectorate of Ruanda from Tanganyika Territory. I am just about in the geographical center of Africa—if not darkest Africa, the heart of Africa all the same.

The rain falls with steady beads, drumming a monotonous rhythm on the roof—a sullen rain that seems set to go on forever. I stare through the windshield, where crazy meandering rivulets drain across the glass, distorting in funny shapes the hut in front—kitchen-to-be—and the aluminum prefabricated structure, my future occasional home for the next 12 or more months. Low-flying clouds roll across the mountain ridge, the acacia trees on top tearing long shreds from their flanks. An unconvincing rumble of thunder attempts to bring life to the dreary weather. The rain has saturated the foliage of the nearby acacia tree, making long runs across its dark bark like wet fingers on a blackboard. A sudden gust of wind shakes heavy drops that clatter noisily on the roof of the car. I stare at the depressing world outside, questioning once more the philosophy that brought me and kept me in Africa. If, at first, it was adventure that lured me, it was the tsetse fly that kept me. The fly, 30 million years ago, roamed the Colorado plateaus before they became the Rocky Mountains, survived the turbulent Pleistocene only in its original African habitat.

Carrier of microscopic trypanosome parasites that cause sleeping sickness in man and domestic animals, the tsetse fly is subject to intensive scientific research. By nature of its transmission, research covers many elements of the African environment, including such components as climate, vegetation, topography, human and wildlife populations. The multidisciplinary aspect of the problem has been responsible for the creation of that fastidious group of tsetse specialists, the glossinologists. These are individuals who occasionally pop up from undergrowth, small "butterfly" nets in hand or eyes glued to the trunk of an acacia tree or peeping under a fallen log. They are bitten hundreds of times by tsetse flies and it seems that only their strong belief in their own immunity keeps them from getting the disease.

Having concluded the tsetse surveys in the Mosso region during the previous year, I am now carrying out similar research in the north-eastern part of Ruanda, called Mutara, named after a previous great Watutsi king. The region has the shape of a triangle, its apex forming the joint borders of Ruanda, Uganda and Tanganyika Territory (now Tanzania). The triangle is cut in almost equal parts by the main road to the boarder post of Kakitumba. It is a rolling land of gentle, grassy hills and wide, dry valleys, in the west grazed by Watutsi cattle, in the east administered by the Kagera National Park. The road follows the twisting contour of the higher crests allowing an uninterrupted view of a seemingly endless savanna, capped by a dome-shaped sky parading orderly, white cumulus clouds. Sudden gusts of wind bend the long stems of *Themeda* grass in successive waves of purple and silver or creating little sand-devils on the laterite road, and carrying the scent of *Gardenia* and *Acacia* blossoms.

The beginning of Kakole Camp was described in my letter to our director, then on business-home leave in the United States.

Kakitumba, April 26, 1954

Dear Professor,

I am at Kakitumba rest house, the extreme northern corner of Mutara. I am writing you by the light of a faithful Coleman lamp, shared by hundreds of flapping insects which, half-burned, fall into my tea.

It is the close of the day, the tsetse flies are fed, I have separated the serum, I am halfway through Swynnerton's *Tsetse Flies of East Africa*, and I am ready for bed. The evening breeze is cooling somewhat the stuffy air of the rest house, but bringing with it the musty smell of the bats living under the roof. Far away a hippo is laughing, silencing momentarily the eternal chirping of the crickets.

Several months have passed since I started working on our "contract" with the "Plan Décenal." It was early February as I sat down at the foot of Kakole Hill, the northern hill of the fly-belt, looking with somewhat moist eyes at the Kagera River, reflecting how beautiful Africa is. C., who was with me, interrupted my dreams by announcing that he was setting off to look for *Acacia compylacantha* seeds or whatever. I said he had my blessings.

We took over the Kakitumba rest house and started our cooking with Kakitumba water. C. promptly developed the most typical diarrhea, so colorfully described in Dr. Jacqué's lectures, with an impressive fever around 40°C. After the administration of huge quantities of sulfaguanidine, C. recovered, in response, he said, to the alternative of dying from sulfa poisoning. We jeeped along and about the hills and one day captured a *Glossina pallidipes*, unreported from these areas. Strong with this new knowledge, we contacted Wilson, the tsetse man across the Uganda border. Unbelieving, he came back with us to make sure the fly was where we said it was. It was. We captured some more in other places, Thus satisfied, Wilson went back to ring the alarm in Uganda and Tanganyika.

In the meanwhile I had all kinds of trouble recruiting local laborers from the nearest village ten miles away. This done, we started building the camp—my third in four years. The site: the place where I first overlooked the Kagera valley with poetic eyes, at the foot of Kakole Hill. We started cutting *Acacia hebecladoides* to be used for poles, *Acacia campylacantha* for beams, and *Acacia seyal* var. *multijuga* for firewood. C. said we had no use for *Acacia milbreadii* or *Acacia senegal*. (Botanists are very picky.) I cast an envious eye towards the Kagera papyrus and the clear water that ran between them both located within the protected areas of the Kagera National Park. Gratefully, we received permission from Mr. Haezaerts to use both, the former for covering the roofs, the latter for a general water supply.

As the building of the camp proceeded at a slow pace and expenses mounted, I had a mild brain wave. During my travel in Uganda I had noted the many prefabricated aluminum huts used in government temporary camps. So I went to see our accountant to ask about the solidity of my budget. "Mmm, mmm," he said. "O.K., O.K." I said, "how about cutting me in for a mere 30,000 francs. Three more camps and we shall start saving by the reuse of the same materials." "Mmm," he said. So I am now the proud possessor of a cozy bungalow.

I had left ten men with Wilson at Mbarara to be trained as flyboys. They came back in good spirits and with enlarged knowledge. They can tell me when a fly had its last meal and when a female fly had its last baby. That sort of thing.

In the meanwhile I had surveyed most of the hills and dales. It seems I am the first white man to climb Kakole Hill. I am not surprised at that. Who but a crazy glossinologist would think of doing so? It was worthwhile, however, because my crude survey map correlated nicely with the aerial photos we received later and it was now possible for me to recognize the types of vegetation and to plot possible fly-rounds.

These last days I have measured on the ground three fly-rounds. The one going over Kakole ridge is the longest, 4,150 meters, and the most difficult. I started on Saturday morning at about nine accompanied by five fly-boys and two "mpagazis." I marked every 50 meters, noting compass bearings, and compared the progress on the aerial photo while reading the altitude and indicating the vegetation types. After dragging on like this a whole day without food and, worse, without water, we finally arrived at the Kakitumba River at five in the afternoon. From here we had still another hour's walk back to camp. Eighty-three poles had been cut and "planted" to mark the "catching stations." Ah, for a good sleep. It was not to be so. Sharp rocks had cut my feet through the rubber soles of my shoes, acacia thorns had claimed large portions of my knees and arms, tsetse flies had had a field day and never fed so well. While we were crawling through thicket vegetation, a large number of caterpillars had attached themselves to exposed skin, leaving behind tiny barbed hairs that started to itch between two and three in the morning.

The following day I measured a second fly-round that samples most of the valley leading to the Kagera River. Much easier than the Kakole round, it is 2,850 meters long. A third round measures 3,300 meters and runs along the northern slope of Kakole Hill. In the meanwhile I have received official authorization to survey areas within the national park. Hence, I shall measure a fourth fly-round along the Kagera River.

The amount of game in these hills is astonishing. Impala are everywhere. Zaghi, who finally came back from leave, says that one day a herd of about 40 cattle walked not more than 30 yards from the camp. Only they were buffaloes. He saw rhino on the Tanganyika side of the Kagera. Hippos are to be heard all day long and during the night. It is therefore easy to collect many blood samples from a variety of game. This is how we stand now:

1. Kakole Camp, consisting of three large huts for fly-boys and other personnel, Zaghi's house and my aluminum hut; a kitchen and the compulsory high fence will be finished by the first half of May.
2. Ten men have received good training and will form the basis of our survey personnel.
3. Three fly-rounds have been measured and will be run from the first of May, to start our scientific observations.
4. We have received permission to work in the park.
5. A number of blood smears have been handed to M.C. from impala, zebra, and topi. I make it a routine to make also "Klatch" preparations from liver, spleen, and heart.

6. Improvement in techniques of collecting serum has given me good quantities and qualities of serum from impala, zebra, and topi. I have produced good antiserum in rabbits from waterbuck and ourebi. This serological work takes most of my time between safaris.
7. The *G. pallidipes* situation is quite confusing. I have captured these tsetse in half a dozen places on either side of the hills. I intend to concentrate on this fly as soon as routine work is well established.

I just finished Swynnerton's 600-page book on tsetse flies. The things not mentioned on tsetses in this book could be put underneath a postage stamp, as Wodehouse would say. A real bible.

Well, dear Professor, I hope you have a good time in dear U.S.A. Imagine this letter being delivered to the busy Lexington Avenue address with the smell of hippo not quite gone from these pages. If you ever stop at Carmel on your way to Belmont, order a walnut chocolate ice cream at "Tom's Cafe." It is delicious!

Cheerio.

From our Center at Lwiro two different roads could be followed to reach Mutara. One skirted the west shore of Lake Kivu and the southern slopes of the Virunga volcanoes, the other forded the southern end of Lake Kivu at the bridge spanning the Ruzizi River outlet. It climbed through the primeval Nyongwe mountain forest and, crossing the Congo-Nile divide, descended into the eastern lowlands. Within a matter of 20 miles or so, both roads were within the 360-mile range from Lwiro. Both roads were equally spectacular and each had its own difficult passages. At first I preferred the northern route because of the dramatic views of the volcanoes, but many times I went the other way which passed our IRSAC Center at Astrida at the one-third point of the way, and could provide help in case of a breakdown or other problems.

Among my diaries I find the description of one of my trips along the northern route.

Thursday, August 12, 1954

I awake and I can see the approach of dawn in the sky. It is 5:30. No use going back to sleep as I am leaving early today on a week's safari. The first rays of the sun are a feeble yellow, foreboding rain. I hear Mutima enter the kitchen and rummage among pots and pans. I shave, dress, gather my toilet kit and pack my bag. At seven the pickup arrives, Narcisse, the African driver at the wheel. He and Mutima stow everything in an orderly fashion, but I know by experience that soon the bouncing over the rough roads will throw everything into utter chaos. The jerry can with kerosene may start leaking in spite of the extra seal made from a piece of inner tubing and then drip onto the top of the basket with potatoes. Inside the "malle-cantine" (picnic basket), the pan could be rubbing a hole in the tablecloth, and when I finally arrive at my destination, still 360 miles away, the butter will have the viscosity of something between S.A.E. 90 and rear axle grease, if by chance the jar is still intact.

It is eight o'clock and we are driving north along the western shores of Lake Kivu towards Goma. The road is slippery, but not too bad so far. Yesterday's rain has dried up somewhat, but in the forest we are now driving through, everything drips, saturated with moisture. Narcisse has problems with the second gear, which has a tendency to jump out at each corner and heaven knows how many times that happens. The road winds its way up away from the shore towards famous Km 113, where it runs through a gap like an advancing army. The cloud hangs for a moment unmoving as if undecided until another gust of wind pushes it on and the lower part tumbles into the valley. As we descend the other side of the pass, the lake is once again visible, now some 1,500 feet below us. The weather has turned for the worse. A dark wall of rain moves slowly across the water towards the shore. Small islands are sharply silhouetted as if drawn with India ink on gray cardboard. We arrive at the dreaded curve of Km 109. Going down, it is not too bad and Narcisse knows the road well. Coming up the road for the first time, however, one is sure to miss this turn and to have to back up for another try. As this maneuver must be carried out on a narrow escarpment bordering the lake 1,500 feet below, it is an unnerving experience.

We arrive at a place where the road is being widened. Loose soil and rocks make the passage very difficult. Just at this moment the rain is upon us in solid sheets of water and turning the loose earth into a series of mud-traps. At one point the vehicle starts sliding slowly towards the precipice. A border of grass and rocks stops the skidding and we breathe easier again. Lower down the same thing happens; this time we slide towards the lake. Again, the skid is stopped by a ditch that, if difficult to get out of, is preferable to the lake.

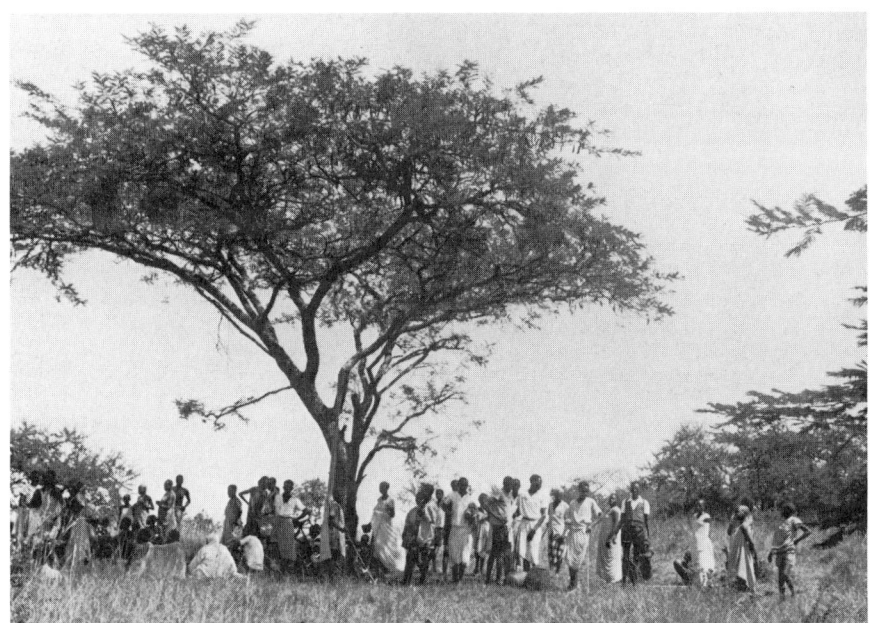
Mutara villagers wait for blood samples to be taken.

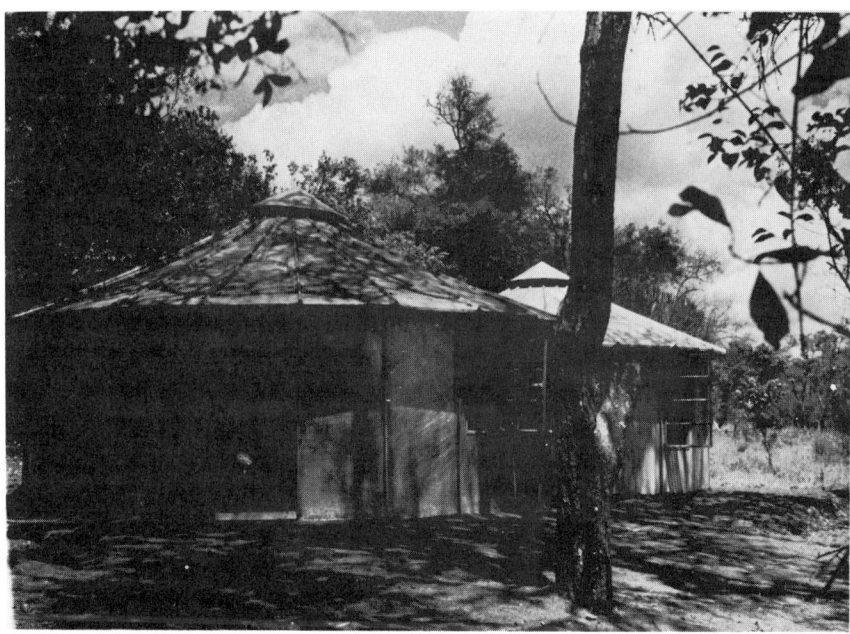
Camp Biharagu at Lake Tshohoha.

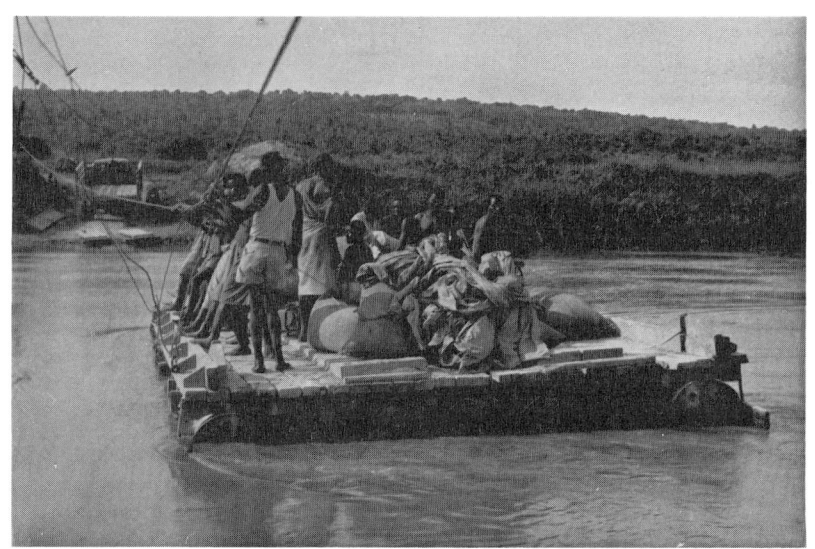
Ferry across the Nyawarongo River.

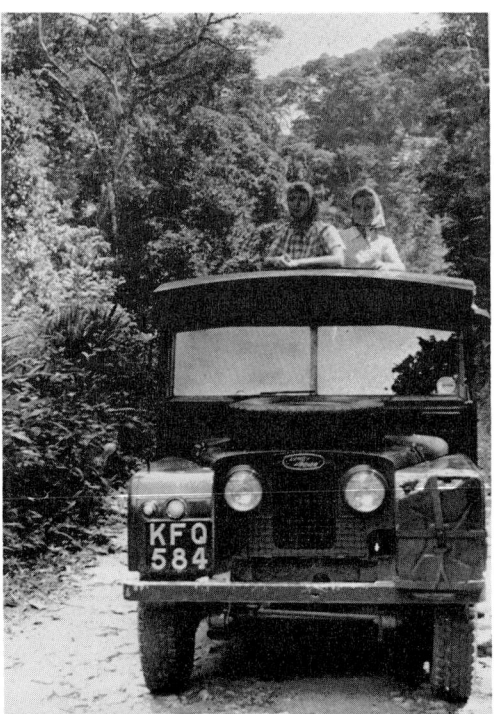
Our faithful Land-Rover. Winnie and Jessie look through the "survey hatch."

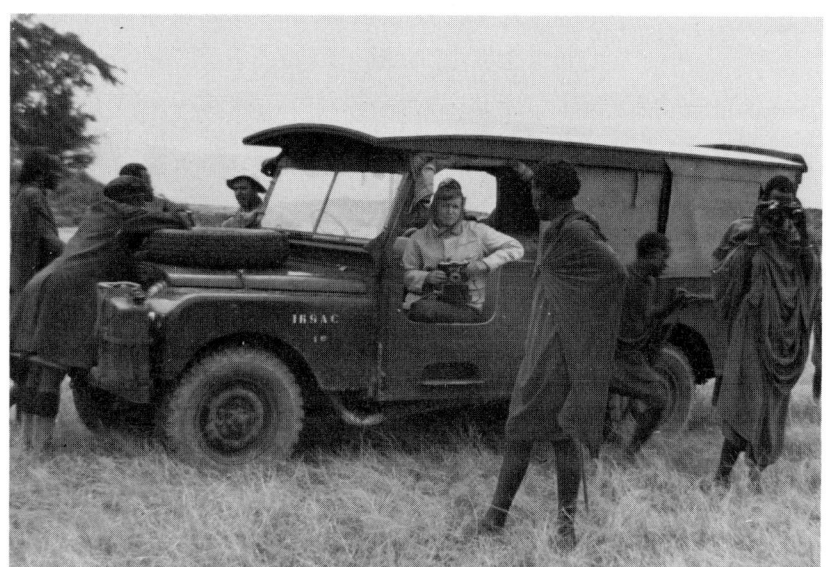
A group of Maasai people in Ngorongoro Crater, Kenya.

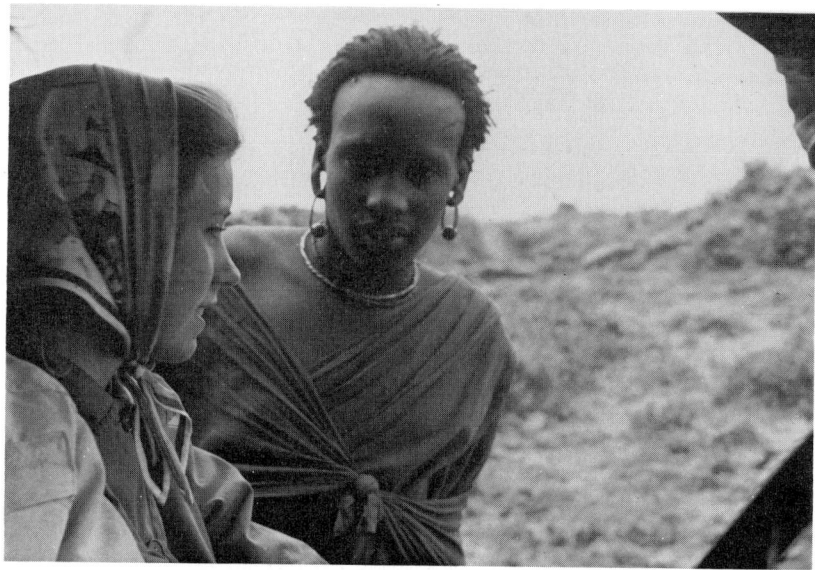
Jessie in serious conversation with one of the Maasai.

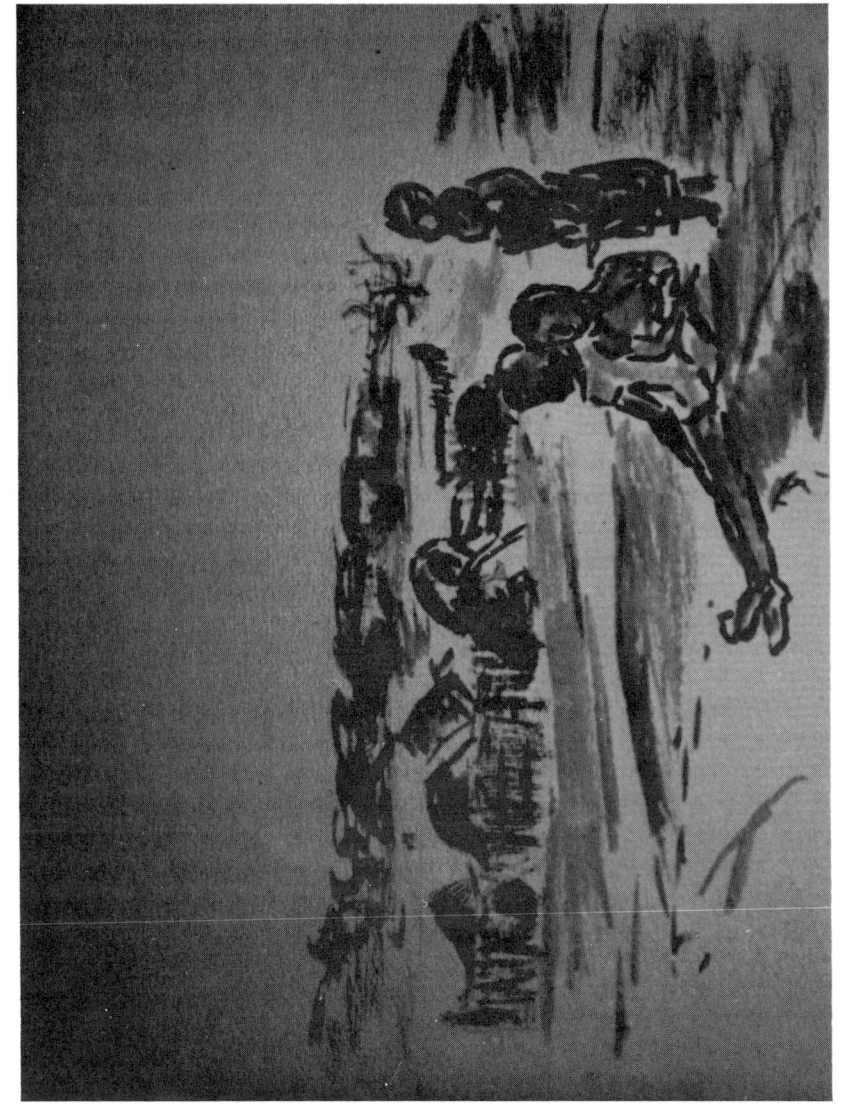

Sketch of some Maasai by Jessica Rice. Used with her permission.

The rain stops and I wish for the sun because I am very cold. My wish is only partly fulfilled: a weak "winter sun" manages to shine for a brief moment. Near Kirotche at a point where a lava flow has cut off a small bay in the lake, one of the volcanoes comes into view. It is the active Nyamulangira. Smoke mixed with condensation rises from one side of the broad, blunt crater and rolls down its western slope. This part of the road has some dangerous "death-corner" curves and we barely escape collision with two trucks coming from the opposite direction. A sign states: "Passage difficile." That is putting it mildly.

From Kirotche onwards, the road has been cut out of solidified lava. Three flows can be distinguished. The one from 1912 is already covered with well-developed typical lava vegetation; the one from 1938 supports the same type of vegetation, but much lower. The most recent eruption in 1948 caused a two-branched lava flow, one of which reached the lake in a huge cloud of steam. These recent flows are still bare of vegetation (1954).

It starts raining again. We reach Goma around noon, just before the closing of the shops and in time to buy bread and a water filter. We have done 110 miles in five hours—that kind of road. I figure, wrongly as proved afterwards, that we can reach Ruhengeri without taking gas at Goma. From Kisenyi, a well-known lakeshore resort on the Ruanda side of the border, we climb away from lake level into the Ruanda highlands. At the altitude of 8,500 feet, the road reaches a wide, flat valley intensely cultivated because of the fertile volcanic soils. To the left the cones of two volcanoes rise abruptly, the Karisimbi and the Migongo. Although close together like Siamese twins, they differ markedly in character. The Karisimbi is topped by craggy, toothy peaks; the Migongo has the classical shape of a perfect cone.

Suddenly the engine dies, we are out of gas. The old truck is using gas like a jet. We find the rubber tube (no safari leaves home without it) and insert it in the reserve 50-gallon gasoline drum. Narcisse sucks the liquid from the other end and plunges it into the tank as soon as the fuel starts flowing. We restock our fuel reserve at the Hindu shop in Ruhengeri.

The road continues to Biumba, another 70 miles, and the countryside changes once more. The dark lava soil is replaced by rosy laterite with high quartz and mica content. The roads cut in these soils are generally smooth and well graded, but still slippery during the rains. They follow the crests of the high plateaus at an average of 6,000 feet as pink ribbons or a pink garter when they span a mountain top. The dark, fertile soils of the high valleys between the crests are much cultivated. Near Biumba, large pyrethrum fields drape the gentle slope of one of the valleys in a display of brilliant white. Biumba, at 7,200 feet, is the highest government post in Belgian Africa. It is also the most expensive, with gasoline costs twice the lowland prices.

We are now on our last lap to the Mutara region. A long descent takes us into a series of beautiful valleys dramatically illuminated by the setting sun and huge white clouds. Gatsibu is the last commercial center. The road drops once more to the level of the lowlands that stretch all the way, north and east into the East African savannas.

It is night when we arrive at Kakole Camp. Zaghi, my African assistant, comes out with a lamp and begins the usual bustle of unloading, putting up my camp bed, exchanging news, starting the pressure stove to boil water, preparing a hasty meal and finally, with the subdued voices of the Africans around a dying campfire faintly in my ears, I turn out the lamp and go to sleep, civilization behind me. I am on my own, sole master of a landbound ship in a sea of undulating savanna.

The next morning, I accompany the fly-boys on their search for tsetse pupae. They are usually found buried at about one inch in loose soil in shaded places, such as underneath fallen logs, at the foot of large trees, under rock outcrops, and so on—places also favored by lions, leopards and snakes. The morning passes peacefully, but is unrewarding since no pupae are found. Later in the day I drive to Gabiro, the Kagera National Park headquarters and residence of the chief warden. I want to inform him about my scientific hunting permit which allows me to kill any animal species of any sex in any numbers. Such a permit, rarely as it may be granted, is still "a thorn in the side" of a game warden. I think it is wise to see the warden in person and explain the purpose of my special permit and to assure him that I shall not abuse the privileges conferred on me by the permit. In spite of our friendly conversation, I can sense his underlying feeling of resentment. Ironically, my permit allows me more freedom with regard to hunting than he has as chief warden of the park. Our common interest in animal behavior prevails, however, and I spend a pleasant and useful afternoon.

Back "home" I prepare chicken soup from a package—a great advance in the art of safari supplies because of the savings of weight and space—and make "instant" coffee, again a great invention. I make a large spill of coffee on the tablecloth. Without thinking, I wipe it off with a napkin and resume reading. One develops crude table manners when alone in the bush. Narcisse, the driver, has appointed himself as my personal attendant. Mutima did not come with me this time as he was needed at home, and perhaps he was the one who instructed Narcisse to look after me. His close attention, however, has become troublesome and embarrassing. When I have a cup of tea, for example, he watches me to see whether I have finished so that he can take the cup away to be washed. When at that moment I pour another cup, he seems disappointed and looks around for something else to do. His eyes light up because he can put away shorts I have negligently thrown out of the trunk in search of cartridges. Finally, he departs. I settle down to write when his head pops in again asking whether he should fill the kerosene lamp. I say no, tomorrow. What about the pressure stove? I say no, tomorrow. He reminds me that I should put away the dinner plates he just washed. I say O.K. He says good-night. I think he is cross with me because I always beat him in setting the table for meals.

The next day was Saturday, a "free" day when personnel are set to small household chores, such as feeding live tsetse flies on guinea pigs. I decide to go hunting. I have arguments with myself about the selection of gear. There is so much I want to take, but am restricted to carrying capacity of the two fly-boys who will accompany me. I settle finally, for the following: a 9.3 rifle, a 12-gauge shotgun, 30 rounds of ammunition, a box with clean glass slides for making blood smears, three big sterile jars and four smaller ones for collecting whole blood, a small box with small tubes for collecting ecto- and endo- parasites, a cyanide killing jar for insects, a compass, a map, two pencils, a first-aid kit, a knife, a pair of forceps, some tags, a camera, a canteen with tea. The next decision is what to wear. Early mornings at 3,000 feet are very cold and damp. It takes only a few hundred yards walking through high grass to become sopping wet from the icy dew. The choice is whether to be miserable during the first two hours wearing light clothes or be extremely uncomfortable during the rest of the day in heavy boots and water-repellent garb. I have adopted the first. I always wear walking shorts, my legs protected by canvas leggings, manfully bearing the scratches and lacerations on knees and thighs from plants with spines, hooks, needles and burns. Further, how is one to be shod? Preferences run from tennis shoes to heavy army boots. I have settled for old shoes conveniently worn for my own comfort. I once tried black high rubber boots, but their weight, rigidity and the heat generated inside them make for very unpleasant footwear. As for the rest, any shirt will do although breast pockets prove handy. Color doesn't matter as it will soon be besmeared, faded and torn. Headdress: here we run into an area of extremely individual tastes. The kind of head cover I have observed surpasses any degree of imagination. In fact, anything goes. During field demonstrations, for instance, one is amazed to see dandified participants come out for the field trip wearing a hat that defies any description, often showing signs and scars of previous rough usage, but worn with endearing affection. I have long since abandoned the pith helmet, such a classic and a must in "old" colonial times, but so unwieldy in my kind of work, and have lately sported various "bush hats" of all kinds and colors.

I left freshly shaven, in clean clothes and with a bouncing stride. I came back dragging my feet, looking like a tramp after a week along the railroad tracks.

The hunt had been fairly productive. As soon as we had crossed the rise on which the camp is built we saw a group of 15 impalas (*Aepyceros melampus*). They had spotted us and moved slowly uphill, not showing fear but clearly on the alert. A big ram with beautiful lyre-shaped horns (the females have no horns) seemed in charge and he walked up the valley. Dropping all pretenses and with a sharp bark, he led a general flight characterized by acrobatic high jumps. The jumps start with the flexing and stretching of the forelegs which, on the rebound are repeated by the hind legs. I don't know whether this is an inherent defensive endowment, but it certainly makes a running aim very difficult.

Soon thereafter, we saw seven elands (*Taurotragus oryz*). As I had already shot two of those animals last year and still had plenty of serum, I didn't bother them. Elands are among the biggest and heaviest antelopes. Judged from my last year's experience, they are also among the toughest. I had shot one from about 100 yards and it dropped immediately. To make certain I lodged another 9.3 bullet in it from 20 yards. This only seemed to excite the animal, which jumped up and made off at a good clip. I had to run after it and put six more bullets into it before it stayed down. An adult bull stands from 5 foot 7 inches to 6 feet measured from the top of its humped shoulder. Both sexes have horns, pointed backwards, spiraled at the base. The weight of the animal averages between 1,500 to 2,000 pounds. They are usually seen in herds of a dozen or so, but once I counted more than 200 as they vaulted one by one across the road not more than ten yards in front of my car, some with an astonishingly high jump. Elands are generally very gentle animals and it seems a pity that no large scale efforts are being made to domesticate such a potentially valuable candidate for livestock. On one occasion I have seen a few elands mix with regular cattle and be driven with them into a corral at the end of the day.

After we left the elands browsing in peace, we saw another herd of impalas. The approach was difficult because we were now in open country. So I tried a shot from 150 yards. I could hear the bullet strike, but no one dropped. Most animals ran off except for one ram which, curiosity taking the better of its fear, stood its ground. He paid with his life. My bullet hit him square in the head, entering one side and coming out behind the horns. As I knelt beside the corpse, perspiration ran from my face both from excitement and from running. I made the usual blood smears, cursing the flies taking full advantage of my inability to defend myself. The Hutu hunter who had joined us earlier in the morning cut the skin of the neck and the jugular vein. Warm blood gushed into my collecting bottle over my hands. The bottles filled, I started collecting ticks. These insects are well embedded under the skin and very difficult to remove whole including the mouth-parts, without which the specimen is worthless. I always found it repulsive to pry the ticks out with my bare hands. I sent the two flyboys back to camp with the dead animal and with most of my gear while I continued to explore with the Hutu hunter.

The sun was now high in the sky. The wide, open rolling hills of the Mutara bathed in light but for the dark patches marking the passage of bulging clouds. At a distance, halfway up the slope of a hill, a herd of some 20 zebras was grazing. They looked up, their curiosity winning over their instinct for flight. Turning their small, quivering ears in our direction, their attitude clearly showed that they were pondering the problem. Suddenly a few animals turned around and trotted off in a slow but pressing gait. Then the rest followed, the sound of hooves dying in the distance. Soon thereafter we came to another small group of zebras and I prepared to shoot one as I did not have many blood samples from those animals. I managed to crawl behind a good cover and selected a big one. It dropped immediately, the bullet striking the base of the neck, coming out the other side, sectioning the jugular vein and the vertebra. When we came to the body, a large pool of blood had already formed underneath the wound and I managed only a quart bottle. I made the customary four blood smears and collected ticks. Between the two of us there was nothing we could do to transport some meat—a great pity because I had tasted zebra meat before and it is delicious. We covered the animal with grass, a futile task because the vultures had already spotted the kill and were circling overhead.

We came across some more impalas and then another herd of zebras. Not satisfied with the previous collection of blood, I selected one of the animals, aiming carefully for the region of the heart. As the bullet struck, the animal suddenly turned its head to the side as if to assess the damage, then galloped full steam in our direction. Astonished by the apparent charge, I felt a moment of panic. The animal stopped abruptly at 20 yards, turned upon itself and dropped dead. The bullet had gone right through the heart. This time I collected a good amount of blood and after the blood smears and the collection of ticks, called it a day.

I wondered how to get the two zebras to camp or at least, as far as I was concerned, the beautiful skin, when six Africans showed up attracted, no doubt, by the shots. Discussions about the problem ensued. They were not inclined to carry any of the meat, figuring, correctly, that later on they could collect most of the meat for themselves. They consented, however, to remove and carry the skins to camp—for a "matabish" (tip) to which I agreed. It was now two in the afternoon and I felt very tired and footsore. While the Africans began the skinning, I sat down in the shade of a large acacia tree heedless to the exposure to ants and other troublesome insects. I was too weary to care. My bottle with tea was empty and I was suffering a terrible thirst. But underneath my large acacia tree the shade was deep, cool and pleasant. I watched the clouds glide over the sun and whip up a sudden breeze. The ants respected this moment of contentment and left me in peace. At last the skinning of the two zebras was finished and I was now faced with the prospects of a two-hour walk back to camp during the hottest part of the afternoon. And then there are the flies. How rosy life on earth would be without the flies. I remember well how once, in Switzerland, I had to push my bicycle up a long, steep mountain road, a heavy rucksack on my shoulders, both hands fully engaged in the strenuous task and being attacked on all sides by hordes of biting horse flies. This is the only time I can remember coming close to hysteria. To the layman there are two kinds of flies: inoffensive ones which hover over ferns and flowers; the bad ones landing on people and causing all kinds of troubles, settling on food with unwiped feet, soiling delicate lacework with droppings and distracting boys and girls from their homework. In the savannas of Africa some flies, presumably seeking moisture and salt, commute between the left and right eye. At each strike, irritation causes eyes and noses to run to the great enjoyment of newcomer flies. One stumbles, perspires and attracts more flies. Then there is the kind that has taken specialization courses and concentrates on nostrils and mouths. A very small fly devotes its life to hovering inside the ear. Besides tickling the hairs, it creates a high-pitched noise preferably at the moment when one tries to track the sound of a moving animal. One group of flies I called the "tethered flies" because of their ability to bounce right back after being chased away as if attached with a rubber band. One way to get rid of them is to leap into a river, if one is available. Personally, I prefer the tsetse fly. Of course, its bite may cause fatal sleeping sickness, but it is a fly with personality, a goal and a determination characterized by its swift flight and speed of attack. It gets down to business in no roundabout way. It lands and without walking all over one's face, pierces the skin with a neat professional touch, takes some blood and in the process may pump a few hundred trypanosomes into the bloodstream, and is off in a jiffy to rest in the shade. It won't bother anyone for the next three or four days until all the blood is digested and hunger or sex urges it back into action.

Hardship is soon forgotten when "home" comes in sight. We rounded the hill and there, below us, was the familiar campsite, gloriously bathed in the setting sun.

Sunday, August 15, 1954

Today I am halfway through my safari and, therefore, it is time to turn the tablecloth. Besides earmarking the midway point it also helps to hide the spots made during the first half. The large coffee spill is showing through, however. It looks like a prehistoric monster with a wide-open mouth.

My first job this morning is to separate my serum from yesterday's blood collections. This takes time, but I was up early so there is still plenty of day left when I ready myself for another hunting expedition. The Hutu hunter who accompanied me yesterday asked to come with me again today. He must have made a good profit from the meat. He tells me he was one of the Mwami's gun bearers. Failing eyesight may be the reason that he became a "free-lancer," for I often spot animals well before he does. He wears a long black overcoat, a badge of office as one of the Mwami's hunters perhaps. How he endures the heavy coat during the hot hours of the day is a mystery to me. He tells me there should be good hunting across the Kakitumba River where, indeed, we can observe a large herd of impalas. We cross the stream over an *Acacia milbreadii* that, its roots undermined by the current, has tumbled onto the opposite bank. As we advance across the flood plain, the impalas keep an equal distance and finally gallop away, out of reach. Rounding a coppice, we flush a herd of about fifteen waterbuck (*Kobus defassa*), including several large males. I risk a shot at 200 yards, which results only in their disorderly flight. We skirt the fringe of the riverine vegetation, but they spot us again and are off. This little game is repeated several more times, leading us across hills and dales. I give up, finally, for they seem to be better at this sort of exercise. The sun has reached high noon, sending shimmering heat waves above the plains and making judgment of distances uncertain. Wearily I tumble into the shade of an acacia tree. Flimsy though its foliage may be, it still filters the direct sunlight and generates an occasional caressing breeze. I empty one of the two bottles of tea and feel better. Not for long.

One of the followers—it is uncanny how even in this isolated area a hunting party soon will attract people apparently from nowhere like flies at the smell of meat or, to put it in a more poetic metaphor, like butterflies to flowers—suddenly points to our right whispering "kiboko" (hippopotamus). Sure enough, a gray mass, which my tired eyes had mistakingly identified as a somewhat unusual boulder, rises not more than 30 yards away. Instead of the hurried flight I anticipate, the animal becomes rather aggressive, turning its massive head in our direction with a deep grunt. Its small, eyes blink in the sunlight, nostrils flapping angrily. I hear a commotion behind me and looking back find only the hunter at my side. The followers have climbed into nearby trees as if the soil had suddenly become unbearably hot. It was, of course, a hot day. The state of affairs has clearly developed into an uncomfortable impasse—although later, much later, the whole scene seemed absurd. I ponder what to do (I do need a blood sample of hippo blood). But as I reach irresolutely for my gun, the tree people keep warning me "hapana pika, bwana, iko nyama mbya" (don't shoot, master, the animal is dangerous). Never having encountered a hippo on dry land, I ask the hunter if the animal can run fast. "Sawa-sawa machua, bwana" (As fast as a motorcar, master) is his reply. The animal has edged a bit closer, now perhaps only 20 yards away. At this range I certainly cannot miss, but I feel that the distance is a bit on the short side for shooting a one-ton animal, I know I cannot drop with a single 9.3 bullet an animal reputed to have "the speed of a motorcar." It is the hippo that finally decides the issue. In a single swift movement it turns around and trots off at a fair pace towards the river. I am relieved with the outcome although, as I later reflected, it would have been a unique opportunity to shoot the hippo out of water and take blood under ideal circumstances and collect ectoparasites.

Altogether a frustrating day.

Those Mutara Days

Nineteen fifty-four to 1956 were altogether exciting years, a period of great discoveries at our Irangi station; my research in the Mutara region opened a whole new world on animal ecology and the intricate yet clear-cut vegetation communities of the eastern savannas. By now I had spent ten years in Africa, but it was the lonely stays in the Mutara, shared only with the wild animals, that made me feel that I was actually becoming part of the African biotope. I walked the acacia groves not as a foreigner but as a denizen. I began to perceive the subtle forces that regulate the equilibrium between creatures who share the same ecological niches, the forces that move them along an evolutionary path too distant to understand. In fact, it was at about that time that my first thoughts about the evolution of sleeping sickness in prehistoric man began to take shape.

In the savannas, tsetse fly distribution and density are closely related to vegetational patterns. I became an ardent student of trees, shrubs and grasses, greatly assisted by the enthusiastic IRSAC botanists, Christiaensen and Troupin. Acacias became my favorite trees because their communities formed the majority of tsetse habitats in the Mutara region. Christiaensen was a frequent companion in my Mutara and later Bugesera safaris.

With Dora kept homebound after the birth of our son in 1953, Winnie or Jessie became occasional companions when my safaris coincided with their school holidays. Jessie was fourteen when she first came with me to Mutara. She was thrilled to see close up the various antelopes, zebras, buffaloes, warthogs and hippopotamuses. She loved Kakole camp and its neat prefabricated aluminum hut. The morning after our arrival, while I was away on a tsetse survey, she painted a lovely snow landscape (in defiance perhaps of our tropical environment). Her effort signaled the talent of the great artist she would become in later life. At that time, I had taken up watercolors again and we had great fun ridiculing each other's compositions while showing with exaggeration the great satisfaction with one's own work.

One day, coming back from Kafunzo across the Uganda border, we were somewhat surprised to find one of the fly-boys in a tree on fly-round III, which ran along the road at that point. When questioned, he replied that he had been chased a moment before by an angry buffalo. Being treed by a buffalo was not uncommon.

Jessie's wish to see a lion was fulfilled in an extraordinary way the night we traveled back home. We had left camp at three in the morning and only a few miles beyond camp saw two beautiful leopards in the headlights. Instead of jumping out of the way, they kept on running in front of the car, their supple, easy strides a show of grace, speed and strength. Finally, one jumped to the left outside the beam of light, the other following suit soon thereafter. As if part of a zoological display of night predators, not long after the leopards' performance, the headlight shone on two adult lions and a cub stretched out in the middle of the road. As I braked, they moved slowly to one side of the road, the cub nervously blinking its eyes as it followed its mother into the dark. What a sight!

"Thanks, Dad," Jessie whispered.

"Not at all, my pleasure," I replied.

The following month it was Winnie's turn to accompany me to the Mutara. As before, we left at three in the morning in order to arrive at my camp 13 hours later. The reason for these early morning departures was that I wanted to make the journey without stopovers, but still arrive early enough in the day to unload and set up camp before dark. On the return trip home I usually left even earlier so as to do most of the driving during the cool hours in order to reduce risks of deaths among the hundreds of tsetse flies brought back in "Bruce" boxes. These flies would be later dissected and examined for trypanosome infections, while some would be fed on laboratory animals in an attempt to isolate trypanosomes in vivo.

Although Winnie never saw the Mutara lions, there was plenty of evidence that they were around, judging from the racket they made during several nights. A hippo was heard munching just outside the fence one night, while during the day a herd of waterbuck was often seen grazing along the Kagera River. One early morning as Winnie and I were taking a stroll along the river, we were suddenly startled by deep grunts. Not more than 20 feet away, inside the tall papyrus reeds a large hippo was lying on its side, its hindquarters partly inside the water. When we crept closer, the animal made an effort to rise, but sank back with another groan. There was obviously something very wrong. But being within the limits of the park, I did not dare to shoot it and end its obvious misery. Instead I sent a message to the park warden informing him of the sick animal near our camp. We went to see the hippo, which we christened "Eulalie," several times that day and the next days until we left, hoping that the warden had gotten my message and would do something about it.

Poignant among Winnie's recollections of her stay in Mutara are the number of jiggers (*Tunga penetrans*) that found their way under her toenails and grew pea-sized before classical severe itching made her aware of them. *Tunga penetrans* is a flea that was introduced into Africa from South America during the previous century. The female flea penetrates underneath the skin, preferably the toenail. There, sucking blood, it develops its hundreds of eggs, growing in the process to the form of a good-sized pea. When left alone, the mature eggs are expelled daily from the entrance of the wound until the insect dies. This may result in severe bacterial infection leading sometimes to the loss of the infected toe. Many Africans in the habit of walking barefoot suffer mutilated feet as a result of multiple jigger infections. Rule one: avoid contact between feet and bare soil. Rule two: be alert and at the first sign have the insect removed. Africans are very skillful in that sort of surgery, performed by means of the sterilized point (flamed with a lighted match) of a needle. I once tried to remove a jigger by myself, causing the egg sack to break. A serious infection followed and had to be treated with penicillin injections. In Winnie's case, the jiggers were detected in time so that they could be removed without complications. The cook performed the surgery.

As mentioned earlier, Christiaensen, a self-taught botanist, was a frequent safari companion. Ten years older than I, he was the quiet type of old colonial. He had given up an association with his brother in a well-known, lucrative toy shop in Antwerp in order to satisfy his desire to study tropical plants in the Congo. He never went back to toys. Somehow he managed to muddle through as a small-scale planter, his latest venture having been an unprofitable coffee plantation on the eastern slope of Mount Kahuzi. It was there that our director "discovered" him and took him on as a technical assistant (botany), in part to work with our appointed botanist, Dr. Troupin, in part to assist me in the identification of the vegetation communities characterizing tsetse fly habitats. Christiaensen was a marvelous teammate. With a vast knowledge of African plants he was also a versed reader of scientific literature and history. He had a jovial tongue-in-cheek wit and found merriment in the most ticklish situations. C. (Christiaensen) was a member of an old, well-established Antwerp family with traceable roots going back two centuries. During the long evenings we had great fun trying to remember and locate Antwerp streets, family names of mutual acquaintances, old Antwerp legends and history. We derived much pleasure in discussing a wide variety of subjects such as geology, landscapes, zoology and botany, both of us being inquisitive readers of these subjects.

The 1950s were years of relatively relaxed international relations—at least as far as we could make out from the news that filtered down to the bush. Moreover, strange to say, we felt relatively secure from international conflicts as if Africa were an island outside world affairs. For us, Africa was really our home, and rare political discussions were more concerned with the present and future of the colony than that of its motherland. Residents of the Congo had no voting rights and politics surrounding them were, therefore, low priorities during social gatherings—unless they touched the future of the colony. I would not have been surprised if, had the colony existed another 20 years, a move for independence *by the white population* could have been a possibility—another Rhodesia.

C.'s association with my tsetse research was a godsend for him. He could study and collect plant specimens to his heart's content while drawing a salary, certainly a more satisfying occupation than that of a struggling planter. C. taught me how to recognize the various *Acacia* trees and other constituents of tsetse habitats. Not versed in botanical taxonomy, my identification of trees was soon based upon photographic memory of shapes and rudimentary morphology rather than by precise recognition of leaves', seeds' or flowers' characteristics. It gave me great pleasure to identify the major plants of a clump of trees from a distance while C. had to examine the same trees from close-by, often to come to the same conclusions as I.

Naturally, many of our discussions centered around tsetse flies. Why was *G. morsitans* found in woodland savanna, in the Mutara region, represented by various species of *Acacia*, while *G. pallidipes* preferred thicket vegetation, and *G. brevipalpis* opted for riverine underwood? I explained that the presence of tsetses is regulated essentially by three major factors: (1) climate; (2) availability of mammalian blood; (3) the presence of shade—all of which translate into: (1) minimum and maximum temperatures, amount of rainfall and relative humidity and their seasonal fluctuations; (2) the presence of host animals; (3) tree groundcover. Except for the climate factor, the two other factors are, to a certain degree, mutually compensatory. Was it possible to characterize a tsetse habitat by a mathematical formula that would incorporate the various degrees of these factors, essential to tsetse survival? Our discussions about these were endless.

I am always surprised, when I read my old diaries, at the number of mishaps, setbacks, adversities and all kinds of hardships so easily submerged and forgotten among the more salient occurrences during a 20-year career. They are, however, so characteristic of life in Africa as I knew it that not mentioning them would border on deceit.

Friday, January 14, 1955

Leave Lwiro at four in the morning in my Plymouth accompanied by C. Arrive Usumbura (now spelled Bujumbura) at nine. Visit various officials trying to borrow aerial photographs of Mutara that would help locate vegetation and densities. None available. Leave Usa (common shortening of Usumbura) at 12:30. Arrive Astrida IRSAC Center at 16:30. Stay overnight at Hotel Faucon.

Saturday, January 15, 1955

Work on brakes and try to borrow a jeep. No dice. Leave Astrida at 9:40. Arrive Kigali at noon. Buy food and other items and leave at 12:45. Arrive at Kakole camp at 17:15.

Sunday, January 16, 1955

Quiet Sunday. Cross Uganda border to buy parafin (kerosene) at Kafunzo. Customs officer warns us that he shot a lion a few days ago, but that the animal had not been found. Chances are a wounded lion is prowling the area. If I tell the fly-boys, they won't go out tomorrow.

Monday, January 17, 1955.

Have made arrangement with Chief Gahitsi for borrowing a small cow to be used as bait animal for tsetse flies, and for two tipoys (carrying chairs) for today's foot safari. Around eight, an old man with a cow arrives, together with sixteen porters with a large basket which, the owner explains, is what is used in Ruanda for carrying "dignitaries." There is no choice but to accept what is available. We send four of the men out to cut two sturdy poles for carrying the contraption—an adequate description as it turns out later. They are back at 10:45, so that it is already late before the lorry is loaded to go and take us to Kijojo where we plan to start our survey. We leave instructions with the driver to wait for us on the road south of the camp where we guess we will emerge from our overland trip. We start our survey by recording the vegetation on both sides of the river Katitumba which we cross and recross several times, making use of the "basket," a scene duly photographed and filmed for posterity. C. decides it is time to make full use of the "basket." It is amusing to see him bouncing up and down from the flexible bottom of the basket like a puppet. I expect him to be seasick any moment. But he says it is restful; first he doesn't have to walk, second, breathing is made easier because each time he descends to the bottom, his sides are squeezed. A threatening sky turns into a wind-and-rain squall, drenching us to the bone. We struggle on as there is no place for shelter. After a short while the sun comes out again and we dry out as quickly as we got wet. We sit down to lunch and are horrified to find that it is already four. We estimate that the main road is still seven miles away. Against all logic we expect and are disappointed not to see the main road from the top of the several ridges we have to cross.

The sun sinks lower—as they say in novels as if that is an unusual phenomenon—and we get into an argument with our guides about the right direction. C. and I feel that we should travel in an easterly direction while the guides want us to go more southwards. As a result, we decide upon something in between—often a wrong compromise.

After climbing several more ridges, we arrive at the top of a high one and observe that had we gone due east, we would have arrived closer to our camp, but only by traversing very hilly country. Had we chosen the more southerly direction, travel would have been easier and we would have reached the main road sooner. It is now 17:45 and the sun touches the horizon—an event phophesied by the aforementioned novels. We correct our direction to S.S.E. With darkness falling and because I am walking faster than C.'s basket bearers, I find myself separated from the main party. I am glad to find, however, that of the two guides who stuck with me, one has my rifle. Guided by the silhouette of prominent trees, we plow on. With the increasing darkness it is difficult to avoid the low thorn bushes. In fact, I don't seem to miss any and soon my knees and thighs feel as if they have been raked by a dozen wildcats and then "cured" with rock salt. We reach an abandoned kraal that I know is not far from the main road. Looming in front of us is a hill which I mistake for Matimba. It proves to be Lugarama, a hill farther north. I change direction and going through a deep depression find myself wading among low thorn acacias, that make me feel that the pack of wildcats has increased considerably in numbers and is taking away what was left of whole skin. The ordeal completely blunts my fear of walking into a pride of lions or leopards. At last we reach the main road. I am completely exhausted, sweating and bleeding. We build a fire, first to guide the other party, second to keep warm, third to give our position to the driver of our lorry. Not long afterwards we hear the voices of the other party and at the same time the approach of the vehicle.

Hot soup and bread restore body and soul and at 9:30 we hit the sack calling it, rightfully so, a day.

Wednesday, January 19, 1955
Covered by the scientific permit according me the privilege of surveying areas inside the park, I decide to make a one-day trip aimed at reaching the Kagera River where it meets her tributary, Kalangaze. The lorry takes us to the village of our "casual laborers." This time we manage to hire two teams with two "carrier baskets," a total of sixteen men. As we are about to start, the K.N.P. guard, a compulsory companion imposed by the permit, objects to our firearms, saying we cannot take them inside the park. Knowing the sensitivity of the chief warden about our presence in the park—even by virtue of a permit by the highest park authority—I do not want to create ill feelings and decide to leave the guns behind in charge of Zaghi, taking with us only the ammunition. We are finally off at nine. It is a pleasant day, not too warm, a fresh breeze rattling the seeds inside the acacia pods. Descending a first broad valley, we find

it occupied by large herds of impalas and zebra. Hundreds of animal spoors mark the muddy bottom. A white deposit, indicating the high salt content of the soil, explains the attraction of this valley for game. The opposite slope is covered with dense vegetation composed of various acacia species. We are soon attacked by hordes of tsetse flies, all *Glossina morsitans*. Although they are of great importance to the completion of my tsetse distribution map, we are glad to emerge on a treeless mountain ridge without flies. An argument ensues about our whereabouts as the name of the hill on our map does not correspond to that given by the guides. Mindful of the previous day's experience, we follow their direction. Reaching the highest ridge after another stiff climb, we come to the edge of a sharp incline with a view down to a dark-green ribbon of dense vegetation: the Kalangaza Valley. Making ourselves comfortable among the rock outcrops and enjoying the peaceful view of virgin country, we have lunch. A search for tsetse pupae brings in only empty shells until one of the boys comes back with a pupa from which a fly is in the process of emerging. One can observe the exertion of the ptilium—a bulge between the insect's eyes used as a tiny ram to break the outer shell of the pupa case and to facilitate the escape of the young fly from its pupae envelope. This organ can still be seen pulsating as I hold the young fly between my fingers.

From our vantage point one can see the Kagera River making a sharp bend eastwards and then south again as it squeezes between the high walls of opposite mountains, the far side being Uganda territory. On our way down the Kalangaza Valley we come upon two splendid roan antelopes (*Hippotragus equinus*). They take off without stopping or turning around, unlike so many other species of antelope when once at a safe distance. Halfway down the valley we are fiercely attacked by hungry tsetses. They leave us when we reach the treeless flat bottom of the valley itself. All around us is wild, undisturbed country. So strong is the impression of pristine terrain that we believe that we may well be the first non-natives to tread this soil, when C. points to a small box hanging from one of the acacia trees. A closer look proves it to be a checkpoint box for park guards on inspection tour. Our "Stanley" image is somewhat dampened by this discovery. We make a rapid sketch of the area, the course of the (dry) Kalangaza and of surrounding vegetation.

We decide to return by another route in order to increase the area surveyed, a route which, the guides tell us, will bring us sooner to the main road and closer to camp. At this point, C. climbs into his carrier basket and I follow suit after one exhausting climb up a high ridge. Soon thereafter, much sooner than we expected, we arrive at the main road at about ten miles from camp. We dispatch a runner to call the lorry and, in the shade of an acacia tree, we enjoy a rest while completing our field diaries. Back in camp at 17:00.

The next three days are less hectic, with C. gathering botanical specimens, and me accompanying the fly-scouts on the different fly-rounds.

Saturday, January 22, 1955

Leave Kakole camp at two in the afternoon. Stop at the veterinary post at Nyakatale and learn from a passing doctor that three sleeping sickness cases have been found in southern Ruanda and that at Muhinga, across the Urundi border, close to 60 cases have been diagnosed in the last two months. Things are heating up. We arrive at about nine in the evening at Kigali, where we find Rajans' store still open to refill the gas tank. Arrive at Astrida around midnight. Drive to the IRSAC Center and leave the newly purchased but non-working Coleman lamp with the *zamu* (night watchman) with instructions for exchange. We eat our last sandwiches on the steps of the laboratory buildings under the scornful eyes of the *zamu*. He is most probably shocked by our unorthodox behavior, which he may find unbecoming as members of the dignified IRSAC Institute.

We leave Astrida at one-thirty in the morning with a long drive before us. Luckily the night is cool, the road is dry and the headlights provide forewarning to other night travelers. After an eternity, the lights of Bukavu appear in the far distance and below us, and we start the descent towards Lake Kivu. I begin to feel groggy, but now so close to home, I do not want to rest. Suddenly I am awakened when the car slides into a ditch. Through good fortune, the ditch is shallow at this point and I soon have the car back on the road and under control. C., who was also asleep, tells me not to drive like a drunk. The shock has killed our sleepiness. We cross the Ruzizi bridge at Shangugu and drive through the silent streets of Bukavu to the shore of Lake Kivu. Another 23 miles will take us to the IRSAC Center at Lwiro. It is four-thirty in the morning and I think it wise to rest ten minutes to make sure that I have my senses back and to unwind—literally—from the 150 miles of twisting Astrida road. We are almost home, but not quite. About halfway a broken tree lies across the road. I manage to drive around it between the coffee trees of an adjacent plantation. Arrive at Lwiro at six. Too late, and too early to go to bed.

My next month's diary starts:

Saturday, March 5, 1955.
The light fades quickly, leaving a pale, pinkish sky, still too bright for observing stars except for Venus on the far horizon. The flaps of the tent rustle gently in the cool evening breeze. It brings erratic gusts of voices of our porters huddled around the campfires. Purplish smoke drifts leisurely across the campsite. Small bats wheel in crazy patterns across the sky. From the perspective of my low camp bed, the scene, framed by the slanted tent opening, looks like a theater stage. This is our first night in the KNP (Kagera National Park) expedition.

Haezaerts, Chief Warden of the park, arrives from his tent, a dozen yards away, and walks over to our camp. The conversation is strained. As he stated when we met him a few hours earlier, though I have received permission to circulate in the park, this does not include C., my companion. C. points out that we are actually *not* inside the park's domain, but in a section called the "annex," not yet officially designated as part of the park and, therefore, not yet under its jurisdiction. True, but H. (Haezaerts) is obviously very upset. He believes that C., a botanist and member of IRSAC, complicates matters: if his monthly report mentions that under cover of my permit I have introduced another IRSAC member, it would look bad and I might even lose my permit altogether. Arguments about legalities are tossed back and forth and the evening wears on. Even an early moonrise looks forbidding and forlorn. Night passes peacefully, however.

Sunday, March 6, 1955
The night brings council and peace. The morning dawns with an enthusiastic sun, the sounds of boiling pots and cracking woodfires, dispersing their homey smell. H. saunters over

with a seeming offering of the peace pipe and tells us that, having thought things over, he has no objection for us to proceed according to plan. We break camp in good spirits.

The whole morning is spent in the survey of the Kalangaza Valley and side branches. A long ascent out of the valleys takes us to a ridge overlooking a wide panorama. Although only noon, the site is too perfect a campsite to be passed up. In great zest we set up camp and note how well it looks against the background of the great cumulus clouds. After a while, however, these clouds darken, sail overhead, and a heavy downpour dampens body and soul. Around five, the rain stops, the western horizon clears and a yellow hue pierces the remaining cloud cover which suddenly opens and reveals a majestic view of the Muravuha volcano some 75 miles away. A moment later, the summits of two other volcanoes, the Karissimbi and the Mikeno, also become visible. The sky colored by various tinges of yellows and oranges and the ghostlike appearance of the three volcanoes make a panorama of unbelievable beauty and awe. In spite of the cold and dampness we keep staring at the spectacle until it disappears with the setting sun.

The campfires are lit, we have supper, H. comes over for a chat. The almost full moon shines unopposed from the now clear sky. It is near midnight. We are at peace with Africa and with each other.

Monday, March 7, 1955

The sound of angry, flapping canvas wakens me early next morning. A full gale is testing the vulnerability of our tent anchorage. The central pole rocks back and forth as if it were the main mast of a threatened ship. All is damp and misery. What a difference six hours can make! How quickly the mood in Africa can change! A cup of hot coffee, compliments of Kiboko, gives us enough courage to step out from under the blankets and peep outside. A mistake. Our spirits take another dive. The weather improves during breakfast, but we decide to wait and see which way the weather will go. Around ten it definitely veers toward the better and we break camp. Fifteen minutes later black clouds come rolling in again, open up and drench our miserable caravan. We follow a deep valley with well-developed and diversified vegetation, including the rare *Euphorbia dawei*. Big acacia trees are covered with "old man's beard"

(*Usnea* sp.). Here are perfect tsetse habitats, but, of course, in this heavy rain no flies are about. The vegetation changes gradually into denser thicket-like communities and finally into uniformly dense cover on the average about ten feet high. C. has nicknamed these a "dreamland thicket." The far side of the valley shows more open woodland and among the trees we see a large herd of some 200 buffaloes, looking as miserable as we are.

During midafternoon, H. and I arrive at the Kagera River. C's party, slower because of his mapping of vegetation types, is far behind. We build a fire and decide to make camp here. The rain has stopped once more. With the arrival of the rest of the caravan the tents are put up and after a change of dry clothes and the intake of warm food, we feel much better. I feel well enough, in fact, to sketch a watercolor, showing the Kagera Valley seen from our campsite, on Kamabake Hill.

That night we all have a copious meal in the moonlight, since C. fails to make the Coleman lamp work. Much more romantic anyway. Croaking frogs along the river make up a background serenade.

Tuesday, March 8, 1955

The tent flaps are pushed aside and the boys bring in the coffee, yellow sunlight streaks through my mosquito net, setting a cheerful note. Good spirits prevail and C. has many wisecracks about the beard I am growing. Promising as it looks to me in the mirror, C.'s description of the stubble would embarrass even the most negligent street sleeper, a "dirty chin" being one of his less offensive remarks.

Having by now developed a well-organized routine, we are soon packed and on our way once more. We follow a broad, flat valley, the Kamabake plain. The vegetation looks like promising tsetse habitat, but I suppose it is still too wet for them to come out. We spot ourebi antelopes (*Ourebia ugandae*) and reedbuck (*Redunca ugandae*). Soon afterwards we start catching *Glossina pallidipes*. Rain starts again, increasing in strength as we move out of the valley and reach the beginning of a track leading to Gabiro and the main road. Our vehicles are supposed to pick up around noon. It is now 10:20. Luckily there is a small hut in which we can shelter from a sudden downpour. Unfortunately, an urgent call of nature forces me to wander outside in search of a suitable thicket, not too wet inside and not already occupied by a lion or buffalo. At eleven, the sun comes out once more and things are warming up and drying out, awakening the tsetse flies. They come out in droves, all *Glossina pallidipes*. Their presence in the valley greatly extends their previously known distribution in this part of Africa. At 11:30, the KNP pickup arrives, but instead of our lorry, only the jeep shows up. The lorry has engine trouble. Back at Gabiro, the KNP headquarters, we borrow H.'s pickup to go back to load our gear left at the hut. In the meantime our driver, with the help of the park's mechanic, works to locate the problem. They have taken the carburetor apart—a favorite pastime of African drivers—and are now purging the fuel lines. C. and I return to Kakole in the jeep, arriving near sunset. With our equipment and food still at Gabiro we are facing the prospect of foregoing the evening meal and even spending the night in a bare bunk at the Kakitumba rest house. Checking the rest house to make sure it is unoccupied, the customs' officer learns about our predicament and invites us for dinner with him and his family. Around ten we drive back to camp and are happy to find that the lorry has been repaired and has returned with all our equipment so that we can make up our beds and stay in our own camp. Funny how in Africa things often work out.

The next two safaris brought our Mutara work to a close. It ended 18 months of detailed observations during which we gathered a wealth of information about two tsetse species, *G. morsitans* and *G. pallidipes*, their distribution, vegetational habitats, seasonal fluctuations, feeding patterns, together with daily meterological data. Based on this information, we drew up a plan to control the flies in the grazing lands by means of the modification, that is, partial clearing, of their woodland habitats. In the meanwhile, the Ruanda-Urundi government had requested IRSAC to carry out similar research in the region south of Mutara, called Bugesera.

Friday, April 8, 1955
I cannot leave early today because my Plymouth needs a new main spring and the lorry is being serviced. Finally off at eleven. Arrive in Bukavu at 13:20. It's too late or too soon to draw money from the bank, which closes between 12 and 2.

Have a sandwich lunch at a local cafe, browse for a while in the bookstore and buy A. Loveridge's *I Drank the Zambezi*. Finally off at 14:30. Light rain starts falling, and we soon meet a very wet road as we start the ascent into the highlands. Thirty miles from Astrida we are held up by a heavily laden lorry trying to get out from a 300-yard-long stretch of deep mud. We wait for more than an hour while the driver and helper apply all the tricks used under the circumstances: scraping the earth around the wheels, piling rocks around and in front of them or providing a firm hold by means of cut boughs and twigs. Slowly the vehicle has inched out from the deepest part of the puddle, leaving me enough room to try passing it on one side. In the attempt I get stuck myself, but manage to get out with the help of a large number of children who had come to watch. Reach Astrida at ten past eight, and spend the night at the IRSAC guesthouse.

Saturday, April 9, 1955

We are glad to see that our lorry has arrived, but our departure is delayed because a shipment from the IRSAC-Uvira center has still to be unloaded. Leave at half past ten. Road good but wet. Reach Kigali at half past one. Meet Dr. Adamanditis, Chief of Veterinary Services, near the Gabiro turnoff. An extremely strongly built chap much respected in the region not only for his imposing physical appearance and his staunch principles but also as one of the rare men who fought a lion and escaped—although somewhat mauled. The lion was shot by another hunter before it could do more damage. Adamanditis tells me that he has received the funds to start anti–tsetse clearings in the Mutara and that the local vet, Liebert, will be responsible for carrying out my instructions. When I want to resume my journey, find out that I have a flat. Change tire. Reach Kakole Camp at half past six.

Sunday, April 10, 1955

Cross into Uganda to have my tire repaired at Kafunzo, the close-by border town with its unavoidable nduka and the usual standby mechanic, owned by the customary resident Hindu. It is said that the Hindu shop owners and traders make a small fortune off the backs of the local native population and may be involved at times in some shady business, but to the lonely traveler on the hazardous roads of Africa, the Hindu nduka is often a *Dar-es-Salaam*, a harbor of salvation.

It starts raining. When will the dry season begin? Back in camp at two. Compose a memorandum regarding the proposed vegetation clearing for tsetse control, with a framework for a timetable and priorities.

It is Easter Sunday.

Monday, April 11, 1955

Rain most of the day. Send the lorry to Kafunzo to repair spring. Spend most of the day on paperwork: polish and add to the outline for vegetation clearing and prepare a presentation I have to make for an inter-regional meeting on the 21st.

Tuesday, April 12, 1955

Fetch my repaired tire and also the repaired lorry. Make survey of various points along the main road where the high density DNP tsetse flybelt spills into the adjacent Mutara pasture lands, which we will have to consider as a priority clearing job. Note other sensitive places where cattle come into contact with flies and mark those among the priorities. These places are further characterized by their basic vegetational composition. Coming down a hill, meet a man barely able to walk, in torn clothes and with a severely gashed back. Says he has been attacked by a leopard. I take him to Nyakatale dispensary and tell the attendant to clean and disinfect the wounds until the arrival of Dr. Pinckers later in the day. Drive back to the main Kakitaumba road where I meet a man carrying a small boy wounded by the same leopard. Take him, too, to the dispensary for treatment. His wounds are luckily not very severe. On the return to camp see many zebras and topis.

Thursday, April 14, 1955

Had another flat tire yesterday and thus another trip to Kafunzo for repairs. Send the lorry to collect both tires while we carry out an experiment aimed at calculating the time it will take to cut trees of various species and thicknesses in order to prepare an estimation of tree/man/hours for the coming clearing projects. Time to cut down an average acacia using a European axe: 12 minutes for *A. hebecladoides*, 10 minutes for *A. senegal*, and 5 minutes for *A. campylacantha* and *A. seyal*. With two tires of my car in for repair and waiting for the lorry to return with them, we are without transport. The day wears on—raining most of the time. Finally the lorry appears at 16:30. As expected, a long confusing and unconvincing story ensues, the gist of which is that Kifita, one of the fly-boys, had taken a bicycle he believed belonged to Samson, our head fly-boy, and was apprehended by the rightful owner with the result that Samson became involved in a shouting and fist match. With the arrival of a native constable, both men were put in jail to calm down. Around 20:00 Samson is driven back to camp by the Hindu trader and he, too, has a heart–rending story to tell. So ends a fruitless day—but not entirely. Around ten-thirty I am awakened by the voice of the custom's officer shouting: "Come quickly, we have killed a hippo!" It proves to be a slight understatement. It transpires that I am to accompany the officer with my heavy rifle to finish off a hippo lying wounded somewhere in the bush. I dress quickly and drive to Kakitumba. I find a gathering of native hunters armed with spears. They direct me towards the decline leading to the Kagera River. Torchlights are flashed hither and thither showing nothing but silent bush sparkling with moisture. I do not feel at ease—an injured animal is always dangerous, whatever the species. I am told, moreover, that there were actually three hippos, one which was seen to go down, and another charging, dispersing the hunters. After a long while, one of the lights focuses on a dark mass. The hippo lies on its flank trying with jerking leg movements to slide down the slope of the riverbank. I approach and from 15 yards put a bullet in the right ear. With a deep sigh and a shudder the animal slides slowly lower on its left side. Hectic moments of blood collecting follow, blood smears are made and a search is made for ticks. During the process I tell Zaghi and the others that I hear the buzzing noise of tsetse flies and to look out for them. No one believes me until my flashlight silhouettes the unmistakable shape on the customs' officer's shirt.

On the way back to camp we are stopped by a small hippo standing in the middle of the road. It shuffles about, looks a few times in the direction of the car, sniffs and waddles some more and finally saunters into the bush. It is two in the morning by the time I have attended to the proper storage of the blood samples and the blood smears.

Wednesday, May 18, 1955

This will be the last routine visit to Mutara. It has been a busy week with the visit of several foreign researchers, including a party from the Smithsonian Institution. As such, preparations for our last Mutara safari have suffered some neglect but we push off in good style at 8:15. The weather has finally turned to dry season norms. Cannot resist to stop and browse at the Bukavu bookstore. C. has received the "Hasselblad" camera he ordered several months ago. Hence, we stop many times in the Nyongwe forest so that he can practice photographing vegetation. We have lunch at Uwinka, one of the highest points along the mountain road to Astrida, and the coldest. A few miles further I have to stop again to change a tire. Reach Astrida at five. The whole IRSAC population is bursting with activity in preparation for the visit of King Boudwijn in June.

We spend the night at the IRSAC guesthouse after an excellent meal at the local hotel-restaurant, Faucon.

Thursday, May 19, 1955

Have my tire repaired. Buy an easy-to-operate camera for Jessie's fourteenth birthday. Off at ten, the big lorry following. Road in excellent condition, not too wet, not too dry. Reach Kigali at 13:00 and tank up. At Nyakatale, leave note for Chief Kijojo asking him to send all his people to Kakole camp tomorrow for a malaria infection survey. Arrive in camp at 18:00. C. lights the lamps and nearly sets the camp afire. The lorry has not yet arrived and we are left without food. I find an old can with baked beans, a leftover from a previous safari. Together with slices of dry bread it has to do for supper.

Saturday, May 21, 1955

The people did not show up for the blood smear session yesterday. A note from Chief Kijojo explains that they will come on Monday. Anxious to get more blood samples from warthog, I go out with Kiboko. Did not find warthog, but shot an impala at 150 yards. Good shot, one would say. Not really because it is a female, while I had aimed at the male just in front. Some marksmanship! Rather hot today, but with that good feeling of dry season weather accompanied by those lovely sudden breezes. The chief game warden, leaving in a few days on home leave, visits us to say good-bye.

Need more blood samples from baboons. I visit the forest gallery along the Kakitumba where the animals are usually found. I encounter two groups, but they are very cautious and I have the opportunity for only two pot-shots, both misses.

Monday, May 23, 1955

Yesterday, back from a long survey in the Nyakatale area and ready to sit down for a sundowner, we hear a big commotion and shouting from far behind the camp. Some time later Kiboko walks in with half a dozen men carrying poles draped with fresh, red meat. The story is that Kiboko had found a freshly killed eland being devoured by a single lion. By making loud noises and threatening with sticks, the lion was packed off long enough to select choice pieces, the lion looking on with spiteful eyes. So the story went.

This morning, about 35 men arrived from Kijojo to have their blood taken for malaria infections. The women have refused to come because they are too busy with the crops and it would take too long to walk to the camp. We propose to drive to the village the next day and take their blood in situ.

Tuesday, May 24, 1955

Off with the lorry at eight and stop at our first rendezvous, where we unload our laboratory equipment. The two tables are installed in the shade of a large acacia tree. Soon the women and children start arriving and we are in business. Each extended finger—the smaller ones forceably—is stabbed with a hypodermic needle and the bead of blood "smeared" onto a glass slide which is then marked by means of a diamond-point pencil. Age, sex, location and the tribe are recorded in a register. Around eleven we move our installation to sample another village farther down the road. The blood-taking session ends with the use of our last one hundredth slide. Some women protest that they were left out.

On the way back to camp from Nyakatale we are stopped by the passage of a herd of more than 200 elands, counted as they leap from one side of the road to the other, some with a very high leap, really astonishing for such large and heavy antelopes.

Wednesday, May 25, 1955

Have barely finished breakfast when a team of Smithsonian Institution scientists drive into our camp, one day earlier than expected. This is their first visit to a real bush camp since landing, a week ago, at Bukavu airfield, fresh from Washington, D.C. They seem impressed by our camp, astounded that it resembles Hollywood's version of life in Africa. They admire especially our comfortable prefab aluminum hut. It has not taken long for Africa to catch up with the "innocents abroad": during the Astrida night stopover, Waldo Schmidt has been bitten in his thumb by a snake and he is still "under the weather" from shock and from the anti–venom injection. I explain our tsetse work. Photo- and movie- cameras are clicking. This is not the first time that we "pass a screen test," but we never made it to the "top ten."

We accompany the team to the Uganda border, where we interpret and help sort out paper work for all the equipment they are bringing in. Decide to follow them for a distance into Uganda and go to see Fred Wilson, the tsetse man on the Uganda side. On the way are stopped by a group of people excitedly pointing to a cobra (*Naja*) they have just killed. Waldo Schmidt looks on from a safe distance. We say good-bye to the U.S. team. Discuss our tsetse clearing plans with Fred while still another tire is being repaired at the Mbarara service station. Arrive back at Kakitumba customs station at 21:00. When I want to switch on the car lights, nothing happens. I drive back to camp the last three miles by the light of the parking lights, only one of which is working, I later discover.

Saturday, May 28, 1955

Today is packing day. Up early and eager to leave. I suddenly feel restless now that the moment has come to wind up the Mutara survey and I am looking forward with great avidity to start research in another region. Pack everything in trunks and boxes. At first glance I estimated that it would require two trips to get everything moved, but as we start organizing the load I wonder whether we couldn't get everything out in a single trip. In our preoccupation for storage space we almost forget to remove and pack the thermo-hygrograph installed the last weeks in "dreamland' thickets.

In the afternoon pay off the local fly-boys and sell small items and small pieces of furniture in an effort to reduce the load further.

We pass a last night in camp. In the distance a lion roars.

Sunday, May 29, 1955

Up early and in full "packing fever." As we load the last items, it looks as if we shall indeed be able to get everything out in a single load. Then Samson arrives with *his* gear, which alone would fill a third of loading capacity. With a sinking feeling we eye the odd-shaped, irrationally packed, bulky bundles held together with bits and pieces of wire and rope. We manage to repack his belongings in a more logical way until we get it all on the lorry, after he has sold two wooden beds, three goats and a bicycle to some of the watching crowd. With a sigh of relief we see the lorry off at eleven. A real success. We now regret that we have accepted dinner at the Noels, the customs' officer's family as we could easily have left at the same time as the lorry. We scrape some food together for lunch and spend the rest of the afternoon at the Kakitumba rest house. The dinner of wild hare, beautifully prepared by Mrs. N., is excellent and largely compensates for the half day's "loss." With most of our bedding packed in the lorry, we sleep without a mosquito net (a fact that does not escape the local mosquito population). Filling in between massive mosquito attacks, C.'s loud snoring makes the rest of my night sleepless.

Monday, May 30, 1955

I am glad when the first light brings relief from the sleepless night. Up at 5:30. Our last breakfast in Mutara and off at 8:00. Arrive at Goma at about three in the afternoon. Remembering that my car has no working lights, we argue whether to risk driving on in the hope of reaching Lwiro before dark—which will depend upon eventual hazards along the road and possible other delays. We look for a mechanic in Kisenyi and adjacent Goma. We learn that at Dahani's we may find someone to help us, but the shop is closed. While debating the situation, Kiboko meets a friend who takes us to a mechanic who finds the trouble in no time: a broken wire connection which is repaired with a piece of electric tape. So we decide to keep going and arrive safely at Lwiro around 21:00.

So ends the Mutara research.

Notes on An Overland Journey Dar-es-Salaam to Lake Kivu

Adventurous spirits die hard. After a six months' home leave in 1956, during which we toured Belgium, France, Switzerland and Italy, we decided to return to our post in Africa the slow way: by train from Antwerp to Marseilles, by ship through the Suez Canal to Dar-es-Salaam, by train across Tanganyika Territory (Tanzania) to Kigoma—an inland port on the eastern shores of Lake Tanganyika—then by boat across the lake to Uvira, and finally by road to Lake Kivu. Government and paragovernment personnel have their air tickets and normal travel expenses paid by their employer, to and from home-leave destinations. In our case, permission for an "out-of-the-way" journey was granted only with the understanding that I would have to pay any expenses outside those normally reimbursed for the direct Brussels-Lwiro travel.

Following the inevitable delays going through customs, immigration and ticket offices, we stepped aboard the *Marechal Joffre* at the Marseilles embarcation terminus around half past ten on the tenth of August. There was a moment of panic when I was told that the eleven seatrunks sent three weeks before had not arrived at the quay. But a few moments later the trunks were located and loaded in time for departure.

Built in 1930, the 14,900-ton *Marechal Joffre* is the oldest ship of the French East Africa Line. It is said that she can do 16 knots. Being the only ship of the line painted entirely in white, she is affectionately referred to as "le bateau blanc" by the "habitués." We later found out that she was always listing one way or the other, sensitive to wind pressure against her high superstructure.

Around noon the last moorings were cast off and the *Marechal Joffre* moved away from the "Old World," bound for the "Dark Continent."

Time went by in sweltering heat as we passed through the Suez Canal and the Red Sea, finally crossing the Tropic of Cancer. During the day we managed to keep cool in the swimming-pool. In the cabin, the temperature was unbearable in spite of the electric fans. To dress for dinner in the evening was an ordeal. I lay in my underwear on my bunk directly below the fan until the gong rang. Putting on shirt and tie, I jumped into my trousers, put on my coat and rushed into the dining-room where the air-conditioner kept the temperature twenty degrees lower than the outside. It felt like walking into an ice-box although the room thermometer read 23°C. These sudden changes in temperatures brought on a bad cold bordering on pneumonia—or so it felt.

Passing Bab el Mandeb, we entered the Gulf of Aden and sighted the port of Djibouti. Once inside the bay the sun disappeared behind a dark-brown smog, possibly the smoke of bushfires. The *Marechal Joffre* had difficulties approaching the quay whether from a strong current or from the shallowness of the water. I had a distinct feeling that once or twice we actually struck bottom. She needed the combined effort of three steam-winches and a tugboat to take her alongside and moor. Four first-class passengers left at Djibouti. They were the ambassador to Sweden and family returning to their post in Addis Ababa. Some time after midnight we cast off and the ship resumed her journey.

By mid-morning, the next day, we were approaching Cape Guardafui, close to shore. An isolated fishermen village came into view, peacefully cuddled inside the sandy saddle of two rocky peaks. Could it be Bereda? Several schools of dolphins appeared suddenly alongside the ship, jumping high across the bow-waves, exhibiting playfully their prowess as if to welcome us to the Indian Ocean. Their demonstration was loudly applauded by the passengers.

It was while keeping away from the weather, inside the lounge, that we made the acquaintance of a Kenya District Officer back from home leave on his return to Fort Hall, his station north of Nairobi.

"The Mau-Mau situation is getting worse", he said, "whole families of white settlers in the highlands have been murdered, including their African servants. All were horribly mutilated. The settlers should leave but few do. Some have been working their farm for three generations and do not want to abandon their toil of 50 years or more. They claim that their land was properly purchased from the colonial government and is legally theirs. The Kikuyu claim that the tribal lands were theirs long before."

The description of a different colonial experience came from the wife of a French administrator on their way back to Tananarive, capital of Madagascar.

"You should see our garden, there is never a season when flowers are not in bloom. At this time of the year the roads are double lines of blood-red flowers of the flamboyant trees planted on both sides. We have a lovely house with a view of purple mountains. And the people, they are so friendly and interesting. Annette, our youngest daughter, loves her school and her schoolmates. We are happy and lucky living in Madagascar."

Around midnight of the 23rd we crossed the Equator. The seas remained choppy with long swells and waves tossed about by the strong winds. Two days later we sighted the coast of East Africa. Soon afterwards a pilot-boat came alongside, bouncing in our bow-waves. The Kenyan flag made us feel close to home. Once the pilot aboard, the ship eased slowly into Kilindi harbor and port of Mombasa, a fine natural deep bay, part of the broad sea-arm that surrounds Mombasa on all sides and makes the city actually an island.

We made fast around eleven and when we heard Swahili words we felt as if we had never left Africa. British officials, very smart in their spotless, starched uniforms came aboard to clear immigration papers. Many passengers left here, having reached "home" or to continue their journey inland by road or train. We would still remain on board for another 24 hours until the ship docked at Dar-es-Salaam. With fascination we watched the activities in the bay and on the quays. Across, the white, sandy shores were covered with natural vegetation and coconut groves, shading clusters of thatched huts. I stared at the African scenery for a long time, feeling that although we might never completely "fit-in", we would regret it forever when we left.

A picture of the approaches to Dar-es-Salaam ("Harbor-of-Salvation") could serve as an advertisement to promote "cruising the tropics." A cluster of dark rocks, at the mouth of the bay, marks the narrow entrance formed on one side by a long peninsula lined with palm-dotted brilliant white beaches. All at once, the narrow inlet opens into a wide crescent-shaped lagoon with a view of the town snugly nestled within its coconut-tree-lined waterfront. As soon as the ship dropped anchor we were in for a busy time. Again, we were lucky to have the help of a representative of the A.M.I. shipping company, (Agence Maritime Internationale), a Hindu who in no time got our papers squared away and our trunks from the hold into a waiting launch. By mid-morning we and baggage were on our way to the shore, slowly swinging away from the lee side of the huge white hull of the *Marechal Joffre*, and into the sun.

After the usual contretemps with customs and immigration, where our knowledgeable Hindu was once more of tremendous help, we settled in the New African Hotel located right on the waterfront. From the terrace we saw the *Marechal Joffre* slowly swinging at her moorings. Against the tropical beach background, the ship looked majestic and romantic. Weighing anchor late that afternoon, she glided effortless out of the bay, past the coconut groves and disappeared from sight. Our last link with Europe was severed.

At the hotel I was caught in the cog-wheels of civilization in the form of: train reservations, invoices, passports, checks, luggage registration, travelers checks. Luckily my Indian friend stood by me like the providential rock but when he showed me the final bill I had to confess I had no money left to pay. He visibly reeled from the shock, his belief in human trust undergoing a severe setback, no doubt. However, when he learned that I was a staff member of the IRSAC Institute he agreed to accept a I.O.U., later to be settled by a bank draft. He came with us to the station and recommended us to the train conductor, a grey bearded, old Indian gentleman, wearing a blue turban. The train consisted of two new first class all-aluminum coaches, a dining car and a long string of second class carriages painted in the classic red E.A.R.H. (East Africa Railways & Harbours). Our coach was marked: "Dar-es-Salaam to Kigoma." Two towns separated by a twelve hundred kilometer journey, from East to Central Africa, from the Indian Ocean to Lake Tanganyika, ending close to where Stanley found Livingstone and uttered the now legendary words: "Dr. Livingstone, I presume?"

The inside of the coaches was most impressive, showing the latest in train-coach furnishings. The compartments were arranged so that they could be used singly or, by opening a double door, be converted into a big saloon. The powder-blue leather seats were deep, soft and comfortable. Movable armrests divided seats for four passengers; when folded turned the seats into most restful beds at night. Above, a second bed could be pulled down. Each compartment had its own wash-basin in stainless steel hidden by a hinged formica top that, during daytime, was used as a small table. The floor was covered with a soft-blue carpet. Sliding panels revealed small cubicles with clean towels, a drinking-water tap, paper cups and wastebasket. A mirror and small individual reading lights completed the functional decor. If I describe the carriages in some detail it is because nowhere in Africa had we ever seen such practical luxury. We had looked to this train journey as an interesting but probably not a pleasant experience. Now it seemed that we were in for a treat.

At precisely 12:30 we started on our 1245 kilometer journey across Tanganyika. As soon as the train left "Dar," we were summoned to dinner by the music of a sing-song gong. The dining car was of a much earlier vintage than the passenger coach but it had a cozy feeling of near pompous elegance; the food was excellent.

The train traversed a dense stand of lowland forest, the last we would see for a while as the land was rising steadily to meet the extensive high savannas. The wood-burning locomotive seemed to labor under the effort.

My desire to travel the overland route via eastern Africa was not without scientific interest; I was most anxious to view some of the classical East African tsetse fly belts, in particular the "Itingi Thickets," a unique large extent of dense vegetation, and the vast areas of "miombo" parkland. The railroad runs through the "Itingi Thicket" near the eastern edge of the Central Tanganyika Plateau. It consists of five to six thousand square kilometers of uniformily dense coppice shrub, three to five meters high. The importance of this vegetation to the glossinologist is that, although surrounded on most sides by tsetse flybelts, the thickets themselves remain free of them. Thought to be too dense for a tsetse habitat, it is, therefore, worthwhile studying as a possible barrier to halt the spread of the fly. On the other hand the surrounding "Miombo" vegetation-cover provides typical tsetse fly habitats in most of East Africa. Composition of miombo varies but is essentially based upon two kinds of trees: *Brachystegia spp.* and *Julbernardia spp.* (or *Isoberlina spp.*) In Tanganyika, *Brachystegia-Julbernardia* woodland covers almost half the territory, about 460,000 square kilometers. The study of tsetse flies has shown that in savannahs, the distribution of the fly is directly related to the pattern and density of the tree cover, vegetation communities which are also the habitat of wild animals from which the fly derives its bloodmeals.

When the next day we crossed typical tsetse fly country I was elated catching my first tsetse *inside* the dining car. Soon afterwards more flies came in and I had a most satisfactory afternoon collecting and identifying them, to the great amazement and joy of the African train staff who must have thought me a bit weird—more so than other white people. Incidentally, trains and road transport may, indeed, play a significant role in the spread of tsetse flies.

We spent two comfortable nights on the train. The first day, towards sunset, we had a marvelous silhouetted view of the Uluguru Mountains rising sharply out of the plains. The train never traveled far without stopping at one of the numerous small stations. At each, hustling and shouting Africans ran alongside the carriages pushing or throwing their bags through the open windows before the train came to a halt. De-training wives carrying small babies and luggage had to push through the assaulting throng in the wake of their husbands who tried to open a path for them to get off. Local onlookers stood watching, gesticulating and shouting when they recognized one of the arrivals. Even greater chaos reigned at the big town stations of Morogoro, Dodoma, Itingi, Tabora and Manyoni. Peddlers selling bananas, ground nuts, palm-oil, small chairs, tables, and wooden spoons had a thriving business. Talking to one of the wood carvers I found out that tables and chairs were made from "Mninga" ("bloodwood" = *Pterocarpus bussei*), the spoons from "Msaki" (*Commiphora ugogensis*).

Early in the morning of the second day the train stopped in the middle of nowhere; only a nearby coppice of Combretum trees relieved the uniformity of the low shrub savanna. My first thought was that the train was held up by an uprooted tree across the tracks. An attendant told me that this was not the case:

"Pishi nataka kamata kuni" (the cook wants to gather firewood), he said nonchalantly. Rail-travel in Africa!

Soon after breakfast we reached Kigoma and the end of our train journey. Kigoma is a small town located at one point of a crescent-shaped bay in the northern half of Lake Tanganyika. The place owes its existence to shipments of goods in transit from the Belgian Congo. A small steamboat of ancient vintage, the "Kivu," plies between Albertville, Kigoma, Usumbura, Uvira and back to Usumbura, towing barges with merchandise to these small harbors. She has room for twelve passengers in six cabins. Depending upon the number of barges in tow, she makes three to six knots.

I was in for more time-consuming sorting out of official documents and confirming passage on the boat across Lake Tanganyika. Again, a shipping agent was waiting for us but he was far less efficient than the one in Dar-es-Salaam. After all, we had arrived in the heart of Africa where things are done in a more leisurely way. The transfer from train to boat of twelve trunks and seven pieces of luggage was especially a strenuous task, it seemed. Other problems arose when I was asked to pay the bill including the one from Dar. I proposed to pay with a check drawn on the bank in Bukavu but the shipping agent declined. He said that the luggage would have to stay in Kigoma until full payment of the total bill. The argument reached an impasse when I said I was not leaving my things behind. At that moment the Belgian Consul arrived and when I proved that I belonged to the IRSAC Institute, he vouched for the payment and we were cleared for "take-off."

The "Kivu," a string of four big barges in tow, left around noon. Slowly, very slowly, Kigoma Bay faded in a muggy dry-season smog. It was the thirtieth of August, my birthday.

The journey across the lake was uneventful. We arrived early the next morning at Usumbura where we let go two of the barges, then crossed the lake for Kalundu on the western shore. Our hope of finding transport from our institute did not materialize. I met acquaintances from our previous stay in Uvira who managed to make a telephone connection with the IRSAC main center at Lwiro asking for transportation to wait for us in Usumbura, where the boat was to return later in the day.

The "Kivu" arrived back at Usumbura around one but encountered great difficulties mooring in the face of a very strong wind that kept her from approaching the wharf. At last we made fast and the procedures of our last baggage transfer began. A station wagon from IRSAC Lwiro-Center had arrived, followed by a van from IRSAC-Uvira Center to load our luggage. Around four we drove off on the last lap of our very long journey.

Elated with the brand-new tarmac road, the driver zipped along at 120 Km/hour through the Ruzizi Valley, onto the Kamaniola escarpment and into the cold Kivu highlands. When we reached Bukavu we left the tarmac road for the last 50 kilometers of our journey, a stretch of typical dusty, bumpy, winding African dirt road. We arrived at Lwiro around eleven, had a cold supper at the guest-house and, tired—and a bit dazed—wondered what brought us back to Africa.

Camp at Lake Tshohoha

For two years I had been using my personal vehicle for my journeys to Mutara and Irangi on the basis of a mileage allowance. But field work in the Bugesera would really require a four-wheel drive, all-terrain vehicle. Even on the relatively smooth roads in and to Mutara I had to replace springs many times as well as tires, not counting innumerable tire repairs. The accountant was getting unhappy paying my monthly car allowances, while I was equally disturbed about my repair bills.

Then, one day, our director, back from one of his trips to attend a scientific meeting in Nairobi, had purchased a second-hand safari Land Rover from one of the hunting companies and I was to fly over, collect the vehicle and drive it back to Lwiro. Furthermore, the vehicle was to be used exclusively for my own field work. This was excellent news. One week later, Dora, Richard, now four years old, and I boarded the DC-3 at Usumbura bound for Nairobi. Another passenger on the plane was Professor P. C. C. Garnham, a famous British parasitologist, with whom I had an interesting conversation about primate malarias.

We stayed three days in the New Stanley Hotel, waiting for the release papers of the Land Rover. Dora had a great time shopping; Richard not so good when one of his "Dinky" toy cars disappeared while he was playing in the lobby. He made such a racket that the assistant manager and finally the manager became involved in the "affair-of-the-missing-toy." From our room on the second floor, we had a view of the Delamere circle, with the statue of the pioneer colonist in the center. (Years later, the statue was removed and the Delamere Avenue became Kenyatta Avenue). The vehicle was released on the third day and we left without further ado. It was a long-base Land Rover 1955 on to which a wooden body had been built, open on both sides, thereby leaving an uninterrupted view from the front as well as from the back seats. The four open sides could be closed by means of canvas curtains, rolled up when not needed. This protection against driving rain was rather symbolic. Behind the back seats was a roomy storage space. A marvelous feature, especially for my kind of work, was the hatch in the roof above the driver's seat. With the trap door open, one could stand up and put head and shoulders through the opening, view the surroundings and use the flat roof as a drawing table. Skylights and hatches have a reputation for leaks. Whether this one conformed to the trend was irrelevant because during heavy rain so much water came in between the canvas curtains accumulating on the sheet metal floor that even a large leak elsewhere would go unnoticed. I loved "my" Land Rover. We spent hundreds of hours together, drove along thousands of miles of African roads, dashed through stubborn undergrowth, emerged from the deepest mud. The engine sang sweetly on smooth roads as if it were humming from sheer contentment. Except for punctures and an occasional bad mood, it never let me down even over the roughest trails. Made to be used in British territories, it had a righthand steering. This would have been awkward in right-hand side traffic, such as in the Congo and Ruanda-Urundi, but as most of my travel was on single-lane bush roads, this was of little importance.

The vehicle and I took to each other immediately and it was in good spirits that I drove out from Nairobi on the road back to the Congo. We spent the first night at the pleasant Eldoret Inn in the Kenya highlands. The following day, on our way to Kampala, we stood in awe before the mighty Owen Falls near Jinja, where the thunderous waters of Lake Victoria force their way through the narrow gorge to start the Victoria Nile. It was probably the last time we would see the Falls as at our next visit construction had already begun on the dam for the production of hydroelectric power. Another 50 miles brought us to Kampala, capital of Uganda, where we booked at the fashionable Victoria Hotel. It was here that three years earlier, as a suspect in a Mombasa murder case, I had spent the night under the surveillance of Lt. Swan. I would have liked to ask him if he had caught the murderer, but to revisit the room where I had undergone one of the most traumatic moments of my life had no appeal.

The next day we drove 270 miles to Kabale, where we spent the night at delightful White Horse Inn. After a cozy English breakfast the following morning, we set off for the last 236 miles to Lwiro. On the stretch of road to Kisoro, we had marvelous unobstructed views of the Virunga volcanoes from various angles from the twisting, roller coaster road. Previous rains were the reason for the exceptional clarity of the atmosphere, which in this area is seldom without clouds or mist. I used the whole of the film of 36 exposures I had just loaded into the camera and regretted that I did not have an extra one, so unbelievably beautiful were the views. Just before Rutshuru I had a first puncture, which luckily could be repaired in town. The rest of the journey was uneventful.

Rewinding the film for mailing, the following day, I discovered that it had not been properly threaded and had not advanced. None of the glorious views had been photographed! Missing those unique views by sheer stupidity has remained one of my greatest frustrations! Other preoccupations would soon claim my attention when, a week later, I started work in the Bugesera region.

The arrival in the Burgesera by tsetse flies seems closely linked to the history of its human occupation. At the time of my survey in 1955, settlements were concentrated along some of the larger lakes and, in the west, in areas bordering the river Akanyaru. The people, Watutsi and Bahima, believed that the invasion of tsetse flies was of recent date, perhaps between 1945–50. In the fifteenth century, Bugesera was an independent kingdom with a dense, pastoral population. Old men remembered that at one time some 60,000 head of cattle grazed the lands "stretching as far as the eye could see." When I started my research in 1955, the cattle population was approximately 7,000. The dramatic drop in numbers was caused by a series of pestilent cattle diseases during the first half of this century: (mouth-and-claw) (1907); anthrax (1920); rinderpest (1934); mouth-and-claw (1936). With the enormous decrease of the herds, followed by human emigration, the unused pasture land and abandoned fields reverted to savanna vegetation which, in due course, became suitable to tsetse flies advancing from adjacent Tanganyika Territory. Moreover, the abandoned lands were repossessed by their original wild animal species, assuring an ample supply of blood for the tsetse.

In 1957, *Glossina morsitans* was the only tsetse found in the Bugesera. But the presence of *Glossina pallidipes* in the Mutara just north, made me believe that the invasion by the latter of the Bugesera would be a matter of time. Indeed, the large, varied communities of thicket vegetation would seem ideal *G. pallidipes* country. They were, in fact, a characteristic feature of the region and were of such great botanical evolutionary interest that

G. Troupin, our botanist, made it the subject of a separate re search project ultimately published in a voluminous scientific publication.

The thickets were a joy to drive through. Located on mostly flat terrain, they formed patterns not unlike a purposely planted labyrinth, the space between the clumps of xerophilic vegetation devoid of other growth but for spare grass cover. Many of the clusters had apparently started around a termite mound—possibly because the cool and moist environment of the mound was a stimulus to seed maturation and young plant growth. Also, in an open landscape birds tend to perch on top of termite hills and may deposit seeds attached to their feet or plumage or in their droppings. The average height of the thickets was about 20 feet. They could be divided botanically into two major groups. One was composed mainly of *Olea*, *Euphorbia* and *Teclea* species, with underbrush pioneer species of *Capparis* and *Acacia*. The second type, usually somewhat taller and occupying more extensive areas, was dominated by *Apodytes dimidiata*. The dense growth and entwining underbrush made these communities impenetrable. They were, as far as I could make out, unsuitable as *G. morsitans* habitats in their pure form. But surrounded by *Acacia* and other woodland vegetation—typical tsetse habitats—the thickets were part of a complex that was puzzling for the botanist as well as for the tsetse ecologist.

The routine Bugesera research started in May 1957. The area could be approached from the south via Ngozi and Kininya, or from the north via Kigali. The northern route was the better one, but one had to cross the river Nyawarongo on a wooden ferry pulled along a cable. The ferry crossing was not always without hazards. When the river was at flood stage, one had to drive through the water, trying to guess where the boards were that served as a loading ramp. When the water level was low, the drive on to the ferry was very steep and especially heavy lorries had a rough time getting on or off. Once across the river, a pleasant drive on a well-formed sandy track traversed dense, solid thickets. This was followed by lovely open parkland. Twenty miles south of the river the vegetation changed into mixed woodland with *Acacia*, *Albizzia* and *Combretum* the dominant tree species. At this point, one started picking up tsetses. A few miles beyond was the village of

Kibugabuga, at the extreme eastern tip of Lake Tshohoha. Two lakes bear the same name. This was Tshohoha north.

It seemed a good place for a base camp. Unfortunately, both rest houses were occupied—one by Mr. L'Espagne, a health officer engaged in a program of prophylactic injections against sleeping sickness; the other by an agronomist, so we had to return for accommodations to Kigali each day of that first week.

The first days were spent in surveying and tracing a first fly-round of 31 times 100 meters. I took on four local young men to be trained as fly-boys. Zaghi was in bad shape during this time with severe diarrhea and a nagging cold. However, we managed to get the program under way before I returned to Lwiro, ten days later.

Lodgings remained a real problem during the first months. The local villagers were not very cooperative in this matter. By July things eased somewhat when I moved the prefab aluminum hut from Mutara to Kibugabuga.

If the fauna in Bugesera seemed less numerous and varied than in Mutara, its flora were certainly more diversified, and its landscape boasted a large number of lakes, many located along the drainage valleys of the Akanyaru and Kagera rivers. The apparent paucity of game in Bugesera could be the result of the intense hunting of past and present human population or it could simply be because the dense vegetation and few large open spaces reduced the opportunity to sight game. Small numbers of game could prompt tsetse flies to feed on humans instead, which could explain the human sleeping sickness outbreak. Related to this, I picked up a story from the locals that confirmed the importance of tsetse feeding patterns. It seems that sometime after World War II, an enormous increase in the warthog population played havoc with the new tuber crops. An intense anti-warthog campaign using arsenic poisoning was successful in drastically reducing the number of warthogs, but it may have resulted in an increased feeding of tsetse on humans, especially considering that the warthog is a major source of blood to savanna tsetses.

By the end of July, five fly-rounds were in operation. Each of the rounds started or ended near a road track accessible to Land Rover. Each sampled different types of vegetation communities. Compiled over a period of almost two years, the figures of captures broken down into the usual categories of males and females, young or old flies, hunger stages, blood contents, and the release and recapture of marked flies gave us an idea of the vegetation communities that were crucial to the fly's survival. Fly-rounds III and V were experimental. Here, I had divided a representative patch of vegetation into 25 squares each of 100 meters. A grid system of rounds sampled each of the sides of each square so that the compiled results provided figures of surface occupation in more detail than those derived from the linear fly-rounds. A special team made records of resting flies on different tree species, giving insight on vegetation preference. For instance, observations in two of the fly-rounds indicated that 24 percent of the flies were seen resting on *Acacia* trees, 31 percent on *Combretum*, 10 percent on *Parinari*, 10 percent on *Rhus*, and 5 percent on *Lannea*, making up 80 percent of the total. The remaining 20 percent were divided among various tree species without any clear predominance.

During their 1957 summer vacations, Winnie and Jessie, each in turn, were visitors to my Bugesera camp. They enjoyed mostly the early morning drives along the deeply shaded sandy tracks. It was then that we saw the velvet monkeys (*Cercopithecus aethiops*) actively collecting fruit in the thickets. The large variety of fruit- and berry-bearing trees must have seemed like paradise to them. At several points along the bush roads that circled the thickets with great abandon, we stopped wherever we wished and walked with unchecked freedom. It felt as if we owned the land.

During Winnie's visit, a leak developed in the oil sump of the Land Rover on our return journey to Lwiro. Had it occurred at the start of the journey in the middle of the bush land, it would have been extremely annoying. Luckily, I spotted the leak as we were about to leave Goma on our last leg to Lwiro. I was able to stop the small hole—no doubt caused by a sharp stone—with rubber cement and a patch of inner–tubing. We arrived without further trouble at Lwiro. When the vehicle was inspected, we also found that the gas tank was leaking!

In August, it was Jessie's turn to accompany me. The house for the head fly-boy, made by men of the local chief from local materials, was now finished, so I could occupy the prefab aluminum hut, staying overnight in camp for the first time. During the evening of the first day we were invaded by hordes of mosquitoes. It was literally impossible to eat our food without constantly slapping all parts of our bodies in an effort to minimize their attacks. A casual collection of mosquitoes that night, all *Anopheles*, consisted of six different species, including *Anopheles funestus*, one of the main malaria carriers in Central Africa. I reasoned that the tremendous number of mosquitoes was due to the bright bundles of light projected in the dark night through the numerous round aeration holes in the aluminum walls.

Three days before leaving Bugesera, we made a dash to the Mutara, where I had to make a few last observations and to see if I could recruit some of my old fly-boys. Leaving camp at six in the morning, we arrived at Nyakatale, Mutara, at ten. A government meeting was in progress, and although I was unofficially invited to attend, I felt that I could not spare the time. We left Mutara at 13:10, after a short survey to complete some parts of my vegetation map, and were back at Kibugabuga at six. Late Sunday afternoon, a passing traveler delivered a message from our director, summoning me back to Lwiro, where I was expected the following morning. I could not leave immediately because the ferry did not operate after sunset. We left at dawn the next day, arriving in Lwiro at dusk. There I learned that I was being asked to participate in another attempt to capture gorillas. On Tuesday morning I left for Utu, back to the rain forest.

"The Lords of the Jungle"

As during previous gorilla operations, it was the Swiss wildlife zoologist, Cordier, who was once again in charge. When the day after my return from Bugesera I arrived at Utu, accompanied by Chardome, my parasitologist colleague, procedures were well under way. We were told that one and possibly two gorilla families had been isolated in a narrow valley and that already a hundred villagers had been positioned to keep the animals within the area. The next morning we were taken to the site, close to a well-marked passable track about 20 miles from Utu. Shouting and hammering guided us to the area being fenced in by means of a high nylon net especially manufactured for this operation. The animals had been sighted from time to time by "scouts" and the fence-net roped in accordingly. The idea was to confine the gorillas to the smallest possible area where, it was assumed, some or most of the animals might be immobilized and captured by throwing large, heavy nets on top of them.

The space within the fenced-off area grew smaller as the day wore on, but was still too large by sunset for attempting more direct action. It was hoped that the animals would not try something rash during the night and would still be inside the fence the following day. When we returned at sunrise, the men, under the direction of Cordier, had further reduced the area and it was clear that the crucial moment could not be far off. Suddenly there was the sound of a wild rush and we all braced ourselves for an unknown onslaught. A dozen gorillas, small and large, burst precipitously out from the dark background and, seeing a wall of higher primates armed with clubs and spears behind a protective net, jumped like trained circus animals into two isolated tall trees, seven in one, five in the other. Curtain—Act I.

Act II began in dead silence. The gorillas, bemused, stared down from their lofty perch at uneasy spectators—would-be captors at a loss as to what to do next. This was absolutely not according to plan. How could one expect to throw nets over gorillas safely roosted in branches of trees 50 feet above ground? We tried to dislodge the apes by making loud noises and violent movements. The animals replied angrily by barking back and making threatening gestures. The game went on during most of the morning, the would-be captors growing more frustrated, the gorillas wondering, no doubt, what the game was. At noon, Cordier made a decision: "We shall have to cut the trees down." Appalled by the idea, but seeing no other solution, we agreed. A "volunteer" was chosen. He was given the best axe and the assurance that we would be ready with blazing guns should, "by any small chance" one of the gorillas decide to come down to hamper his tree cutting activities. We all admired the man who went inside the net and approached (stealthily it is true) one of the trees. The animals looked down as if they could not believe their eyes. They went silent, but started behaving nervously. They moved up and down the branches to survey the approach from all angles as if trying to figure out what it meant and how that changed the rules of the game. Could it be that he wanted to join them in the tree? They were quite intrigued.

Act III started with a loud bang as the axe was brought down with a mighty swing. All hell broke loose. Gorillas fell over each other in an effort to scramble to safety higher up. For the first time they seemed to realize their predicament. This was a game no longer. This was serious stuff. Loud cries of protest underscored their concern. Bang number two increased their restlessness and their wild gestures of disapproval. The tree cutter gaining confidence in the apparent disarray of the animals, took heart and let go with some more powerful swings, each time raising his eyes to observe the effect. At the fourth bang that shook the whole tree, one large male gorilla started down the trunk but stopped short at about ten feet from the ground. Here, holding fast with both feet, he started a rapid ratatat, pounding his chest with fast drumming hands—a splendid performance that made the woodcutter jump 20 feet away from the tree, ready to beat the hundred-yard dash record. Thus satisfied and admired by the rest of the troop, the plucky gorilla retreated, back to his consorts. "Well done, Dad. Good show," one could imagine his family cheering.

The tree cutter, now somewhat reassured, called the bluff and went back to his activities. This whipped up the enthusiasm of several other eager villagers and soon the forest resounded with treechopping. This seemed to stimulate the courage of some gorillas, several of whom came down to repeat the performance of the first aggressive one. None ever came lower than the first animal, however, perhaps not realizing that the noisy hammering would eventually bring them down to earth. We prepared for this eventuality, readying the nets and warning the men with the poles that they were to be used to pin the nets down once an animal was inside, not to clobber it.

Act IV. With a loud report, both trees came down almost simultaneously, followed by a rain of screaming gorillas. The scene inside the enclosure showed an unbelievable melee of net-throwing *Homo sapiens* and side-stepping *Gorilla gorilla* that would have delighted a choreographer, that is for those animals that had the ability to put up a fight. Many had been dazed or knocked half unconscious in their fall, however—a few had died. The able-bodied showed great fighting verve, which was admirable after a 50-foot fall, but in the end they were unable to resist hordes of spirited captors brandishing large poles and throwing ensnaring nets. No gorillas escaped. When the dust cleared, unfortunately, three gorillas lay dead, killed in their fall, three died later that night; six survived the ordeal.

For most of the performers, higher or lower primates, Act IV was the final act—but not for the parasitologists. M.C. and I worked the whole night carrying out autopsies on the dead gorillas by the light of three Coleman lamps. Blood was collected for genetic studies and for later examination for blood parasites; specimens of all organs were preserved in formalin, including eyes; the intestines were opened, examined for intestinal worms, and preserved in a mixture of alcohol and glycerine; subcutaneous tissues were examined for filarial worms; hand, finger and footprints were made on special white paper; ticks, mites and other ectoparasites were collected. When at three in the morning we had "processed" the first three D.O.A.'s, the other three had died and we started all over again well beyond sunrise.

The gorilla capture was carried out for three reasons; first, the F.I.S. film ("The Lords of the Jungle") sponsored by King Leopold III, in which the gorillas play a main role, second, Cordier's contract to capture and deliver live gorillas to world zoos, finally, our own, that is, IRSAC's scientific interest in studying the gorilla's "life-cycle," promoted by our director, Dr. vanden Berghe.

A huge stone-walled enclosure had been built for that purpose at Tshibati, IRSAC's experimental animal farm high up the mountain at the same life zone level as that of the wild mountain gorillas of the nearby Kauzi Fauna and Flora Reserve. It was here that a mature couple, male and female gorillas from the Utu expedition, were kept for long-term studies. The wall enclosed a natural landscape of boulders, vegetation and a small stream. Slits and small holes in the wall enabled undetected observation and photography. It was during the constant watch that the birth of a young gorilla was witnessed. Unfortunately, and strangely, the infant was killed by its own mother soon after birth for reasons no one could fathom. It was described by an observer (L. vanden Berghe, *Folia Scientifica Africae Centralis*, (IRSAC's own publication): vol. V, no. 4, 1959.)

The birth of a male gorilla occurred on October 26, 1959 at 12:15 p.m. Barely interrupting her meal, the young mother reclined on her left side, raised her right thigh and delivered her young within five minutes. Now in a sitting position, she sectioned the umbilical cord, whereupon the young gorilla started moving lively between her mother's thighs. The mother then took her young and brought one of its feet to her mouth, thought to be that of the classical gesture of licking. Before we could intervene, the mother had sectioned the foot, soon followed by that of a hand, while the skull was perforated by one of her canine teeth. It was possible to retrieve the young, too late, however, to save its life.

Cordier's camp in Utu also saw the birth of a young gorilla, but the baby was soon neglected by the mother. It was nursed with bottled milk by Mrs. Cordier and grew into a healthy gorilla baby whose portrait appears in the *National Geographic* magazine, January issue, 1960.

The IRSAC gorilla work attracted international attention and several eminent zoologists came to visit the Tshibati farm, among them Dr. J. T. Emlen and Dr. G. Schaller; the latter became well known for his book: *The Year of the Gorilla*.

One of the first notes on gorilla ecology by L. vanden Berghe, which appeared in *Fo.Sci.Afri.Center.*, vol. IV, no. 2, 1958 reads:

Groups of mountain gorillas in the region of Mount Kahuzi consist on a average of 20 individuals. One group of 34 was observed once, however. Each group has only one adult male, two or more females and a variable number of young of various ages. Adolescence arrives not before 12 to 15 years. Females probably do not produce more than 6 to 8 young. The adult male sleeps in a sitting position at the base of a tree, while the female and the youngsters sleep on a platform of twigs and leaves in the fork of the lower branches. Beds are remade every night in the same area. Gorillas sleep on the average 6 hours during a moonlit nights and up to 10 hours on dark nights. They are inactive and at rest between 10 a.m. and 3 p.m. They feed twice a day, in the morning and at the end of the day. Their food is essentially vegetarian, mainly the stems of large leaves. They are often seen eating the marrow of banana trees in abandoned fields. The young gorillas drink with their faces close to the water surface. Adults dip hand and forearm (right or left) in the water and drink the liquid running from the hairs—like gibbons.

Of all the primates, gorillas are certainly the least arboreal. The family group is dominated by the large adult male. His despotism is further enhanced by the apparent absence of hierarchy among the females and the young. Young males, rarely females, imitate their fathers in certain gestures, such as the rapid drumming of the chest with the open hand—not the fist—when excited. They will also slap their thighs, legs or feet but also the ground, a tree, and so on. The dominant male rejects young adult males from the group, either by killing or otherwise. This must be the origin of solitary males or groups of males.

Gorillas will rather flee than fight. "Flee diarrhea" is common.

IRSAC's interest in primates was not confined to gorillas. As part of our commitment to the interregional pool of correlation maps, we started to compose a distribution map of primate species and local variations in our areas. My wife played a patient role in this endeavor, carefully extracting essential data from the rough notes of Dr. Rahm, our Swiss zoologist, or those of Dr. Pirlot, who was conducting a general faunistic survey and was particularly interested in intraspecific variability.

Our gorilla studies, and those by other researchers, showed that the gorilla is not the savage man killer once believed to attack on sight, but rather a mild-natured primate who wants to be left alone.

The Last Camp

With three fly-rounds well south of Kibugabuga and with my increased interest in the dry forest as a possible tsetse habitat, I decided to set up another camp, this time on the shores of Lake Tshohoha south.

On 19 February 1958, I started out from Lwiro in the Land Rover followed by the lorry loaded with a secondhand prefab aluminum cabin, oval in shape and roomier than my first one. With me were Zaghi and a cook, Ramono, who was to be stationed permanently in Bugesera as cook-houseboy. I intended to recall Samson because I had become increasingly dissatisfied with his work. Also the new square fly-rounds needed strict supervision, a task for which I could trust only Zaghi. When I told Samson of my decision, he was dismayed, but not terribly upset or surprised. He begged me to keep him on the payroll for another two months so that he could look for another job. This I did.

A number of fly-boys were by now working in the vicinity of two villages near the southern lake and I decided to choose one of these villages Biharagu, as the site for the new camp. I learned that an old track skirted the lake and joined a bush road higher up. It was a long detour to Biharagu and the track was in a shocking state of repair, but the driver of the lorry managed to get the vehicle close to a possible campsite. In the meanwhile I had received the full cooperation of the villagers and they started cutting a new road along the passage I had intended to make with the Land Rover. I chose a lovely spot to put the cabin with a view of the lake, still within the shade of a row of tall trees. The following day I started wrestling with blinding aluminum panels, stays, traverses, window- and doorframes, ill-matched bolts and nuts. By noon I had the walls set up. By that time my tea was finished. Defying all my principles of hygiene, I accepted a large bottle of local "pombe." It tasted like weak beer that belied its alcoholic contents, but was gratifyingly refreshing. While I stood precariously on a chair on top of a 50-gallon drum, brazenly helped by the effect of the pombe, the roof went up during the afternoon hours. That night I slept in my new camp.

A few days later the aluminum hut in Kibugabuga was transported to Biharagu camp, where it was connected to the larger cabin by a passage made of two side panels. In the middle of this complicated operation a pouring rain turned the red earth into what looked like a blood bath. But the job had to be finished. On top of everything else, I made a mistake in the number and sequence of the panels. This was discovered only when I was putting on the roof and I realized that I had one space too many. We now had to shift the whole hut into the correct position. The unctuosity of the quagmire made this task relatively easy. The rain kept coming down all afternoon, converting the construction site into a glutinous red slush. Many aluminum panels bore streaks of hands that seemed to have belonged to persons making a last desperate effort to cling to something solid before being swallowed up into a red morass. When the last bolt met the proper nut, the rain stopped. I sank on to one of the clean chairs, wet and miserable throughout. Gone was the glory of Africa.

The next day, when everything had been cleaned and leveled, the camp looked very attractive indeed. I now had a spacious living room and an uncluttered bedroom with two camp beds, leaving enough room for personal trunks and other gear. A small table with a washbasin and towel rack, another small table between the beds, a number of shelves along the walls, and a long wire from the roof to hang the lamp made a very comfortable lodging as far a bush camps go. The furniture of the living room consisted of a large table, four folding chairs, wall shelves, two "stands" made from posts, sticks and twigs for storing equipment and food. The four legs of the food stand rested in tins filled with water to prevent ants and other unauthorized creatures from getting to the food before we did. One day we found the trunk containing the food reserve crawling with ants. Following their trail we discovered that a dry leaf spanned the distance between the outer side of the tin to the leg of the stand and supported heavy ant traffic, occasionally interrupted by panicking ants going the wrong way. Whether the leaf had been transported by the ants themselves or by a providential wind we did not know.

The measuring of the 25 squares of the special fly-round using only a compass was a cumbersome exercise. One day, as I was tracing a second square fly-round, one of the villagers came running breathlessly to tell me that the V.G.G. (Vice Governor General) had arrived at Kibugabuga and wanted to see me *sasa hevi* (immediately). "Darn it," was my first reaction, "I am hungry, thirsty, perspiring, scratched and my work for the day is still far from finished." But one could hardly ignore the summons of the highest Ruanda-Urundi authority. Before dashing off I hastily introduced Zaghi to the art of the compass, its uses, merits, pitfalls and history. Jumping into the Land Rover, I arrived at Kibugabuga rest house in a cloud of dust, noting with some satisfaction the cloud drifting towards the dozen or so immaculately clad officials. In a way, it was moment of glory. Here I was, an obscure biologist lecturing on tsetse flies, land use, and cattle ranching to some of the most distinguished high-ranking officials. The meeting lasted an hour, the V.G.G. thanked me and I dashed back to "my square." When I arrived, Zaghi had just finished the sides of the last square and it came out perfect. Good old Zaghi. (Zaghi was killed by his own countrymen during the skirmishes in Stanleyville following the Congo independence movement in 1960).

About 20 miles northeast of Biharagu lies the village of Mulehe, perched on top of a low hill called Nemba, the headquarters of a small tin mine company working some pits lower down in the Nyawarongo-Kagera valley. It contains few offices, a small workshop, the inevitable nduka and, important to me, a gasoline pump. One day, the manager told me about the funny shaped stones he kept finding in certain places on the upper slopes of the hill. I decided to investigate. And indeed, it didn't take me long to pick up an odd-shaped rock, clearly man-made, a perfect prehistoric hand axe. As I walked around the crest of the hill and found more artifacts, I realized that they were dispersed at pretty well the same level, circling the hilltop like a necklace. When, later, I showed my collection to the late Dr. L. S. B. Leakey, he suggested that the site might have been a "workshop" at the shores of a lake the level of which was much higher than that of the present-day lakes. He thought the tools possibly belonged to the Sangoan industry, dating from around 50,000 B.P. I donated one box of the artifacts to the Corydon Museum (now The National Museum of Kenya), but kept a box of specimens for myself. One of the hand axes lies on my table, used as a paperweight. As I pick it up, it rests comfortably in the palm of my hand. Closing my fingers, I feel the urge to tighten my grip and to use the blunt point as a hammer. Did the craftsman who made the tool derive the same satisfaction? To hold the tool gives me a funny feeling. I love my hand axe.

Dr. Troupin, the botanist, deeply interested in the Bugesera vegetation, became a frequent visitor to my camp. We shared many adventures, one involving a top-heavy canoe trip on the lake. Canoes seem to be my bane. One day, on my way back to Lwiro, I met Troupin halfway on his way to Bugesera. He told me that he had been informed that the V.G.G. had approved our proposal for a forest reserve. He persuaded me to return with him to Bugesera because he wanted my advice as "the most traveled person in the Bugesera." T. (Troupin) was driving a new Peugeot station wagon. When, near Kabgay, he broke a rear spring, I doubted his choice. It was temporarily repaired in Kigali by inserting a spring retrieved from an old vehicle dump. We arrived at Biharagu camp without further incident, having visited a deep abandoned well on the way, there, someone in Kigali told us, sterile wives were disposed of . . . a long time ago. The next day we visited the southern shores of the lake on foot and by canoe. We discovered a square-shaped peninsula of about one-by-one-mile big, covered with dense, representative vegetation. The place seemed a possible choice for the proposed reserve. Bordered on three sides by the lake, its limits would be easy to define, while a series of posted signs or eventually a fence would delimit the reserve on the land side. Afterwards we drove to the Kindama area, where I showed T. a strange forest consisting predominately of *Apodites dimidiata* trees. He said that he regretted that I had showed him the place because now he wasn't quite sure which of the two sites would be the most suitable. I proposed that he should make a strong case to have both sites accepted as a reserve. I departed the next day for Lwiro, leaving T. behind with his dilemma.

Three weeks later we both returned to Bugesera for more surveys and to make a vegetation inventory of the square fly-rounds. It was during this period that I started to speculate whether tsetses are attracted to certain colors or perhaps sensitive to contrasting light patterns. In the past, controversial reports indicated that tsetses preferably attack Africans because of their dark skin and they were, therefore, more prone to contract sleeping sickness than light-skinned individuals. Yet the flies certainly showed no dislike towards me and fed on me with indiscriminate abandon. Most of us agreed that movement was the primordial attraction to tsetse flies and I suspected contrasting light played a role. One of my early experiments was to test color attraction. Two-by-two-foot wooden panels were painted in primary colors, then coated with a sticky substance (birdlime was one) and hung on a cable among the vegetation. Difficulties in finding the right adhesive prevented bringing these experiments to an interpretable conclusion. (Several years later, similar experiments I carried out in other parts of Africa were more successful.)

The question of contrasting light and light intensities remained fixed in my mind until one day we acquired two registering light meters which measured differences in light intensities by means of two light meter cells, each recording readings every ten seconds on a revolving paper roll. We ran trials in the Mutara along an old fly-round for which we had two years' fly density data. Various technical difficulties, adverse weather and pressure of time—it was the last month of my stay in Africa—prevented us from coming to a conclusion.

One of my major concerns was whether fly-free areas in the Bugesera were in danger of being invaded by advances of flies from the infested areas and, if so, whether it could be prevented. I made several surveys at the periphery of the present flybelt to check on this. One of these distant surveys, south of Bugesera, ended in an unpleasant way. H. Vander Borght, a fellow IRSAC health officer, and I had been working around Kibungu, where most of the sleeping sickness cases had been diagnosed. We stayed at a dilapidated rest house at Rugari. Except for the nearby Catholic mission, it is an isolated and little traveled area. Before leaving, we decided to visit the falls of the Ruvumu River on the Tanzania border. The falls had been seen by few; and these had proclaimed their great beauty. It was a road without issue, so we would have to return to Rugari. We left all our equipment at the rest house and set out in the IRSAC station wagon with driver Joseph at the wheel. The track was in a shocking state of repair and badly overgrown in most places. It followed the desolate, deep-cut valley of the Ruvumu River, the slopes too steep for human occupation. At a point where the track made a sharp left bend, it crossed the river on a plank bridge that made us all hold our breaths until, with a great sigh of relief, we reached the other side in spite of the groaning protest of the crossbeams. Our relief was short-lived. No sooner had we reached the other side than the right front wheel sank into a deep hole, bounced back and the bottom of the car hit with a loud thud a high stone in the center of the track. I feared the worst. Joseph crawled underneath the vehicle and confirmed my suspicion: the oil was running out of a hole in the crankcase. Of all the breakdowns, this is one of the most fatal. There was nothing we could do but abandon the vehicle. We removed our few personal belongings, Joseph hid tools and accessories under the seats, unscrewed the spare wheel from underneath the car, put it inside, closed the windows and locked the doors. It was eleven in the morning.

By road we had logged something like 60 kilometers since we left Rugari, a 12-hour walk if we stepped lively. We hoped to find a shortcut at some point to reduce the distance. But with Rugari located on top of a high hill, we knew that any shortcut would be going straight up. I have followed with great sympathy and almost physical participation the dramatic narratives of long marches by explorers and stranded travelers. Our experience cannot compare to that of those brave men and women, but our walk seemed bad enough. Soon our water bottles were empty and our bananas and oranges consumed. We walked as in a dream, not caring for anything but to put one foot before the other. H. developed blisters and walked in great pain, which he tried to alleviate by putting leaves inside his shoes. Joseph seemed the least affected. We found a shortcut, but as predicted, the path went straight up. We arrived at the rest house at eight in the evening, having walked nine hours with few rests out of fear that once the rhythm broke, we would lack the courage to go on. We estimated that we had walked about 45 kilometers, 5 kilometers per hour—not a bad pace!

The following morning Joseph went back with the mechanic and the pickup truck from the Catholic mission, and with a good supply of engine oil. It transpired that the damage to the oil sump was less substantial than we had thought and they managed to patch up the hole with soap and layers of tape so that the vehicle could be brought back under its own steam. On arrival at Rugari, the repairs still held and we decided to fly on our luck and leave forthwith for the IRSAC—Astrida mechanic shop. We bought a good supply of engine oil and checked underneath the car every so often. We arrived in Astrida without further trouble. In our imagination we had expected the breakdown to set us back at least a week, incurring expenses for towing, costly repairs and an unpleasant interview with the director of the Astrida IRSAC Center. As in the past, things seem to sort themselves out in Africa.

Our work in Bugesera became a kind of government pet project and was eventually included in a documentary film about the "Ten Year Plan." The government interest helped Dr. Adamantidis, director of the Ruanda-Urundi Veterinary Services, find enough funding to pay for a flight in the government Cessna across the Mutara and Bugesera regions. We proclaimed that this would allow us to identify potential tsetse flybelts and compare our observations with the aerial photographs. So one day we stood on Usumbura airfield before a beautiful twin-engine Cessna-Apache shining brightly in the early March morning. With the pilot and Adamantidis in front, Dr. Marsboom, a new vet, and I in the back seat, we took off at a rate that felt like 2 g's. Soon we were high over the mountains. The plane seemed to fly by itself and I thought that I could take the controls if they had let me. It seemed so easy. To demonstrate her abilities, the pilot took the plane in a steep dive and buzzed a dairy farm in one of the valleys and then pulled sharply up again. When our stomachs had returned to their normal positions, the three of us eagerly stated that we had been convinced by that one test.

The comparison between observations of the terrain below and the aerial photos proved indeed extremely useful later on in the planning of the anti–tsetse campaign. This we stressed emphatically in our report, hinting that additional flights might be needed to observe in more detail certain crucial areas. We had all fallen in love with the elegant Cessna.

The growing attention for the Bugesera was not confined to that of the local government. As part of a general common flybelt that included parts of Uganda and Tanganyika Territory, we had several joint strategy sessions with colleagues from British East Africa. Engineers of Dutch firms came to have a look at the Bugesera and, based upon their long and successful experience in land reclamation and development, proposed programs for the rehabilitation of agricultural and grazing lands. Representatives of insecticide manufacturing companies converged on Kigali, carefully avoiding tsetse contact. One exception was the visit of Dr. Rudolph Geigy, of the famous Swiss company and director of the Swiss Tropical Institute. Dr. Geigy was personally very much interested in tsetse fly biology and ecology. He himself had conducted research on the subject at the Geigy sponsored field research station at Ifakara in Tanzania. He and two of his assistants—one of them, Dr. U. Rham, who was to join later the IRSAC Institute—accompanied me on a tour of the Mutara and Bugesera regions and, later, the Irangi forest.

Towards the end of 1958 I was ready to discuss our findings and suggest possible antiglossina action. We had a first meeting at the Residency in Kigali, presided by the Resident-Adjunct, Mr. Regnier. My proposal for the anti–tsetse campaign was accepted with little change. The new D.O., Mr. Ducenne, accepted with admirable enthusiasm the task of carrying out vegetation clearings. He mentioned the several trial runs he had already made, using various methods. Another meeting, held in the afternoon, was to discuss plans for the Mutara. Before the start of the discussion, Mr. Haezaerts, chief warden of Kagera National park, read a letter from Mr. V. Van Stralen, director of all national parks, in which he granted permission to extend tsetse control into the Kagera Park in crucial areas of tsetse contact. His choice of words clearly indicated the great pain he felt in according this concession and that, personally, he did not believe in anti–tsetse clearings.

The following day a dozen people packed in three vehicles visited my camp in Biharagu and the nearby fly-rounds. We drove to Kindama, where I explained the potential danger of extension of the flybelt into adjacent not yet infested areas and that those sensitive places should be high on the list of priorities. The aerial photos were, once more, of great value in explaining the situation.

On the third day, the meeting was held at Nyakatale in Mutara, where I had lunch with ten other "specialists." We visited the two priority areas marked for immediate clearing operations. One of the areas was the vegetation salient inhabited by tsetse that projects into the park—and into the heart of Van Stralen. Again with the help of the aerial photos, I proposed that the clearing of the salient be confined to Nyaruwanga Hill on the Mutara side up to the park's limits, which coincided with the main road, and to wait one year to see if this partial clearing would be sufficient to reduce trypanosomiasis in cattle of that area. Everyone was happy with this modification which avoided, for the time being, the thorny problem of intruding into the park.

I returned to Kigali that same evening where I arrived around nine. I was washed out.

The exact extent of the Bugesera flybelt kept bothering me. Why did tsetses appear 20 miles south of the ferry and not north? My explanation was that the dense thicket vegetation was unsuitable for *Glossina morsitans*. But I often questioned my own answer. Surveys carried out in the west along the banks and swamps of the Akanyaru River, for instance, showed a number of large areas of woodland free of tsetses which, normally, should be buzzing with flies. These areas were in all instances separated from the central flybelt by open spaces of cultivated or fallow fields. It seemed to me that, at present tsetse-free, these areas could not remain so for very long and that sooner or later flies introduced by human and cattle movement from fly-infested areas would promote further dispersion.

To test my theory, I had one of the fly-boys ride a bicycle along the road from my Kindama camp all the way to the shores of the Akanyaru swamps. The bicycle was fitted out with a screen coated with a sticky substance. The number of flies caught was recorded every 500 meters. During the 74 runs, each 2,500 meters long inside the recognized flybelt, 538 flies had been caught; against 75 flies caught during the same 74 runs outside the flybelt over 5,500 meters each, a proportion of 20 to 1. It showed, however, that flies were present outside the main flybelt, most probably those that had followed the bicycle.

Another test to assess tsetse dispersion was the barrier I had set up at Nyamata, a village surrounded by fields, but located within dense thicket vegetation about halfway between the ferry and the northern limit of the main flybelt. People, cattle and vehicles moving from the flybelt were examined to see if flies followed them. On the average, close to 100 tsetses a quarter of which were females, were collected each month in this way. These would have been able to produce a number of offspring and, by sheer accumulation, could have started a colony in suitable vegetation outside the main flybelt.

The number of reported sleeping sickness cases increased as more and more inhabitants were examined. Four cases were found in villages within our fly-rounds. When one of our fly-boys came down with high fever, I took him immediately to the hospital. It proved to be malaria, not sleeping sickness. One case was found in Mulehe on Nemba Hill, where I used to collect stone artifacts. And I began to wonder whether prehistoric man had been a carrier of sleeping sickness.

The last but next Bugesera safari started with an official bang in the form of a meeting with fifteen higher officials, representing the departments of agriculture, veterinary services, development and resources, health and social welfare, geology, botany, national parks and wildlife management, and meteorology, presided over by Mr. J. P. Harroy, Vice governor General and Governor of Ruanda-Urundi. After the meeting, Dora and I and three other IRSAC members and their wives were invited for a lunch at the V.G.G.'s residence, where the discussion about the Bugesera continued—to the great vexation of the ladies, no doubt.

While the rest of the IRSAC people, including Dora, returned home, I continued my journey to Mutara, where I had to discuss the anti-tsetse campaign with the local vet officer. With no more camp at Kakole Hill, I intended to stay at the permanent IRSAC camp at Mimuli. This camp had been built near the Kakitumba River to replace my old Kakole camp and allow the continuation of scientific presence in the area, which IRSAC had suggested to make into a natural reserve. The Mimuli Camp consisted of several prefab aluminum structures: a large living room, a study room, a dining room, a large bedroom, a bathroom and a separate kitchen. Several huts made of local materials and in local style provided lodging for permanent and visiting personnel.

I once spent a memorable day there. It was at the time of King Leopold's visit. The day after that first abortive gorilla capture, the director had sent me full haste to Mumuli. The king had expressed his wish to visit Mutara and it was suggested that the royal party would stop over at the camp for lunch. A team under the supervision of the workshop manager had been dispatched to spruce up the place, including the installation of curtains on the windows, cushions for the camp chairs—that sort of thing. The people who used or were about to use the facilities were delighted. For the same occasion, a small overnight cabin had hastily been built at Uwinka giving the best panoramic view of the Nyongwe mountain forest along the Astrida road. Besides the copious lunch snacks that would have satisfied a hungry football team, the supplies sent to Mimuli included a most gratifying array of different liqueurs, besides, of course, all kinds of beer and a wide selection of nonalcoholic beverages. As noon came (the party was expected at eleven) and passed without a dust cloud announcing the approach of the royal caravan, it became clear that there was a fly in the pie or a tree across the road, more likely. We waited. No one would ever reproach us of having abandoned our battle station. One o'clock came and went. To squander time, I started experimenting with various cocktail mixtures—one of my hobbies. Volunteers were willing tasters of each of the experimental formulas. Out of all this came a wondrous drink, later christened "Royal Mimuli Fizz." (For those interested, here is the formula: one part grapefruit juice, one part orange juice, one part pineapple juice, two parts peach brandy, two parts gin, one part soda water.) The Royal Mimuli Fizz is fairly inoffensive as cocktails go. However, the tasting of many prior trial concoctions made the finally approved formula a bombshell. Although ultimately disappointed by the non–arrival of the royal guests, (explained much later by a change in their itinerary), we realized that it was just as well, and that fate had kindly spared us from the woeful moment of facing and greeting the royal visitors and entourage with one hand on a chair for support. We were seven and there were only four chairs.

But to go back to my arrival at Mimuli that evening, tired and late. I found no houseboy nor guard. There was no light. Nothing stirred. The place seemed abandoned. Furious, I unpacked my own Coleman lamp, lit it and discovered that there was no water, not in the main reservoir nor in the water filter. I had counted on food stored in one of the trunks, but they were locked and there was no one to hand me the keys. I was forced to break the padlocks so that, at least, I could get to the supply of soda water.

I left early the next morning; still no one was in sight. I went to see the chief. He said he did not know why the camp was without guard or houseboy that he would send his askari (policeman) until things could be sorted out.

After discussing the anti-tsetse campaign with the vet in Nyakatale, I returned to Mimuli and spent a second night there without seeing a soul.

Passing Kigali the following day on my way to Bugesera, I thought about having a haircut, but the only barber I knew had left town. Inquiring about another barber, I was directed to the center of the busy marketplace where, among dozens of squatting women displaying various foods in gunny sacks, a straight chair was standing with the word "coiffeur" painted in white on the back. As I hesitantly approached, a scrubby man appeared asking if I was ready for a *kata nyeli* (cut hair). His shabby looks, the smell of pombe and the flat box he opened showing barber paraphernalia of doubtful vintage and cleanliness made me shudder. But in an illogical spirit of integration I manfully sat down preparing myself for some kind of ritual. The barber deployed with a flourish a piece of cloth, tying the ends behind my neck. I refrained from looking down on the cloth, guessing the worst. Moreover my attention was diverted towards the crowd gathering around me, composed of both sexes, ranging from crawling toddlers to shuffling elders. There is little doubt that I was the first white—and possibly the last— to have his hair cut in this fashion, thereby turning the routine market day into a center of entertainment and elevating the barber's image to that of a multiracial cosmetologist. He made the most of the opportunity by attending to the smallest details, at times standing before me to eye his art critically, snipping a hair here or there, striving for perfection. During the procedures I tried to keep a solemn face gazing *through* the onlookers rather than *at* them with, I hoped, a noncommittal expression—as if the marketplace was my preferred spot to have a haircut.

I was anxious to wind up my many years of surveys and research and to conclude my work with a proper assessment of our findings and to present a logical proposal for tsetse fly control in the Mutara and Bugesera regions. The desire to close this chapter in my life was related to the fact that Dora and I had come to the long-thought-out decision to leave Africa. I had informally notified my director of my intention of resigning at the end of my contract in August 1959 and of emigrating to the United States. I knew he was sincere when he expressed his deep sorrow and disappointment. I felt the same way. We had known each other for 18 years in scientific collaboration as well as socially. He was more like a friend than a boss. But Dora and I had discussed and debated our future for many months, concluding that we owed it to our daughters to give them a chance for higher education—they were now 17 and 18 years old—and an opportunity for a lifestyle different from that in the colonies. As for my profession, that is, medically-related biological research, I hoped to make a living at one of the American universities or research institutions. Indeed, my first inquiries had been encouraging. Since we set our departure around mid-1959, the end of my present contract, it was imperative that I bring my work in Mutara and Bugesera to an acceptable conclusion and start writing up all scientific observations and recommendations in a formal publication.

My last entries in the Bugesera diary read:

Wednesday, March 4, 1959

Arrived yesterday evening. Camp in good shape.

Start paper work first thing in the morning, collating results of fly-rounds and write introduction to report. Vet officer Marsboom arrives at 12:45 and we work on some maps. As he is going to take over part of our research, Wasso, one of my lab assistants, demonstrates the technique of tsetse fly dissections under the microscope. While engaged in this work, his hut bursts into flames. In the wink of an eye the roof is engulfed. One of the fly-boys manages to throw Wasso's belongings outside before they burn, apparently missing a 100-franc bill on a shelf. The roof of the nearby kitchen is hastily torn down out of fear that the fire will spread to the rest of the building and the camp. After the flames have been put out, we find half-molten panels from the prefab hut. Wasso confesses that he used the spare panels as shelves.

Thursday, March 5, 1959

To Kindama. Pay off the extra labor and some of the local fly-boys. Spend the rest of the time preparing report and completing scenes for a 16mm film about our work, which I started several months ago with the cooperation of the local chief and the health officer.

Friday, March 6, 1959

Splendid cool weather all day. Tour the Gihinga area with the health officer. After our return, he makes out health certificates for my personnel returning to Lwiro next week. After he leaves, I walk slowly along square grid V, probably for the last time. I try to imprint in my memory the trees I have marked and examined so many times from close-by for tsetse flies. A few tsetse follow. They will be sorry, too, that I am leaving. I was such a good source of blood! I reach a depression filled with water from the previous heavy rains. Tsetse are now very active and biting. Ah well, it will be their last meal on me!

Sunday, March 8, 1959

Go visit Chief Bulenge to arrange for filming later in the day. Rather an excuse to drive about on the sandy tracks for the last time in my life. Tracks that I have come to know so well. Some I have measured laboriously and patiently when tracing my fly-rounds. I see clusters of trees I have learned to associate with aggressive tsetses, the glade where I once saw the rare roan antelope, the thicket where, one day, I sat for hours observing game and tsetse while trying to understand their affinities and the spot where, one night, I ran over a civet cat and later saw a leopard.

The chief gives me a hunting bow and half a dozen arrows with iron heads. Both are much larger than the forest bow I received from Makoda, the MaBudu headman near Pawa, almost fifteen years ago.

Monday, March 9, 1959

This could be the last entry in my Bugesera diary. A wonderful, nice day with a beautiful sky. The lorry arrives at ten. Loading is the usual African affair of incongruous odd-shaped bundles, intermingled with assorted furniture, including a door, the whole topped with large baskets of loudly protesting chickens. At 11:15 the vehicle leaves for Kindama to pick up the remaining fly-boys. From there they will drive to Astrida and, the next day, to Lwiro.

Now alone, I putter about, completely lost and downhearted after all the excitement of the previous months and with sorrow for having to close a happy chapter and leave this region that I have come to love dearly.

Near sunset, heavy rain squalls alternating with bursts of sunshine paint wondrous skies and the glittering trees in yellows, oranges and reds. Pink-colored smoke rises from the damp roofs of faraway huts. The dark silhouette of a canoe and a late fisher glide across the golden waters of Lake Tshohoha. Then night covers all . . . "and though fortune may forsake me . . . sweet dreams will ever take me . . . home." Where is home?

The Last Safari

Many months earlier, between 11 July and 10 August 1958, still within the period of active research in the Bugesera, our long East African safari deserved to be the suitable ending to our long African experience, an icing on the cake, a flourishing "trait-de-plume."

At this time, we had gathered a wealth of data on the tsetse fly populations in Mutara and Bugesera and we felt that it would be useful to discuss our findings with colleagues of other institutions such as the "East Africa Trypanosomiasis and Tsetse Research Organization" (E.A.T.T.R.O.), one located in Tororo, Uganda; the other in Old Shinyanga, Tanganyika. I received authorization to visit these centers as well as the "Colonial Pest Research Unit" (C.P.R.U.) near Arusha and the "Malaria Research Station" in Amani, both in Tanganyika. My wife and five-year-old Richard did not accompany me as the 2,500-mile-long journey in the open Land Rover over some rough and uncertain roads, with the strong possibility of spending a number of nights in the open, was not expected to be a comfortable one. Moreover, Dora, at that time a research assistant in the zoology lab, had been put in charge of a project on rodent distribution when her boss left for Canada. But the planned trip fell within the girls' school holidays and they were only too eager to come along. Winnie, then 18 would be a useful standby driver able to take the wheel if needed. Both she and Jessie were also promising photographers.

Friday, July 11, 1958
Leave Lwiro at 7:40. Reach Muhinga, via Astrida and Ngozi, at 17:00. Too late to see the customs officer at Ngara, still 15 miles the other side of the border. Decide to camp at the side of the road. During the maneuver of backing the Land Rover into a space between trees, a loud shout from Jessie makes me slam on the brakes, thereby avoiding backing into a deep, large hole that would have swallowed the vehicle whole. Not a very good start! As my stomach returns to its former position, I find another spot where we finally settle for the night. This means reshuffling the cargo so that the three of us can stretch out on a

relatively even platform in our blankets. This we do with a lot of grumblings, groans and protests.

Saturday, July 12, 1958

Wake up with the first light and glad to stretch out from an uncomfortable position. Dense fog swirls around the campsite, chilling our already cold bones. Quickly we leave for the 15-mile drive to the customs post at Ngara. This is not a through road, so we have to drive back to reach the main road. At this point, we start the descent into the lowland savannas of eastern Africa with their miles of typical "miombo" vegetation, a uniform parkland of evenly spaced trees of the same height dominated essentially by *Brachystegia, Joulbernardia* and other woodland tree species. These communities are found in two large but separate areas of 75,000 square miles. This type of woodland looks so orderly that one has the impression of driving through an orchard or the park of a wealthy landlord rich enough to afford a well-kept chase over countless miles.

We stop briefly at Tinde, home of the well-known "Trypanosome Research Laboratory," where we meet Dr. K. Willett, who is carrying out long-term experiments on trypanosome transmission. Past Tinde, the road winds through some marvelous rock formations which outlined against the setting sun create the effect of some kind of primitive temple of an ancient cult. Soon thereafter we reach Shinyanga, the goal of our second day.

Shinyanga is a small commercial center on the railway from Tabora to Mwanza. Just north of the town lies the famous Williamson diamond mine. Not that the mines are of world-shattering importance. It is the romance of Mr. Williamson's discovery that is being retold many times over a beer in the local pubs and at the tsetse research station where Williamson used to work. It is said that, one day out on a survey, he was marooned by torrential rains and floods and decided that it would be wise to camp on higher ground until the next morning. To make sure that the Land Rover would not slide down the slope, he blocked the wheels front and aft with large stones. The next morning he woke up in bright sunlight, glad for his decision of the previous evening and preparing to drive back to Old Shinyanga. As he removed the stones from underneath the wheels, one caught and reflected the sun in an unusual sheen. The rock contained an almost pure diamond that weighed in at around 150 carats. The days of tsetse research were over for Williamson.

We had arrived at Old Shinyanga, headquarters of E.A.T.T.R.O., an hour after sunset and had been immediately invited to join a dinner party at the Johns. After dinner we were taken to the guesthouse, where we thankfully hit the sack. It had been a very long day.

Sunday, July 13, 1958

After a wonderful night's sleep, we breakfast at the Glasgows. Dr. J. P. Glasgow is the new chief entomologist, replacing the late Dr. C. N. H. Jackson, who died three years ago. We are shown the research laboratories housed in an old German fort built in 1912. I had visited the research center six years earlier. Not much has changed since then. That same morning we climb "Commemoration Hill," where a number of bronze plaques bearing the names of deceased colleagues have been affixed to some of the boulders in a superb cluster of rocks. The one for Jackson reads:

> In memory of
> Charles Herbert Newton Jackson
> O.B.E. - D. Sci.
> 1905 - 1955
> A distinguished scientist
> and most generous friend
> whose enthusiasm and
> love for Africa
> will long be remembered.
> For 27 years his work
> inspired his colleagues
> and now remains
> an abiding monument
> of scientific achievement

An earlier commemorative plaque on one of the rocks reminds us of the deaths in 1938 of B. D. Burtt and C. F. M. Swynnerton in an airplane crash while on a tsetse flu survey not far from Shinyanga.

Besides the typical tsetse woodland, harboring the two species *Glossina morsitans* and *Glossina swynnertoni*, the country surrounding Old Shinyanga—the EATTRO people insist on the

"Old"—is especially remarkable for its forest of baobabs (*Adansonia digitata*). The baobab is a grotesque, voluminous tree with a large swollen trunk 60 to 70 feet in girth, 40 to 60 feet high. In spite of its tremendous main stem, the branches taper rapidly, giving the impression of a number of crooked, stout arms which gave rise to the African legend that the tree, one day drawing the disfavor of God, had been planted upside down, the roots pointed into the air. The baobab thrives in the drier areas of most of Africa, its flowers brilliant white, waxy and pendulous, rapidly turning brown and shedding quickly. The fruit is oblong or egg-shaped, five or more inches in length, three or more inches in diameter. The astringent taste of the pulp delights baboons and elephants. Many baobabs are estimated to be several hundred years old. The pulpy core of the old trees is often burned out by bushfires that do not kill the tree, however. The cavity created is used as shelter by many kinds of animals and sometimes by man.

Monday, July 14, 1958

I take the Land Rover to the workshop for inspection. Long discussions take up the rest of the day. The complexity of the tsetse problem and the degree and quality of research can be judged from the topics discussed: water loss in active and resting flies; differences in fat contents in flies from control and uncontrolled areas; the site of resting flies at night and during daytime; the dependency of savanna flies on warthog blood; estimation and dynamics of tsetse fly populations in an isolated peninsula of Lake Victoria; marking and recapturing methods; the role of the antenna and body spines; vegetation types crucial to tsetse survival; the role of predators such as the jumping spider in tsetse densities; age determination of female tsetse by dissection and examination of the ovaries; methods of raising tsetse in the laboratory; soil temperatures and the survival of tsetse pupae, and so on.

Impressed by the venerable baobab forest, Jessie makes several excellent sketches of the area. In late afternoon, I play tennis with Bursell, Johns, Mr. and Mrs. Southon. Dinner at the Bursells.

Tuesday, July 15, 1958

Leave Old Shinyanga at 9:10. The road to Nzega is bordered by flat, monotonous country covered by large expanses of "gall acacia" on "black cotton soil." Gall acacia (*Acacia depranolobium*), also called whistling thorn, is a small tree, 5 to 15 feet high, with gray or dark bark. The straight thorns are often fused and inflated at the base, forming a globe or gall. These extraordinary aberrations are the result of an excretion by certain ants who use them for shelter. They enter the globe through a single small hole. A strong wind will cause the holes to emit a weird whistling sound, repeated across the low woodland like the passage of moaning ghosts.

Beyond Nzega, the road dwindled to a mere trail. We had been informed and warned, when we reached the Sekenke swamps, to look for the trail by following sticks or knotted tall grass—an original way to mark a road, I thought. The reason for this was that the passages on solid ground shifts with the season and "one had to read the road as one went along." We approached the swamps—an extension of uniform tall grasses that stretched as far as we could see—with considerable concern. Our finding of knotted grasses, however, gave us a certain degree of confidence, confirming that my advisers had not "pulled my leg." Albeit, the signs were not displayed at regular intervals and one often had to guess where the next knot might be. Many times I went on blindly, hoping the next knot would not be far off. On other occasions, I had to change direction when I felt that we were driving on unstable soil. What if we got stuck and sank lower in the mire with no help in sight? We hadn't passed a single vehicle so far, and I was not surprised. The passage of the swamps, perhaps ten miles wide, seemed ten times as long and it took us almost two hours of four-wheel driving. At last, the ground grew firmer—reluctantly, I had the impression—with still a few soggy patches as a reminder. With the last knotted grasses behind us, we reached a track visible by the passage on solid ground of motor vehicles without the help of braided grasses. It led straight to Sigida, where we arrived half an hour before sunset. We booked into the only hotel. From the outside it looked rather dismal, an impression that did not improve when we were shown our room, the only one available, we were assured. It had sagging ceilings and peeling walls. As if out of desperation, someone had started painting one wall in aquamarine blue, but, realizing the futility of the effort, had abandoned the project at the door. A naked bulb hung from the middle of the ceiling, but had been diverted, no doubt by an enterprising traveler, over the twin beds by means of a string attached to a nail in the wall. A third bed against the opposite wall sported a nightstand fitted out with a lopsided light that did not work. We discovered the bathroom at the far end of a corridor, its poor lighting gratefully hiding the details of the facility.

But we made a joke of the whole situation. After all, we had passed the test of the swamps.

Wednesday, July 16, 1958

As we entered the dining room early the following morning, the Hindu owner and his wife were already seated at one of the corner tables. He asked if we had had a pleasant night and we assured him that we had never slept better. He showed great surprise. We had the classic eggs, bacon and sausage and strong tea and were halfway through our breakfast when the door to the rooms opened and the room boy, balancing a silver platter on his widespread hand, came to our table and, presenting the object lying on top, said to Winnie and Jessie: "nguo yako, me nazania Mem-sahib" ("your garment, I believe, Miss"). On the platter lay a dainty pink panty which Jessie, blushing like a fierce sunset, snatched up mumbling "Akisanti." Winnie and I had great difficulties keeping a straight face. The story is being retold to this day.

Leave Sigida shortly after eight. Bitterly cold and foggy. Some thirty miles after Sigida we start having beautiful views of Mount Hanang (11,215 ft.), unfortunately frequently hidden in fog-clouds. We stop at a swift, icy mountain stream to fill our water cans. The road is in a terrible state of repair, getting worse and muddier as we proceed. Wide potholes have been filled with large, rough stones. A breakdown in these parts would be disastrous as no one else seems to be using this road. We pass a group of huts that could be Dongobesh. Houses are of the pit dwelling type, partly buried in a dam of black earth, the roof made of soil, only two feet above ground at the rear. Blue smoke filters through cracks and clefts, indicating that the dwellings are inhabited. Two women come outside at the sound of the laboring Land Rover. Not sure whether this rough track is actually part of the official road network, I shout: "Mbule, iko wapi?" ("mbule, where is it?"). They point in the direction where I thought it should be and thus encouraged we plow onwards. The village of Mbule does not look less shabby than Dongobesh. Ten miles beyond this point the road climbs on higher ground, followed by an immediate improvement of the road surface. We have occasional views of a long, narrow lake that, I guess, must be Lake Eyasi. Soon afterwards we reach Karatu. I am grateful for the gasoline station, which relieves me of drawing from my 50-gallon reserve fuel. We reach Lodoro Gate at the entrance of Serengeti National Park five minutes after closing time, so we have to put up for the night at the gate's rest house.

Thursday, July 17, 1958

Drizzle and soft rain all night. Up at half past six and off near eight. Thick fog. Soon after we drive into the park, a buffalo crosses in front. It, too, has trouble with poor visibility. Road, very slippery, 12 miles long, winds its way to the lodge at 8,000 feet. Book a very nice, warm and cozy cabin for the night. After disposing of some of our gear, drive down the other side of the rim into the bottom of the Ngorongoro crater, accompanied by the park's guide. With a diameter of around 30 miles, it is the largest crater in the world, so huge that at the bottom it doesn't look like a crater at all, but just an undulating grassy plain with distant high slopes. A hazy sun and whirling mist-clouds on top of the rim draw changing patterns across the tall grasses bending in the wind. We drive through herds of wildebeest and zebras as if we were ranchers inspecting our stock. We come close to two rhinos that, the guide tells us, are usually docile if not pressed. The guide seems to know his territory very well and takes us to many beautiful spots where large herds of wild animals are peacefully grazing. In a far corner of the crater we come upon a group of a dozen Maasai warriors armed with spears. As soon as we stop, they swarm around us, asking the guide what we are doing in this part of the Ngorongoro. While the leader talks to the guide, the others inspect the inside of the Land Rover and the different gadgets we carry. One is intrigued by my field glasses. When I show him how to use them, pointing to a far-away zebra, he literally can't believe his eyes. Waving his hands in front, making sure the animal has not closed the distance, he jumps with delight. Two of the warriors are especially intrigued by Winnie's and Jessie's fair hair. They feel the texture as if to convince themselves it is real, and babble excitedly. Another has discovered the outside rear mirror of the car and studies his own face intensely. When we decide to break up the party, I have difficulties persuading the chap with the binoculars to hand them back to me. Finally I drive off at the moment when a friendly meeting is turning into exaggerated familiarity bordering on aggressiveness.

It is now late afternoon, time to find the main track when the guide suddenly points to two female lions intensely watching a herd of zebras from a low rise. Under the guide's direction I drive to within ten feet of the animals. They seem more intent upon bringing home the evening meal than being bothered by a silly Land Rover and, after a cursory glance, return to their observation. After our initial nervousness, the excitement wears off and we start a casual discussion with our guide about plans for the next day. As we drive off, one of the lions turns its head with an expression that seems to convey "good riddance."

Friday, July 18, 1958

Up at 6:30. The cabin boy has already lit the log fire. It feels congenial. The guide arrives at eight and we are off again, descending the 20-mile twisting road into the crater. After a while the fog thins and soon the bottom of the crater appears bathed in sunshine. Instead of driving farther into the crater we take a track to the north leading towards the Olduwai Gorge. It is rough going and some parts, treacherously sandy, wind through some fascinating wild country. A group of giraffes are resting in a thick acacia grove. The sun is out in full strength. We arrive at the gorge and drive to a site close to where the Leakeys have been finding stone tools and hope to find, eventually, fossils of prehistoric man (one year later they did discover a perfectly preserved "human" skull dated at 1.8 million years of *Zinjanthropus bosei (Australopithecus bosei)*. The Y-shaped gorge was cut over thousands of years by ancient watercourses through 300-foot deep sediments that had filled an ancient lake including volcanic materials from the nearby Ngorongoro volcano. We walk some distance inside the hot gorge bottom, I with a trace of emotion at the thought that I am standing at a place where once some distant ancestor trod.

From the entrance of the gorge we drive another ten miles up a trail that climbs towards the immense expanse of the Serengeti Plains. We turn around and drive back towards the crater at a place marked by a tall dune of black volcanic ash which, the guide says, moves around with the wind. On the way back meet many more giraffes. We are back at the lodge at one. Pack and leave for Arusha. The sandy track skirts the northern shores of Lake Manyara. Take gasoline at Campi ya Nioka (Snake Camp). Here the track changes into an excellent two-way tarmac road all the way to Arusha, which we reach at 16:40. Asking for the C.P.R.U. at one of the shops, we meet one of its members, Mr. Forster. We book at the Safari Hotel and for the first time in many days enjoy the luxury of a hot bath, ample room to unpack and wash clothes, large beds with real mattresses, and an excellent dinner.

Saturday, July 19, 1958

Visit the "Colonial Pesticide Research Unit" located eight miles outside Arusha. My visit to this research center concerns tsetse fly control and is, therefore, one of the main objectives of the trip. It is here that various insecticides and methods of application are studied and tested, not only for tsetse flies but for many other insects of medical and agricultural importance. Research is carried out in the laboratory under experimental conditions as well as in the field under natural conditions. To study the biological effect of various chemicals on tsetse flies, a colony of *G. morsitans* is kept. The long-term maintenance of the fly under artificial conditions, however, meets with many difficulties and setbacks. At the time of my visit, insecticide applications by aircraft were being studied, especially the use of the ULV (Ultra Low Volume) applications, in experimental blocks of tsetse habitats.

Sunday, July 20, 1958

Visit and photograph Arusha's marketplace, a colorful picture dominated by Maasai people. They are not easy to photograph: either they get angry or ask for money.

Monday, July 21, 1958

The day passes in discussions with C.P.R.U. members: R. Foster, P. J. White, D. Yeo, L. Lloyd and G. F. Burnett, the director.

Tuesday, July 22, 1958

Leave hotel at eight, town at eight-thirty. Excellent tarmac road allowing occasional wonderful views of the snow-capped Mt. Kilimanjaro, Africa's highest peak at 19,340 ft., and of Mt. Meru at 14,978 ft. Tarmac ends ten miles beyond Moshi, but the road is in good condition, mostly quartzite sand, although corrugated in some parts. The crest of the Para and later of the Usambara mountains are constantly visible in the far distance as the road winds through the wide valley of the Pangani River. The tarmac starts again near Korogwe. To balance the bonus, the engine begins to misfire and to lose power, especially when going uphill. With the help of two Hindu truck drivers, clean pump and carburetor both clogged with water. In spite of the cleanup the engine does not run as it should. No doubt, the source of the water is in the reservoir itself and constantly fed into the carburetor. Reach Muheza with difficulty. Locate an African mechanic familiar with Land Rover engines who changes the engine firing time. The engine runs somewhat better and it is with some confidence that we start the 18-mile winding road uphill to Amani, the Malaria Research Unit, our stop for the day. Glad to reach the top at 18:30. By sheer luck, the first house we stop at for information is that of Dr. Gilles, well-known mosquito specialist, whom I wanted to meet. He directs us to the guesthouse where we spend the night. That night we are invited with him to Captain (R.A.F.) Allen's house.

Wednesday, July 23, 1958

With Dr. Gilles, we drive to Muheza to witness a release of *Anopheles* mosquitoes which have been marked by radioactive phosphorus incorporated into the larvae's diet. Afterwards we collect mosquitoes resting inside houses in a nearby village. Later they will be taken to the darkroom where, in contact with photographic paper, the ones emerged from previously released radioactive larvae will show by a black spot.

Thursday, July 24, 1958

Together with Dr. Welch, a botanist, we visit a small pond, the site of research carried out by Dr. Pringle, fresh-water ecologist on snail transmitters of human schistosomiasis. He has recently returned from a schistosome control project in the Middle East. That night we are all invited to his home for dinner, an occasion for him to show off some truly beautiful carpets he brought back from Iraq.

Friday, July 25, 1958

Leave Amani at eight. After 25 miles engine overheats. Inspection shows the loss of the fan belt. Luckily I have a spare, but have a hard time putting it on. Arrive at Tanga and the coast of the Indian Ocean around ten. At this point we turn north to cross into Kenya, 40 miles later. The road follows the shore allowing occasional glimpses of the beaches, a splendid combination of waving coconut palms, brilliant white sand and the transluscent turquoise water turning purple in the distance. Arrive in Mombasa via the Likoni ferry (Mombasa is an island) by three in the afternoon. We spend the night at Nyali Beach Hotel, north of town.

The next several days are divided between sightseeing, shopping in Mombasa and relaxing on the beaches. I have always enjoyed my visits to the coast of Kenya and this time is no different. Mombasa pleases me with the romantic atmosphere of its old town quarters, their narrow, twisting streets and alleys, punctuated by emerging minarets, the sunny façades of the quaint houses with their musty smell of time, their picturesque balconies of carved lattice, and for the old harbor, anchorage of spirited dhows, their port-of-call for the last 2,000 years. A visit to Fort Jesus is, of course, a must. The well-preserved fortress, built by the Portuguese in the latter part of the sixteenth century, was the scene of many furious battles and long sieges between the Portuguese garrison, the Muslim inhabitants and their Arab leaders. In 1698, after a three years' siege, the fort fell to the Arab army from Oman, ending the Portuguese ascendency over Mombasa and that part of eastern Africa.

Another 70 miles north of Mombasa lies Malindi, a pleasant town well known for its lovely wide beaches, its casual luxurious hotels, the historic streets and buildings and the extensive ruins of nearby Gede, an ancient Arab town that flourished in the fifteenth century.

Wednesday, July 30, 1958

Leave Nyali Hotel a bit after eight. Traverse Mombasa and the causeway onto the main road to Nairobi. Tarmac for the next 50 miles changes into a wide, well-graded red-earth road. Take gasoline at Voi, where we turn west on the road to Taveta, a narrow, rough dust-road improving somewhat after 20 miles. Cross into Tsavo Park for a few miles and then into Tanganyika. Lots of game, including elephants, close to the road. Reach Moshi early afternoon. We had planned to spend the night here, but as it is still early, decide to push on. On leaving the town almost collide with the rear of the car in front when it suddenly brakes and swerves, apparently to avoid hitting a goat. It is midafternoon when we reach Arusha, so decide to continue, turning north on the main road to the Tanganyika-Kenya border. Spectacular views of Mounts Kilimanjaro and Meru. Arrive at the border and Namanga at sunset. Ask for a room in the only hotel which looks like a transformed farmhouse. The hotel is fully booked, but they find us a small but comfortable room and an extra camp bed for me. After a quick evening meal we enter a spacious place typical of the colonial farmer's living room: low beams, whitewashed walls, sturdy dark wood furniture and a large, square hearth with a roaring wood fire. Only the Dalmatians are missing. We are invited to make part of the half circle of hotel guests, three white hunters and two German girls, facing the warm glow, nursing large mugs of beer and listening to hair-raising hunting stories. A very pleasant evening and later a wonderful restful night.

Thursday, July 31, 1958

Up shortly after five. We cross the gate into Amboseli Park at six. Dusty but well-graded 45-mile-long road takes us to Tokai lodge, where we are given a guide. We see rhino, buffalo, impala, Grant's gazelle and ostrich. From Observation Hill we spot two lions devouring a dead elephant. The snows of Kilimanjaro are not to be seen this morning. In trying to take a shortcut through bushy undergrowth mixed with fallen branches to have a closer look at a group of about seven elephants, get entangled in a mass of bushes, dead trees cemented together with unwielding vines. My efforts to get the Land Rover across a fallen trunk fails and the engine stalls. In the meanwhile, the elephants are closing in. One of the elephants trumpets, the others get nervous. The guide urges me to get going. Winnie and Jessie are silent, but the expression in their wide-eyed stares would fill two chapters. After the second attempt I manage to get the engine going. I slam the four-wheel drive into gear and with some rocking back and forth bring the rear wheels across the fallen palm trunk which, with a splintering snap, gives way and the vehicle bounds forward, free once more. Back on the relative safety of the main track we treat the incident as a huge joke (if one can believe the nervous laughs). Returning to the lodge, we find a group of people staring from a safe distance at the underside of a Land Rover. A python has wound itself around the drive shaft, or vice versa, and no one knows what to do about it. For one thing, it cannot be shot as we are inside the park reserve. Second, how does one get a python to unwind? The question remained unanswered as we left the lodge on our way back to Namanga for lunch. A few miles before Kajiado, halfway along the 100 miles to Nairobi, a large bird nearly knocks out the windshield when it collides full force with the speeding vehicle. As we approach Nairobi, the weather clears and we enjoy some spectacular views of the mountains that form the eastern ridge of the Rift Valley. Reach Nairobi at four-thirty. Find the New Stanley Hotel partly demolished "for remodeling," the sign says. We find rooms at the "Equator Inn." After this long and eventful day go to see the film: "This is the night."

Saturday, August 2, 1958

Yesterday was a day of shopping while the Land Rover was left with Cooper Motors for servicing.

This morning met Dr. P. Glover and are invited to tea the next day at his home in Kabete. In the afternoon visit the Coryndon Museum (now National Museum of Kenya). Meet the director, Dr. L. S. B. Leakey, British archaeologist famous for his work and findings on prehistoric man at the Olduwai and Ologesailie sites in the Rift Valley. I leave him a box with the stone artifacts I collected last year in Nemba Hills.

Sunday, August 3, 1958

Some more shopping in the morning. A very pleasant afternoon tea at the Glovers. Phil Glover was engaged for many years in tsetse fly research projects in relation to wildlife conservation as a government zoologist. Later we all go to visit the new airport at Embakasi. We are impressed by the style and size of the complex. In the evening see the film starring Pat Boone: "Bernardine."

Tuesday, August 5, 1958

Yesterday was a Bank Holiday. It's useless, therefore, to stay in Nairobi for shopping although our list has not been exhausted. Leave Nairobi at nine on the road to Uganda. Nairobi lies on a 5,000-foot-high plateau, part of the eastern rim of the Rift Valley. The road follows the escarpment for 40 miles, then plunges rapidly to the bottom of the valley, 2,000 feet lower. When the crest-road is not hidden in clouds, rather rare, one has a marvelous view of the plains below and of the 9,000-foot-high extinct Longonot volcano. Ten miles along the valley lies Lake Naivasha, home of the pink flamingos. Another 43 miles will take us to Nakuru, but before reaching the town we make a loop to the left to visit the archaeological site near Lake Elmeneita. A dark haze generated by distant bushfires hides most of Lake Nakuru as we pass the town in early afternoon. Molo and Highland Hotel, our overnight stop, is only 30 miles away, high up the mountain at 8,100 feet. A steady drizzle, later turning into a steady downpour, makes everything look cheerless and brumal. Even the rooms feel cold in spite of the log fire.

Today it is still foggy and damp although the rain has ceased. Winnie and Jessie go for an hour of horseback riding. But I am glad to leave this cold and morose place for Kisumu, a sizable town at Kavirondo Bay on Lake Victoria. We stop only for gasoline. Passing Kakemega, we cross the border into Buganda at Busia and arrive in Tororo in late afternoon. This will be a two-day stopover as I am to visit another E.A.T.T.R.O. research center.

Wednesday, August 6, 1958

Besides the EATTRO research station and the nearby cement factory, Tororo is famous for "the rock," a huge granite monolith that rises steeply from the surrounding plains. It is inhabited by barking baboons during the day and laughing hyenas at night.

Have a morning session with several scientists: K. R. S. Morris, who specializes in trapping devices to catch tsetse flies alive; G. R. Jewell, experimenting in marking tsetse flies with luminous paints so that their resting sites can be studied at night; B. D. Renninson, interested in sampling methods and attractants; R.D. Pilson studies tsetse population dynamics; M. Cunningham is devising methods to preserve *in vitro* trypanosome strains isolated from various animals.

The girls idle their time away with the Jewells at the local sports club, especially enjoying the large swimming pool.

The food served at the hotel is of rather poor quality and during the last night Jessie is very sick with a stomach ache. The echo of laughing hyenas is heard from the rock.

Thursday, August 7, 1958

Leave Tororo for Kampala. Jessie is still not well. Arrive in Jinja, but the Owen Falls are no longer: the Jinja dam now regulates the water flow from Lake Victoria into the Nile, producing hydroelectric power for a large part of the country. See immigration at the police station and inquire about Lt. Swan, my nemesis of five years ago. It gives me some comfort to learn that he is no longer serving in Uganda. When asked why I wanted to see him in particular, I reply that we shared memories during the Mau Mau uprising.

Friday, August 7, 1958

I meet A. G. Robertson, who is in charge of a pilot tsetse eradication program in the Karagwe district across the Kagera River from my previous Mutara research area.

This will be our last chance to shop in East Africa, so we make the most of it by visiting the numerous Hindu shops that line the main arteries of town. To celebrate our last day here, we spend the evening in company of Robertson at one of the night clubs. Goodbye East Africa.

Two days later we were back in Lwiro, having spent the previous night at Kabale's "White Horse Inn." We had traveled 2,392 miles. We had seen Africa's highest mountain, its largest lake, its most diverse wildlife and the site of early man. For myself, I had met with the most knowledgeable scientists in the areas of my research and made many acquaintances who became lasting friends.

Farewell to Africa

The forest has given way to vague shrubland—so gradually and imperceptibly that it takes a while to realize that we are already flying across the Sudan. The sun has disappeared behind a curtain of rising dust long before it will set behind the horizon. The earth is fading into a blur of dark gray, covered with a veil of blue haze. A sudden reflection of the sky on a small lake; just a flash. Probably my last glimpse of Africa. I still cannot explain why I am not feeling a stronger emotion. Is my decision to leave Africa, after almost 15 years, so momentous that my feelings are dulled? Is it because subconsciously I fancy that I shall return some day perhaps? Or is it that only my body is leaving while my mind is still wandering the wide savannas or the depths of the rain forest?

The four engines of the DC-6 drone on, on and on—eager and faithful, so it seems. In the darkening sky the cowlings glow a dark cherry red. The wings rock with a slow, gentle rhythm. I close the curtains. A symbolic gesture, that. I recognize one of the stewards as a relative of the Michel family. He invites me to the pilot's cockpit, fascinating and weird with all those green flourescent lights. One red light comes on and switches off again. Nothing to worry about, I presume. It is most frightening to see the faintly visible nose of the aircraft plunge into nothing, glide into empty space with no limits, nothing to judge by. One almost expects something to appear at any moment that would lend some sense of perspective. Only darkness and the feeling of movement. Well, everything is under control, as far as I can judge. How could it be otherwise? A wonderful machine, the DC-6. By the way of conversation, I ask my friend the steward where the radar is.

"We haven't got one on this ship," he smiles.

How remarkable, I comment, that the navigator can find his way among all those stars.

"The weather is closing in," is his cheerful reply.

I make a last effort to have him corroborate my sense of security by observing that, at least, the engines are running smoothly.

"We have trouble with number two," he says. "Magneto cut out a moment ago. Hope the stand-by will last till we reach Cairo."

Thanking him, I regain the safety of my seat. Can I hear number two laboring?

Dora and the children had left Lwiro a week ago, flying to Mombasa to board one of the Castle Line ships bound for Europe by the way of the Cape of Good Hope. Their good-bye to Mutima had been an emotional scene, both parties close to tears. After all, Mutima had been part of the family for 14 years. He had seen the girls grow up from children to young ladies, had known Richard from birth till he was six. My good-bye to Mutima, yesterday, had been equally painful but brief when, suddenly, he turned around and walked away never to look back again.

From my seat I try to organize my thoughts, but I seem to go through a dream over which I have no control. Things started happening as if I had given a push to a ball on an incline—poised there for some time—and suddenly I cannot stop its momentum. I only know it started with my decision to leave Africa and to emigrate to the United States. But I still do not completely grasp the importance of this decision since things are moving faster than my thoughts. Yesterday, at this time, I was still at Lwiro in the house we had occupied for the last six years. In a moment I shall land in Cairo, number two willing. Tomorrow Brussels and a few days later New York.

Early this morning, my connecting flight to Stanleyville, a DC-3, left Kamembe field on the Ruanda side of Lake Kivu, divided into the Ruzizi valley, my early stamping grounds, and deposited me at the northern tip of Lake Tanganyika, site of the new Usumbura airport. Another connecting flight, a DC-4, would take me to Stanleyville. It was during this change of planes that my last African adventure occurred. As I was about to board the waiting plane, (we had run late) the metal box containing 600 color slides popped open, spilling all on the runway. With the help of the SABENA stewardess I managed to get all the slides back in the box and boarded, the last passenger. One more glimpse of Lake Tanganyika, the Mitumba mountain range, the forested western slopes—with somewhere Irangi and my rash observation tower, the hazy Congo River, and a bumpy landing at Stanleyville.

I have a long wait at the SABENA guesthouse, where I meet Maandag, an old friend from the hockey club I have not heard from for more than 15 years. I am paged by the ticket office and fear the worst because I have heard that all flights are fully booked. It is only to ask me whether I would be willing to give up my seat on the three o'clock plane in favor of a lady who would then be able to travel in company of her husband who was given the last seat on that flight. In exchange, I would fly on the two o'clock plane, the only difference being that this flight would stop over at Libenge. The sound of that place makes me shudder. It is here that Dr. Zanetti met his death in the SABENA air disaster on Friday, May 13, 1948.

Libenge lies on the left bank of the Ubangi River, which at this point forms the border between the Belgian Congo and French Equatorial Africa. The airstrip has been cut out neatly from the surrounding forest, leaving a long, rectangular red scar. At its approach, the DC-6 sinks ever lower over the cauliflower canopy, gingerly it seems, the widely balancing wings trying to compensate for the updraft and, when all hope seems lost, drops its tail behind the last *Gilbertiodendron* and settles on the unpaved airstrip in a cloud of red dust. The aircraft comes to a halt in front of a single small building painted bright yellow, perhaps to help the pilot locate the airfield. The building smells of bats and stale tobacco. It resounds of cha-cha-cha music and bouncing ping-pong balls. After half an hour we board again. The temperature inside the cabin must be close to the threshold of vertebrate survival. The pilot manages to get the plane in the air before the end of the runway. For him, it must be quite an experience to see those tall trees rushing towards him at 100 mph, and wait until speed and lift make the plane airborne, allowing the wheels to pass the highest trees without dislodging the toucan's nest.

Of course, we made it to Cairo. And when after an hour of waiting in the cold and stark transit room, we lifted off the runway, I knew I had left Africa.

Our decision to leave Africa proved a wise one, if only for the events that followed. We had left the Congo in August 1959. Less than a year later, the country exploded in a frenzy of independence movements that, instead of joy and a new beginning, resulted in bloody political and tribal rivalries that would last intermittently for several years. It left the country morally and financially weak and ended in a draining dictatorship. The tone was set for things to come when, during the independence ceremony, the sword of King Boudewijn was snatched from his side by a Congolese bystander, counting no doubt upon a huge profit when sold on the black market.

For many of us colonials, as well as for the many visitors who had enjoyed the enchantment and hospitality of the country, it felt as if an edifice, lovingly, patiently and conscientiously built from scratch, had been wantonly destroyed. As for ourselves, we remembered those fascinating years mostly with memories of dancing and chanting MaBudu, the fireside tales of Mutima, the mustiness of the forest, the cry of the bolikoko, the sulfurous scent of the green ants, the soft winds of the savanna swaying the themeda grass, the fragrance of the acacia blossoms, the silhouette of the languid giraffe and, yes, the buzz of the tsetse fly.

Epilogue

Twenty-five years have passed. A few years ago I had an article published that recapitulated my feelings after two decades of maturation. It was written to release the pressure of my thoughts and I am grateful to the editor of *The Explorer* (1983) who published it and for his permission to quote excerpts.

"Many hours have I squandered, sitting inside a tree-thicket in the vast woodlands savannas of the no man's regions between Rwanda-Burundi and Uganda and Tanzania. The afternoons were hot, the air seemed to lack oxygen, insects were crawling freely inside my shirt and leggings, perspiration dripped from my brow into my eyes, to the great delight of the gnats that gratefully sipped the salty moisture. No one ever discovered me in this foolish position, not that I feared such an unlikely event. I was all alone in my little kingdom; the thicket was my castle. The enemies were all around me, most of the time inconspicuous but for an occasional buzz and a zoom.

"The reason for my strange conduct was my great enthusiasm and dedication to tsetse research. I doubt that this will alleviate the somewhat uneasy impression my behavior may have created in the reader's mind. I assert that my seeming idleness was not in conflict with the mandate of my research project. My watch inside the thicket was part of a personal plan aimed at solving the long-debated question about the resting sites of tsetse flies. This is a somewhat precipitous way to describe my position, both physically and figuratively. Here, I should like to make a suggestion. If by ill chance you meet a glossinologist during a social gathering, *do not* bring up the subject of his trade unless you are comfortably settled in an armchair, your drinking requirements properly attended to, and willing to listen to a two-hour monologue.

"*Glossina*, commonly known as tsetse flies, carriers of the dreaded sleeping sickness or African trypanosomiasis and of nagana, causing heavy losses in livestock, are know only in Africa. Many methods have been tried to pry into the most intimate aspects of the lives of tsetse flies. Such knowledge would help make insecticide applications more efficient, less expensive, quicker and longer lasting, would reduce ecological side effects or would lead to other means of eradicating 'the scourge of Africa.'

"Tsetse control had been carried out by aerial spray, catching the fly on the wing, so to speak, or by ground application of residual insecticides, both methods aiming at the dispersion of the insecticides where contact with the fly would be the greatest. Hence the purpose of my thicket watch: finding those parts of the vegetation where the fly spends most of its time resting, when not busy feeding or, in the case of the males, on a sex spree. Hundreds of articles have been published, each adding to our knowledge of fly behavior and to the methods of control. Inconclusive as some of these papers may be, they are often fascinating reading to the glossino-ecologist who appreciates the description and intimate details of the fly's reproduction cycle, the intricacies of feeding patterns, the complexities of fly-host relationships, the delicate affinities with vegetation communities, the long-term effects of rain and drought, the controversies of early or late bushfires, the preference for certain game animals, the role of pastoralism and nomadism, the consequences of human behavior and migration, the history of human settlements. Many of these ecological gems are spiced with dry personal humor or, at times, with barely hidden disappointments. Archaeological discoveries are mentioned casually. Detailed maps, called sketches, plot areas never trodden by man before.

"The recollection of my vigilance inside the thickets brings back pleasant memories. I remember how passing clouds darkened the sun and generated a soft breeze that would rustle the trifoliate leaves of *Rhus*, sway the delicate, spiny foliage of the wild *Asparagus*, and force the moisture-loving gnats to take refuge on the lee side of the trees. The heavy late afternoon atmosphere would make me feel drowsy and induce a pensive mood that took me back to my earlier years of research in the tropics, many spent in different African regions. My early field stations were built from mud and thatch. Some were deep in the rain forest, some were in hot savanna country, some were lapped by the swift waters of a river or hedged by the shores of a placid lake. In later years, more sophisticated comfort was possible with the use of prefabricated aluminum huts.

"Sooner or later, my camps would be visited by other scientists often to start their own subject of research. Some of the early camps attracted so much interdisciplinary interest that permanent structures were built, replacing previous tents and huts. I always had high hopes that the impromptu visitor, whether a biologist, sociologist, geologist or botanist, would contribute information that would help piece together a comprehensive ecological picture.

"I have seen many scientists come and go, sometimes spending only a short time in the area, walking off with pertinent and vital information that was subsequently lost for lack of communication, like walking off with an essential piece of a puzzle. As the years went by, I began to realize that even the fitting of individual pieces of the puzzle would be an enormous task—as more data accumulated, the complexity of the ecosystem became increasingly apparent, its ambiguity unpredictable.

"True, we achieved a few individual successes, triumphantly heralded in scientific publications, ephemeral glories now yellowing on the shelves of library stacks, such as a mammalogist who came out of the forest, muddy and hungry, and proposed that the local *Colobus* monkey be given subspecies status because of its peculiar coloration; a botanist who plotted a detailed vegetation map in a five-hectare forest square; a series of platforms that were built at different heights along the enormous trunk of a 120-foot *Gilbertiodendron dewevrei* tree for comparative mosquito catches; the testing of the blood meals of the rare tsetse fly, *Glossina vanhoofi* which showed that the flies fed almost exclusively on bush pig; blood smears of wild animals that led to the discovery of a new *Plasmodium* (malaria parasite) in the brushtail porcupine. Interesting and important as these findings seemed at the time, they were so many drops in an ocean of unknowns.

"It was during an ecological study of the tsetse fly populations in a particularly curious wooded savanna in the Bugesera region of eastern Ruanda that I started my observations of tsetse resting sites. The region had become extremely unpopular because of the sudden and severe outbreak of sleeping sickness. People and their cattle were leaving the area for higher country unfortunately already overpopulated and overgrazed. Besides being found in the classical *Acacia* woodland, *Glossina morsitans*, the tsetse fly responsible for transmission of the disease in this area, was also found in large tracts of dry forest composed of tall and dense clumps of various tree species mixed with almost impenetrable scrub. Many of the tree species were more than 60 feet tall. Areas covered by this dense vegetation were sometimes as large as city blocks. From the air they looked like islands in a sea of grass. According to the botanist, this vegetation was evolving towards its climax that would eventually completely cover the whole area, strangling the pioneer species that had started the process.

"The use by *G. morsitans* of dense thickets was contrary to its classical behavioral pattern so well described by my peers. It was for this reason that I decided to find out why this thicket vegetation seemed so attractive to the local fly population.

"I kept watch inside the thicket for many days, silent and attentive, hoping to learn whether, where and why tsetse flies would make use of this type of vegetation. Astonishingly, I was never bored, but rather enjoyed the feeling of having become a temporary denizen of a closed ecosystem. As I grew more familiar with the surroundings and more at ease in my adopted niche, I also began to notice things. The thickets, seemingly lifeless, drooping and drowsy under the hot sun, were in fact lively communities. From considering myself the dominant species, I came to feel like a presumptuous intruder in a strange world, awkwardly disturbing an organized assemblage, perhaps upsetting the routine of hundreds of creatures. The casual tangle of leaves, twigs, creepers, saplings and bractlets became to my roving eyes, highways of various insects, moving about with purposeful determination, intent on getting things done. The deep track hollowed out from the sandy soil by repeated use by a larger animal, possibly a rodent, skirted such obstacles as a sharp-edged twig or a low-hanging thorny branch. How familiar to the animal was this trail, how important to its life and tasks, and how equally important to the survival and spread of ectoparasites that depend upon the animal's passage, or to the female mosquito waiting for a blood meal. To my left a dangling spider web, the recent death trap of an innocent butterfly, sways in a breeze; a green beetle scurries the floor for leftovers; a fire ant searches frantically for its lost trail.

"From a casual outsider who had crawled inside the thicket, I had now become part of its daily melodrama, a world in which each trembling of a leaf was a major event, the slightest breeze a storm, and the tiniest object a landmark or an obstacle. An independent microcosm that sustained thousands of creatures, an ecological entity subject to all the challenges of evolution and the hazards of extinction.

"In this research it seemed important to me to bring myself as close as possible to the conditions experienced by the insect, physically and conceptually. Hence my thicket watches.

"I am afraid, however, that my temporary participation in the melodrama was too superficial, too insignificant, and too brief for me to grasp the delicate intricacies among the players, let alone analyze their interdependence. And even had a tsetse fly landed in front of me, I would have been at a loss to know why.

"The thickets are still there, awaiting the next puzzled ecologist, unless bulldozers have leveled the terrain for cotton and the tsetse flies have been eradicated."

INDEX

Abiengama, author's work at 75–82, 114–115
Adamanditis, Dr. 351, 384
Antwerp 3, 8, 12, 20, 93
"anyota" secret society, 146
Astrida 204. *See also* IRSAC

bamboo. *See* forests
Bantu, history 26–28
bilharzia. *See* schistosomiasis
Boudewijn I, King 286, 409
Budubudu, author's work in 85–88
Bugesera, history 368
    author's work in 384–390
Burton, Sir Richard 179, 199
Burtt, B. D. 394

Casati, Gaetano 27, 50
caste system. *See* class differences
cattle population 368
chaulmoogra tree 61–62, 146
Chapin, James 27, 249, 278, 287
Chardome, Marcel 20–21, 227, 237, 261, 266, 373
    photograph 238
Chrysops flies 116, 290
class differences 104
Colonial Pesticide Research Unit 400
Congo Red Cross 12, 16, 70, 119
Cordier, Charles 303, 308, 373, 376
Cordier, Emy 376
    photograph 45
Costermansville, description 158–159
COTONEPO 81, 85, 86
Cunningham, M. 405

dance, native 30–31
DDT 190, 192
De Paepe, Dr. 120, 121–123 passim, 125
Dubois, Professor 161

East Africa Trypanosomiasis and Tsetse Research Organization 392
electricity 135–136
Emlen, J. T. 376
European Red Cross 47

filaria worms 116, 290
Foundation Internationale Scientifique 305, 375
forests 60–61, 164, 198, 282
    bamboo 256–257
    tropical rain 277–278
    development 277

Garnham, P. C. 366
Geigy, Rudolph 385
Gerardi, Dr. 16, 25, 46, 106–111, 150–151
glossinology. *See* tsetse fly
gorillas 373–377 passim
    photograph 45, 244
gugu-gudu (tom-tom) 59

Hansen, Gerhard 71–72
Hore, Edward Coode 179
houses, colonial 47–48
hunting 89–102, 194–195
huts, native 51–52

Institute for Tropical Medicine 10, 12, 250
IRSAC 20, 180–181, 186, 377
    Astrida station 192, 199–201
    Elisabethville station 192
    Irangi Field Research Station 279–285
    Lwiro 173, 192, 246–254 passim
    Mabale station 192
    photograph 173
    Uvira station, 167, 172, 185–188, 192, 195
insects 139. *See also* mosquitoes, termites

Jackson memorial (photograph) 175
Jewell, G. R. 405
jungle yellow fever 94, 261, 266
Junker, Wilhelm 27

Kibali-Ituri region, description 26
kilns, brick 59
kitabu (native document) description 57–58
Kivu province, description 156–157
knives, description 31–32

Lake Tanganyika, description 178–179
Lambrecht, Frank L.
    birthplace 3
    parents 4–8
    marriage 10
    training xiv, 10, 12, 192
    photographs ii, 174, 176, 243, jacket
Lambrecht, Dora 10, 133, 134–136 passim, 141, 142, 143, 377, 389, 392
    photographs 41, 239
Lambrecht, Jessie 133, 142, 338–339, 371, 394
    diary 184
    photographs 41, 173, 175, 327
Lambrecht, Richard 247, 366
    photographs 239, 245

Lambrecht, Winnie 133 142, 339–340, 371
    photographs 41, 173, 133, 142
Lang, Herbert 27, 234
Leakey, L. S. B. 380, 399, 404
Leopold, King 243, 305–314 passim, 375, 387
    photographs 242, 243
Leopoldville, description 19, 103
lepers 46–49 passim, 148
    photograph 44
leprosy, treatment 61–62, 74–75; history of 70–73
Liliane, Princess 243, 308–314 passim
    photograph 242
loa loa. See filaria worms

Maasai 398, 400
    drawing of 328
    photograph 327
MaBudu people, description 27, 28–30
    huts 32–33
    photographs 34, 36, 37, 39, 42
malafu (native drink), 79, 80–81
malaria 77, 161, 189, 191, 299
Mangbetu people, description 26–27
    photographs 35, 42, 43
Mau-Mau 359
monkeys, description 92–98, 266, 280, 298
Morris, K. R. S. 405
mosquitoes 190, 191, 192, 261, 280, 281, 288, 372, 401
    anopheles gambiae 190
    anopheles funestus 190
    anopheles implexus 215, 216
    anopheles pharoensis 190
    anopheles pretoriensis 190
    aedes simpsoni 266
Mosso, description 208

nagana, defined 209
Nepoko region, description 103–104, 105

onchocerciasis 290

Pawa Medical Center 12, 24–25, 161
    description 46–48 passim
    photograph 44
pigs, wild 90, 91, 92
Pilson, R. D. 405
Pirlot, Paul 261, 266, 278, 377
plasmodium 413
    plasmodium atheruri 299
    plasmodium berghei xv, 22, 189, 190, 293
posho (market) description 53–55,
punishment, native 55–56, 80
Putnam, Patrick 261–263
Pygmies 26, 77, 86–87, 262–265

religion, Christianity 145–147
Renninson, B. D. 405
river blindness. See onchocerciasis
Rock, Joseph F. 62–63
Rodhain, Jerome 12–13, 70, 93
Ruanda, description 198
Rudahigwa II, King 171, 181
    photograph, 173

Schaller, G. 376
schistosomiasis 255, 401
Schweinfurth, Georg 27, 50
Shinyanga 223–224, 393
soap making 120
soil, type 121
Speke, John H. 179, 199
Stanleyville, description 22–23,
Swerts Dr. 111, 163, 205
Swiss Tropical Institute 385
Swynnerton, C. F. M. 224, 320, 323, 394
    memorial 175
syphilis 77, 109–110

tattooing 30
termites, description 51, 64–68
    photographs 38, 43
    swarming 68
tipoy 31, 139
    photograph 41
trains, in Africa 362–363
trees, description 60–61
trumbush 31
trypanosomiasis 77, 208, 223, 385
Trypanosoma 209, 221
    trypanosoma lewisi 296
    trypanosoma rhodesiense 210
Trypanosome Research Laboratory 393
tsetse fly 77, 208, 209–210 passim, 215, 224, 314, 319–320, 335, 342, 352, 362, 368, 370, 371, 381, 382, 386, 394, 400, 411–415 passim
    Glossina morsitans xv–xvi, 215, 217, 341, 345, 350, 368, 369, 386, 394, 400, 413, 414
    Glossina fuscipleuris 215, 222
    Glossina brevipalpis 222, 225, 341
    Glossina swynnertoni 224, 394
    Glossina vanhoofi 288, 290, 298, 300, 413
        photograph 244
    Glossina papalis 267, 288, 289
    Glossina fusca 267
    Glossina pallidipes 321, 341, 349, 350, 368
    Glossina tabaniformis xiv
    catching stations 283–284, 322
    pupae 330

ulcer, tropical 77
Usumbura, author's work in
  181–182

vanden Berghe, Louis xiv, 20, 167,
  171–172,190, 192, 237, 249, 250,
  278, 375, 376
    photograph 172, 243
Village Agricole d'Isolement de Lepreux
  73, 146

Vincke, Ignace xv, 189, 190, 191, 192, 214,
  292, 293, 294
    photograph 174

Willett, K. 393
Wouters, Fred 117, 121–125 passim, 147
    photograph 40

yaws 77

Zanetti, Dr. 24, 57, 106–111; death, 162